T0294606

Pain/Palliative Care

Editors

SEAN C. MACKEY
RONALD G. PEARL

ANESTHESIOLOGY CLINICS

www.anesthesiology.theclinics.com

Consulting Editor
LEE A. FLEISHER

June 2023 • Volume 41 • Number 2

ELSEVIER

1600 John F. Kennedy Boulevard • Suite 1800 • Philadelphia, Pennsylvania, 19103-2899

http://www.theclinics.com

ANESTHESIOLOGY CLINICS Volume 41, Number 2
June 2023 ISSN 1932-2275, ISBN-13: 978-0-443-18338-6

Editor: Joanna Collett
Developmental Editor: Arlene Campos

Anesthesiology Clinics (ISSN 1932-2275) is published quarterly by Elsevier Inc., 360 Park Avenue South, New York, NY 10010-1710. Months of issue are March, June, September, and December. Periodicals postage paid at New York, NY and at additional mailing offices. Subscription prices are $100.00 per year (US student/resident), $386.00 per year (US individuals), $478.00 per year (Canadian individuals), $740.00 per year (US institutions), $936.00 per year (Canadian institutions), $100.00 per year (Canadian student/resident), $513.00 per year (foreign student/resident), $498.00 per year (foreign individuals), and $936.00 per year (foreign institutions). To receive student and resident rate, orders must be accompanied by name of affiliated institution, date of term, and the *signature* of program/residency coordinator on institutions letterhead. Orders will be billed at individual rate until proof of status is received. Foreign air speed delivery is included in all *Clinics'* subscription prices. All prices are subject to change without notice. POSTMASTER: Send address changes to *Anesthesiology Clinics,* Elsevier Health Sciences Division, Subscription Customer Service, 3251 Riverport Lane, Maryland Heights, MO 63043. Customer Service (orders, claims, online, change of address): Elsevier Health Sciences Division, Subscription Customer Service, 3251 Riverport Lane, Maryland Heights, MO 63043. **Tel:1-800-654-2452 (U.S. and Canada); 314-447-8871 (outside U.S. and Canada). Fax: 314-447-8029. E-mail: journalscustomerservice-usa@elsevier.com (for print support); journalsonlinesupport-usa@elsevier.com (for online support).**

Reprints. For copies of 100 or more of articles in this publication, please contact the Commercial Reprints Department, Elsevier Inc., 360 Park Avenue South, New York, NY 10010-1710. Tel.: 212-633-3874; Fax: 212-633-3820; E-mail: reprints@elsevier.com.

Anesthesiology Clinics, is also published in Spanish by McGraw-Hill Inter-americana Editores S. A., P.O. Box 5-237, 06500 Mexico D. F., Mexico.

Anesthesiology Clinics, is covered in *MEDLINE/PubMed (Index Medicus), Current Contents/Clinical Medicine, Excerpta Medica, ISI/BIOMED*, and *Chemical Abstracts*.

Contributors

CONSULTING EDITOR

LEE A. FLEISHER, MD, FACC, FAHA
Robert D. Dripps Professor and Chair of Anesthesiology and Critical Care, Professor of Medicine, Perelman School of Medicine, University of Pennsylvania, Philadelphia, Pennsylvania, USA

EDITORS

SEAN C. MACKEY, MD, PhD
Redlich Professor, Chief, Division of Pain Medicine, Stanford University School of Medicine, Department of Anesthesiology, Perioperative, and Pain Medicine, Neurosciences, and (by courtesy) Neurology, Palo Alto, California, USA

RONALD G. PEARL, MD, PhD
Dr. Richard K. and Erika N. Richards Professor, Department of Anesthesiology, Perioperative and Pain Medicine, Stanford University School of Medicine, Stanford, California, USA

AUTHORS

ANUJ K. AGGARWAL, MD
Clinical Assistant Professor, Department of Anesthesiology, Perioperative and Pain Medicine, Stanford University School of Medicine, Stanford, California, USA

OMAR KHALID ALTIRKAWI, MD
Department of Anesthesiology, Perioperative and Pain Medicine, Stanford University School of Medicine, Palo Alto, California, USA

MEREDITH J. BARAD, MD
Clinical Associate Professor, Department of Anesthesiology, Perioperative and Pain Medicine, Stanford University School of Medicine, Palo Alto, California, USA

MEREDITH BROOKS, MD, MPH
Department of Anesthesiology, Cook Children's Health Care System, Texas Christian University School of Medicine, Fort Worth, Texas, USA

DANIEL J. CLAUW, MD
Professor, Departments of Anesthesiology, Psychiatry and Internal Medicine-Rheumatology, University of Michigan Medical School, Ann Arbor, Michigan, USA

LUANA COLLOCA, MD, PhD, MS
University of Maryland, Baltimore, Maryland, USA

RENA ELIZABETH COURTNEY, PhD
Salem VA Medical Center, Virginia Tech Carilion School of Medicine, Salem, Virginia, USA

BETH D. DARNALL, PhD
Professor, Department of Anesthesiology, Perioperative and Pain Medicine, Stanford University School of Medicine, Redwood City, California, USA

JESSICA ESTHER DAWSON, MD, MPH
Department of Anesthesiology, Perioperative and Pain Medicine, Stanford University, Stanford, California, USA

RYAN DERBY, MD
Department of Anesthesiology, Perioperative and Pain Medicine, Stanford University, Stanford, California, USA

GENEVIEVE D'SOUZA, MD, FASA
Department of Anesthesiology, Perioperative and Pain Medicine, Stanford University, Stanford, California, USA

DAWN M. EHDE, PhD
Professor, Department of Rehabilitation Medicine, University of Washington School of Medicine, Seattle, Washington, USA

JENNIFER HAH, MD MS
Department of Anesthesiology, Perioperative and Pain Medicine, Stanford University, Stanford, California, USA

DANIEL HECHT, MD
Department of Anesthesiology, Perioperative and Pain Medicine, Stanford University, Stanford, California, USA

YASMINE HOYDONCKX, MD MSc
Department of Anesthesia and Pain Management, University of Toronto, Toronto, Ontario, Canada

ALICE HUAI-YU LI, MD
Department of Anesthesiology, Perioperative and Pain Medicine, Stanford University, Stanford, California, USA

MARK P. JENSEN, PhD
Professor, Department of Rehabilitation Medicine, University of Washington School of Medicine, Seattle, Washington, USA

JAMES S. KHAN, MD, MSc
Department of Anesthesia and Pain Medicine, Mount Sinai Hospital, University of Toronto, Toronto, Ontario, Canada

LYNN KOHAN, MD
Department of Anesthesiology, University of Virginia, Charlottesville, Virginia, USA

ELLIOT KRANE, MD, FAAP
Department of Anesthesiology, Perioperative and Pain Medicine, Stanford University, Stanford, California, USA

ALBERT HYUKJAE KWON, MD
Stanford University School of Medicine, Redwood City, California, USA

THERESA R. LII, MD, MS
Clinical Postdoctoral Scholar, Department of Anesthesiology, Perioperative and Pain Medicine, Stanford University, Redwood City, California, USA

SEAN C. MACKEY, MD, PhD
Redlich Professor, Chief, Division of Pain Medicine, Stanford University School of Medicine, Department of Anesthesiology, Perioperative, and Pain Medicine, Neurosciences, and (by courtesy) Neurology, Palo Alto, California, USA

SUSAN MOESCHLER, MD
Department of Anesthesiology, Mayo Clinic, Rochester, Minnesota, USA

JANE S. MOON, MD
Department of Anesthesiology and Perioperative Medicine, University of California, Los Angeles, Los Angeles, California, USA

LEE HUYNH NGUYEN, MD
Department of Anesthesiology, Perioperative and Pain Medicine, Stanford University, Stanford, California, USA

EINAR OTTESTAD, MD
Department of Anesthesiology, Perioperative and Pain Medicine, Stanford University School of Medicine, Palo Alto, California, USA

KAYLA E. PFAFF, BA
Department of Anesthesiology, Perioperative and Pain Medicine, Stanford University, Stanford, California, USA

NITIN PRABHAKAR, MD
Division of Physical Medicine and Rehabilitation, Department of Orthopedic Surgery, Stanford University, Stanford, California, USA

SCOTT PRITZLAFF, MD
Department of Anesthesiology and Pain Medicine, University of California, Davis, Sacramento, California, USA

JAMES RATHMELL, MD
Department of Anesthesiology, Perioperative, and Pain Medicine, Brigham and Women's Health Care, Boston, Massachusetts, USA

VAFI SALMASI, MD, MS(Epi)
Department of Anesthesiology, Perioperative and Pain Medicine, Stanford University School of Medicine, Palo Alto, California, USA

MARY JOSEPHINE SCHADEGG, MA
Salem VA Medical Center, University of Mississippi, Salem, Virginia, USA

VINITA SINGH, MD, MS
Division Chief, Emory Pain Division, Director of Cancer Pain, Co-Director of Pain Research, Associate Professor, Department of Anesthesiology, Emory University, Atlanta, Georgia, USA

JOHN A. STURGEON, PhD
Clinical Assistant Professor, Department of Anesthesiology, University of Michigan Medical School, Ann Arbor, Michigan, USA

NATACHA TELUSCA, MD, MPH
Department of Anesthesiology, Perioperative and Pain Medicine, Stanford University, Stanford, California, USA

ABDULLAH SULIEMAN TERKAWI, MD, MS(Epi)
Department of Anesthesiology, Perioperative and Pain Medicine, Stanford University School of Medicine, Palo Alto, California, USA

LEI XU, MD
Department of Anesthesiology, Perioperative and Pain Medicine, Stanford University, Stanford, California, USA

Contents

ANESTHESIOLOGY CLINICS

FORTHCOMING ISSUES

September 2023
Geriatric Anesthesia
Shamsuddin Akhtar, *Editor*

December 2023
Perioperative Safety Culture
Matthew D. McEvoy and James Abernathy, *Editors*

RECENT ISSUES

March 2023
Current Topics in Critical Care for the Anesthesiologist
Athanasios Chalkias, Mary Jarzebowski, and Kathryn Rosenblatt, *Editors*

December 2022
Vascular Anesthesia
Megan P. Kostibas, and Heather K. Hayanga, *Editors*

September 2022
Orthopedic Anesthesiology
Philipp Lirk and Kamen Vlassakov, *Editors*

SERIES OF RELATED INTEREST

Critical Care Clinics

Foreword

Pain Management: Critical Advances in Both Perioperative and Population Health for All

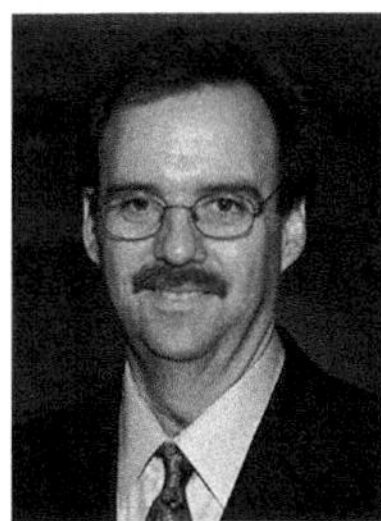

Lee A. Fleisher, MD
Consulting Editor

Over the past two decades there has been intense interest in pain management while addressing the opiate epidemic and the unintended consequences of attempts to irradicate pain in the hospital setting. The COVID-19 pandemic has led to a worsening of the opioid epidemic and exacerbation of health disparities. It is therefore important for anesthesiologists, as both perioperative and chronic pain practitioners, to be educated and involved in this important part of our practice. We also must be aware of the way we can contribute to population health, and pain management is a critical component. These important factors are the rationale for commissioning an issue on pain management, which includes articles as diverse as education, health disparities, and complications of interventional techniques.

In order to commission an issue on pain management, I was able to engage two amazing colleagues from Stanford University. Ronald Pearl, MD, PhD is the Dr Richard K. and Erika N. Richards Professor of Anesthesiology, Perioperative, and Pain Medicine. He was Chair of the Department from 1999 to 2021. Dr Pearl completed his MD/PhD at the University of Chicago and multiple residencies at Stanford University. He is board certified in internal medicine, anesthesia, and critical care. He has had an extensive research career in critical care and held numerous leadership positions. Sean Mackay, MD, PhD is the Redlich Professor and Chief of the Division of Stanford Pain Medicine. Dr Mackay completed his MD/PhD from the University of Arizona. He is a physician-scientist trained and experienced in neuroimaging, psychophysics, public health, health policy, patient outcomes, and medical education with a focus on

Anesthesiology Clin 41 (2023) xiii–xiv
https://doi.org/10.1016/j.anclin.2023.05.008
1932-2275/23/© 2023 Published by Elsevier Inc.

pain management. He also has held numerous leadership positions. Together, they have invited a stellar group of authors on this topic.

Lee A. Fleisher, MD
Perelman School of Medicine at
University of Pennsylvania
3400 Spruce Street, Dulles 680
Philadelphia, PA 19104, USA

E-mail address:
Lee.Fleisher@pennmedicine.upenn.edu

Preface

Pain Management: Optimizing Patient Care Through Comprehensive, Interdisciplinary Models and Continuous Innovations

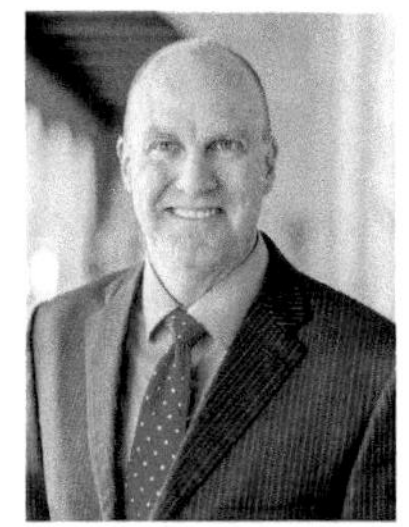

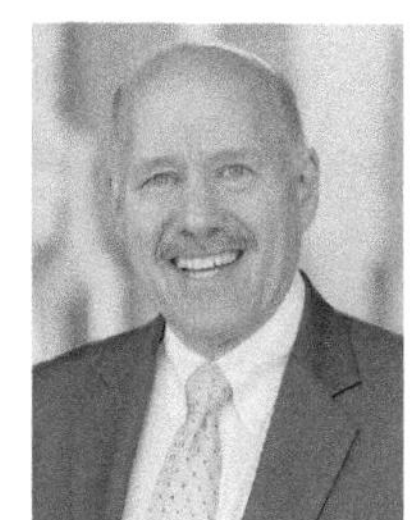

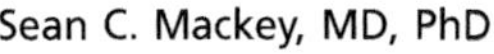

Sean C. Mackey, MD, PhD Ronald G. Pearl, MD, PhD
Editors

Inadequate treatment of pain represents a public health crisis in the United States. An estimated 50 to 100 million US adults suffer from chronic pain (CP), with a tremendous annual cost of over $500 billion annually, representing one of the most prevalent, costly, and disabling health conditions.[1,2] The most impacted and highest-need CP patients have been defined as those with high-impact chronic pain (HICP) by the Health and Human Services *National Pain Strategy* (Co-Chair, Dr. Mackey). HICP is "associated with substantially restricted work, social, and self-care activities for six or more months"[3] and affects an estimated 20 million US adults.[4]

The National Pain Strategy (NPS) advanced several underlying principles, including "chronic pain is a biopsychosocial condition that often requires integrated, multimodal, and interdisciplinary treatment, all components of which should be evidence-based" (**Fig. 1**). Since the release of the NPS in 2016, which was also the last year pain management was featured in *Anesthesiology Clinics*, clinical pain care has advanced on multiple fronts, which we highlight in this issue. We discuss novel uses of ketamine, the emerging field of biased opioid agonists, psychological approaches, and ultrasound-guided procedures. We also present an "old new treatment" in blinded pain cocktails used to reduce or optimize opioid treatment safely. Combining all of these and other therapies in a team-based approach has been shown to yield the most optimal results. Here, we present an exemplar of team-based care with an article on the Veterans Administration's approach to pain management.

Anesthesiology Clin 41 (2023) xv–xvii
https://doi.org/10.1016/j.anclin.2023.03.011 anesthesiology.theclinics.com
1932-2275/23/© 2023 Published by Elsevier Inc.

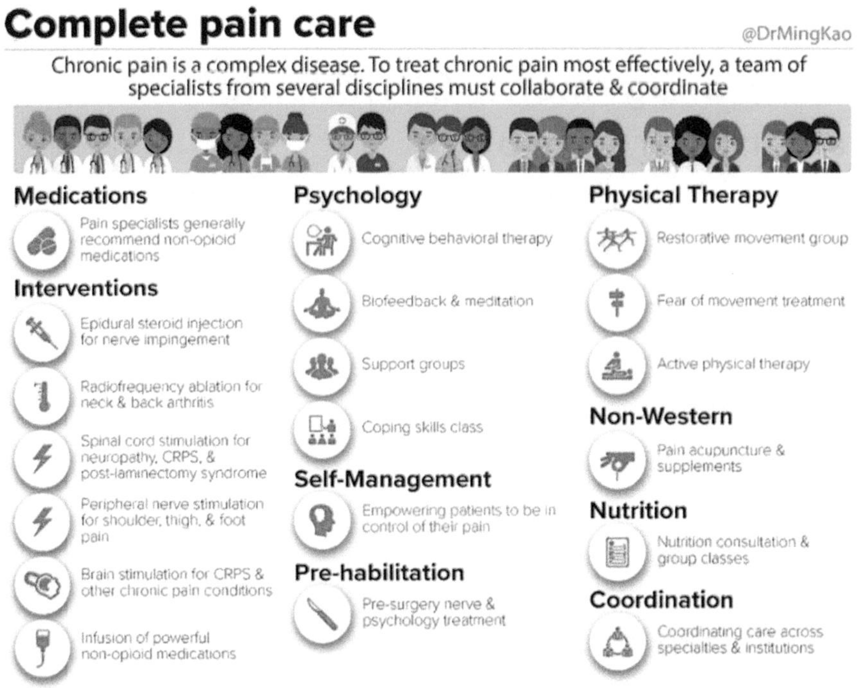

Complete pain care @DrMingKao

Chronic pain is a complex disease. To treat chronic pain most effectively, a team of specialists from several disciplines must collaborate & coordinate

Medications
Pain specialists generally recommend non-opioid medications

Interventions
Epidural steroid injection for nerve impingement
Radiofrequency ablation for neck & back arthritis
Spinal cord stimulation for neuropathy, CRPS, & post-laminectomy syndrome
Peripheral nerve stimulation for shoulder, thigh, & foot pain
Brain stimulation for CRPS & other chronic pain conditions
Infusion of powerful non-opioid medications

Psychology
Cognitive behavioral therapy
Biofeedback & meditation
Support groups
Coping skills class

Self-Management
Empowering patients to be in control of their pain

Pre-habilitation
Pre-surgery nerve & psychology treatment

Physical Therapy
Restorative movement group
Fear of movement treatment
Active physical therapy

Non-Western
Pain acupuncture & supplements

Nutrition
Nutrition consultation & group classes

Coordination
Coordinating care across specialties & institutions

Fig. 1. Components of comprehensive pain care.

In the NPS, we noted, "Every effort should be made to prevent illnesses and injuries that lead to pain, the progression of acute pain to a chronic condition, and the development of high-impact chronic pain." Specifically, many pain conditions start with an injury or surgery. Indeed, surgery is a significant contributor to CP. Here, we present a relatively new model for perioperative care, that of "transitional pain services" that position between traditional acute and chronic pain services. We also discuss optimal assessment and treatments of perioperative peripheral nerve injuries.

In the NPS, we noted the need to improve skills and competencies in pain management. Here, we present an update on pain medicine training in the United States and the strides made over the past couple decades. In addition, there are significant disparities in assessing and caring for those in pain. The NPS advocated "to improve the quality of pain care and reduce barriers for all minority, vulnerable, stigmatized, and underserved populations at risk of pain and pain care disparities." We provide an update on the state of disparities in pain medicine in the United States. One of the key messages of the NPS was that "better data are needed to understand the scope of the problem and to guide action." One of the challenges facing pain research (and all clinical research) is that the gold-standard randomized controlled trial often does not generate generalizable findings to impact health care directly. Indeed, there is a growing interest in pragmatic clinical trials (PCTs) and generating high-quality data within a clinical setting to inform practice better. Here, we present an article outlining the current and future opportunities for PCT and how to use a promising digital health platform called a "learning health system" to optimize the care of patients.

Finally, we thank Dr Lee Fleisher, Arlene Campos, and Joanna Collett for supporting this issue. Specifically, we want to thank Dr Fleisher for his role as Chief Medical Officer and Director of the Center for Clinical Standards and Quality for the Centers for

Medicare and Medicaid Services (CMS). In the NPS, we called for "reimbursement incentives and payment structures that support population-based care models of proven effectiveness, especially in interdisciplinary settings, and encourage multimodal care geared toward improving a full range of patient outcomes." We are pleased that CMS recently released new targeted billing codes to reimburse clinicians for CP management. These codes are an essential step in advancing comprehensive pain care.

We have made much progress since releasing the NPS in 2016. Much more work remains to achieve the vision put we put forward. That being "Americans ... would recognize chronic pain as a complex disease and a threat to public health ... significant public resources would be invested in the areas of preventing pain, creating access to evidence-based and high-quality pain assessment and treatment services and improving self-management abilities among those with pain. ...[I]ndividuals who live with chronic pain would be viewed and treated with compassion and respect." It is an exciting time to practice in this field and to impact the lives of the individual patient, their families, and society as a whole.

Sean C. Mackey, MD, PhD
Division of Pain Medicine
Stanford University School of Medicine
Department of Anesthesiology, Perioperative
and Pain Medicine, Neurosciences, and
(by courtesy) Neurology
1070 Arastradero Road
Suite 200, MC 5596
Palo Alto, CA 94304-1345, USA

Ronald G. Pearl, MD, PhD
Department of Anesthesiology
Perioperative and Pain Medicine
Stanford University School of Medicine
300 Pasteur Drive, Room H3589
Stanford, CA 94305-5640, USA

E-mail addresses:
smackey@stanford.edu (S.C. Mackey)
rgp@stanford.edu (R.G. Pearl)

REFERENCES

1. Von Korff M, Scher AI, Helmick C, et al. United States National Pain Strategy for Population Research: concepts, definitions, and pilot data. Pain 2016;17(10):1068–80.
2. Institute of Medicine (US) Committee on Advancing Pain Research, Care, and Education. Relieving Pain in America: A Blueprint for Transforming Prevention, Care, Education, and Research. Washington (DC): National Academies Press (US); 2011. PMID: 22553896.
3. National Pain Strategy Report - A Comprehensive Population Health-Level Strategy for Pain (2016) https://www.iprcc.nih.gov/node/5/national-pain-strategy-report Accessed April 12, 2023.
4. Dahlhamer J, Lucas J, Zelaya C, et al. Prevalence of chronic pain and high-impact chronic pain among adults—United States, 2016. MMWR Morb Mortal Wkly Rep 2018;67(36):1001–6.

Emerging Field of Biased Opioid Agonists

Anuj K. Aggarwal, MD*

KEYWORDS

• Opioids • Agonists • Perioperative medicine • G-protein coupled receptors
• Pharmacology

KEY POINTS

- The search for a drug with the analgesic effects of opioids without the adverse effects has been ongoing ever since the isolation of morphine from opium.
- Biased opioid agonists represent a new approach to activate G protein rather than β-arrestin pathways selectively, the latter being implicated in many of the adverse effects of opioids.
- Oliceridine, approved by the US Food and Drug Administration in 2020, is the first biased opioid agonist for clinical use available in the United States.
- Experience with oliceridine and the larger history of opioid development presents lessons for the need for scrutiny regarding safety and abuse potential of opioid derivatives.

INTRODUCTION

Taken for granted today, certain concepts in drug pharmacology have had profound influences in the way scientists and clinicians approach research, development, and use of drugs. Such concepts include the drug-receptor theory and the illumination of the function of G-protein coupled receptors (GPCRs); the latter work resulting in the 2012 Nobel Prize in Chemistry. To date, more than 800 GPCRs have been identified in humans, approximately 350 of which have been deemed as potential sites of therapeutic drug action; more than 500 US Food and Drug Administration (FDA)-approved drugs target GPCRs, and as of 2021, nearly 60 compounds in clinical studies target GPCRs.[1] Opioid receptors, one of the largest targets in modern medicine, are GPCRs, and the challenges faced by American and other societies from opioids present one of the largest issues facing drug therapeutics, medicine, and society as a whole.[2]

The concept of ligand bias, also referred to as functional selectivity, is a more recent conceptualization in pharmacology, which has the potential for profound implications

Department of Anesthesiology, Perioperative and Pain Medicine, Stanford University School of Medicine, Stanford, CA, USA
* 450 Broadway Street Pavilion A 1st Floor MC 5340, Redwood City, CA 94063.
E-mail address: akaggarw@stanford.edu

Anesthesiology Clin 41 (2023) 317–328
https://doi.org/10.1016/j.anclin.2023.02.001
anesthesiology.theclinics.com
1932-2275/23/

for the development of new medications.[3,4] The core concept of ligand bias is that some agonists, particularly at GPCRs, can stabilize different active conformations of the receptor than other agonists resulting in variable downstream molecular signals, and thus effects.[5] For opioids, this concept refers to variable downstream signaling, given that the activation of opioid GPCRs triggers 2 main transducing pathways, G proteins and GPCR kinases/β-arrestins.[6,7] The interest in ligand bias, and thus, in pursuing biased agonists, is predicated on the belief that desired effects compared with adverse effects may be mediated by separate signaling pathways resulting from GPCRs. This, in turn, sparked interest for opioid development: does ligand bias have the potential to lead to fulfilling the long sought-after goal of an opioid without adverse effects? It would be remiss to mention that diacetylmorphine, resynthesized by Bayer in the 1890s and then marketed as heroin, a safe and nonaddictive substitute for morphine, belays the perils and promises in the search for a safe opioid, one that has been repeated time and again.[8]

OPIOID RECEPTOR

Despite opioids being among the oldest and most widely used medications in the world, the term opioid itself did not originate until the 1950s followed by the discovery of the opioid receptor in the 1970s.[9] Although much progress has been made, questions and gaps remain regarding the exact mechanism and function of the opioid receptor and its downstream effects in humans. As mentioned, opioid receptors are GPCRs with 3 subtypes: delta (δ), kappa (κ), and mu (μ). In clinical practice, most opioid agonists target μ-opioid receptors which, when activated, result in both G protein and β-arrestin signaling.[10]

μ-opioid receptors, the target of traditional opioid analgesics, signal through activation of G proteins resulting in changes to neuronal function secondary to G-protein signaling mechanisms. At the presynaptic levels, neurotransmission is inhibited through inhibition of voltage-gated calcium channels, whereas on postsynaptic neurons, activation of G-protein coupled inwardly rectifying potassium channels results in hyperpolarization and thus inhibition of neurons.[10] Research has given us a more nuanced and complicated understanding of G-protein signaling secondary to the μ-receptor, including the ability of various kinases to, via phosphorylation, recruit and bind β-arrestin proteins to μ-receptors. This recruitment of β-arrestin proteins itself has been thought to lead to G-protein-independent signaling, although the downstream molecular mechanism remains an area of active research.[4,11]

Research has shown that ligand binding to the μ-opioid receptor can lead to differential activation of G-protein signaling compared with β-arrestin signaling.[12] This significance was highlighted by early research demonstrating differential physiological effects attributed to G protein versus β-arrestin signaling. The physiological effects of euphoria, drug dependence, and in particular, analgesia were attributed to be secondary from G-protein recruitment, whereas the physiological effects of nausea, vomiting, constipation, and respiratory depression were demonstrated to be secondary from β-arrestin recruitment.[13] This differential in physiologic effects due to differential molecular pathways from the μ-opioid receptor led to the pursuit of a biased opioid agonist, which would allow for analgesia through G-protein recruitment while reducing adverse effects associated with β-arrestin recruitment. However, these statements represent an oversimplification of the data, and understanding where this understanding stems from may be beneficial in understanding biased agonists and inform the discussion of specific agents.

The first demonstration of the physiological differences from potential G-protein selective agonism of μ-opioid receptors was in 1999, when improved analgesic effect of morphine was demonstrated in β-arrestin knockout mice with subsequent studies in 2005 showing these knockout mice had reduced gastrointestinal effects and respiratory depressant effects including decreased tolerance in comparison to morphine in mice with intact β-arrestin signaling.[14–16] These results were promising given that opioid-induced respiratory depression is the most common cause of death in opioid overdose and the large morbidity of gastrointestinal side effects from opioids. Early promising research showing this differential between G-protein-mediated physiological effects (analgesia) and β-arrestin-mediated physiological effects (nausea, vomiting, constipation, and respiratory depression) spurred the pursuit of G-protein-biased μ-receptor opioid agonists. Data in the intervening years, however, conflicted with the findings from global β-arrestin knockout models, implicating G-protein signaling directly in respiratory depression as well as in gastrointestinal effects.[10]

A deeper look into the data that emerged after the initial studies are important to inform discussion surrounding current candidates and drugs with biased opioid agonism as a proposed mechanism of action. The focus on the μ-receptor is corroborated by knockout studies showing that μ-receptor rather than δ-receptor and κ-receptor in opioid-induced respiratory depression.[17] This is further correlated with the expression of μ-receptors within neuronal network within the brainstem; studies eliminating the expression of μ-receptors from preBötzinder (preBötc) neurons and Kölliker-Fuse (KF) neurons, areas responsible for respiratory control, reduce morphine-induced and fentanyl-induced respiratory depression in animal models.[18–20] Further studies have shown that the effects of opioids resulting in respiratory depression at these neurons seems to be through μ-receptor G-protein-coupled inwardly rectifying potassium channels, with some research suggesting that voltage-gated calcium channel inhibition on presynaptic neurons is also involved in respiratory depression particularly for preBötc neurons.[10] Further, KF neurons have been found to be hyperpolarized through μ-receptor G protein inwardly rectifying potassium channels, inhibiting inspiratory drive.[21] As stated, these findings conflict with the hypothesis developed based on the knockout models that opioid-induced respiratory depression is not G-protein mediated but rather β-arrestin mediated. In fact, subsequent studies did not demonstrate changes in morphine or fentanyl-induced respiratory depression in β-arrestin knockout models.[22] A similar complicated story regarding mixed roles of G protein and β-arrestin pathways for opioid-induced gastrointestinal effects has emerged.[10]

It should be kept in mind that the hypothesis of differential physiological effects from G protein versus β-arrestin transduction from μ-receptor agonism stemmed from knockout models. However, β-arrestin is a widely expressed protein. In knockout models, many global systems, not just those limited to the μ-receptor will be affected and complicating interpretation of the early results and potentially resulting in unknown phenotypes. Attempts at creating models with more selective elimination of β-arrestin signaling exclusively for μ-receptors through modification of μ-receptor phosphorylation and the ability of β-arrestin proteins to bind to the specific receptor itself still demonstrated respiratory depression in the setting of opioid agonism, implying a more complicated picture of the molecular signaling steps that result in respiratory depression stemming from agonist activity at μ-opioid receptors.[10]

The initial promise of G-protein selective signaling, through a biased agonist at the μ-receptor, was based on promising data from β-arrestin knockout models. These results led to intense interest in the development of a “better” opioid, one with the analgesic efficacy of traditional opioids (morphine as the most common prototype) with an improved safety profile. However, subsequent data and studies painted a more complicated picture regarding specific physiological effects and the role of G-protein signaling and β-arrestin proteins. This pattern, of initial promise and findings, to be later complicated by other studies and findings, foreshadows the clinical development biased μ opioid receptor agonists, and demonstrates our expanding understanding of the molecular basis of opioid-induced physiological changes and the need for scrutiny when making presumptions of physiological effects from proposed molecular mechanisms of action.

Oliceridine and the Approval of the First Biased μ-Opioid Receptor Agonist

In 2020, the FDA approved oliceridine as the first opioid with labeling listing it as a biased opioid agonist. Oliceridine was approved for "the management of moderate to severe acute pain in adults, where the pain is severe enough to require intravenous opioid and for whom alternative treatments are inadequate," further the approval noted oliceridine was for short-term use in hospitals or controlled clinical settings, not for at-home administration.[23] Initial studies of oliceridine revealed a 3-fold preference for G-protein signaling on the activation of the μ-opioid receptor compared with β-arrestin in comparison to morphine or fentanyl.[24] Additional studies in animal models showed higher potency than morphine in regard to analgesic effects.[24]

Despite achieving approval in 2020 by the FDA, the drug was initially outvoted in 2018 due to concerns of Qt prolongation and findings from early clinical studies.[25] In early clinical studies, oliceridine produced subjective feelings similar to other opioid μ-agonists in humans, indicative of potential misuse potential along with conflicting studies noting gastrointestinal effects, tolerance, and addictive properties in animal models are also similar to traditional μ-opioid agonists.[26–28] The clinical description of oliceridine is based primarily on 2 phase 3 clinical studies, APOLLO-1 and APOLLO-2.[29,30] In APOLLO-1, respiratory depression was dose dependent for oliceridine and similar to morphine, which differed from earlier phase 2 studies showing improved respiratory adverse effect profile in comparison to morphine. However, APOLLO-1 did demonstrate decreased respiratory safety events in comparison to morphine.[31] In addition, APOLLO-1 showed decreased use of rescue medication for nausea and vomiting.[29] APOLLO-2 showed similar results regarding gastrointestinal and respiratory adverse effects as APOLLO-1. However, the respiratory depressant effects, although still dose-dependent, were not significantly different to placebo in APOLLO-2.[30] One reason for these results may rest on the previously discussed complexity regarding G protein versus β-arrestin-induced physiological changes. However, to further complicate the picture, other potential theories have been advanced, challenging the notion that oliceridine is a biased opioid agonist at all.

One notable feature shared by oliceridine with many of the currently described biased opioid agonists is that they seem to be partial agonists when measured in vitro.[32] This has raised the question, and perhaps, controversy, whether the improved adverse effect profile of oliceridine is explained from the partial agonist effects rather than the proposed biased recruitment of G-protein signaling over β-arrestin signaling. Although not compared head-to-head, the results of oliceridine do mimic the benefits seen with buprenorphine, a partial μ-opioid agonist with no known analgesic ceiling (similar to oliceridine) but with decreased respiratory and gastrointestinal effects compared with traditional μ-opioid agonists (also similar to oliceridine).[33–36] Why is the exact pharmacodynamic nature of oliceridine, and other lead candidates, so unclear?

Part of the challenge has been the high-fidelity characterization of the pharmacodynamic effects of biased μ-opioid receptor ligands is limited by methodological challenges. Oliceridine, as previously stated, was initially found to have comparable efficacy to morphine regarding G-protein activation, a finding like that of other G-protein-biased μ-opioid agonists.[10,37] However, further experimentation showed that oliceridine, along with the other agents, seemed to have lower efficacy than morphine. So why the discrepancy? Assays used to measure G-protein signaling are not highly sensitive to differences among various agents secondary to reserve receptors and the amplification that occurs with G-protein signaling, allowing even low-efficacy agents to reach the maximal reading on an assay.[10,38,39] This may pose the question of the methodology of measuring β-arrestin pathway signaling; as discussed, oliceridine was noted to have increased G-protein activation compared with β-arrestin signaling. Unlike G-protein transduction, in which the signal is molecularly amplified, β-arrestin interacts directly with the μ-opioid receptor, resulting in a protein–protein interaction without amplification, allowing more accurate measurements between agents regarding β-arrestin signaling.[38]

The importance of these methodological challenges becomes clearer when we consider the implications. If we have an agonist that has low-intrinsic efficacy, when measured against other agonists to compare its G-protein signaling, the low-efficacy agonist may demonstrate a maximal signal on the G-protein activation assay. However, when this same low efficacy agonist is run against the same agents in a β-arrestin assay, the low-efficacy agent demonstrates reduced recruitment of the β-arrestin pathway due to the ability of the assay to detect and quantify these differences more accurately. Therefore, oliceridine, and other candidates proposed to be biased μ-receptor agonists, may well be low-efficacy agonists when compared with morphine rather than biased agonists, showing high G-protein activation comparable to that of morphine but significantly lower β-arrestin recruitment, even though the findings are simply due to the nature of the 2 disparate assays.

Researchers have worked to develop assays to better characterize the pharmacodynamic nature of these agents. These newer studies have shown that oliceridine, and potentially other lead candidates characterized as biased μ-opioid agonists, seem to be partial agonists, serving as a potential explanation for the lower intrinsic efficacy.[32,40] An understanding of the methodological challenges and the observations from the APOLLO trials, raises questions on the proposed mechanism of action of oliceridine and potentially other agents. The importance rests on the presumed safety due to the mechanism of action. An examination of tramadol, an older opioid, helps illuminate the complicated nature of these questions.

Tramadol's metabolite, desmetramadol, was identified as a G-protein-biased μ-opioid agonist with the parent molecule possessing serotonergic and noradrenergic properties.[41] Approved for use in the United States in 1995, tramadol is the second most prescribed opioid in the United States. It has long shown less respiratory depression, including in overdose settings where studies have demonstrated that most cases of overdoses did not demonstrate respiratory depression.[41] Why tramadol does not seem to produce respiratory depression has prompted significant research into its pharmacodynamics. Desmetramadol has shown decreased efficacy for μ-opioid receptors but this does not seem to be a complete explanation when attempting to explain the lack of respiratory depression in cases of overdose.[41] Research has shown that desmetramadol spares β-arrestin activation, leading to the theory that desmetramadol may be a biased μ-opioid agonist, resulting in its increased safety profile. However, this finding must be considered with the issues discussed before assay methodology and the conflicting results surrounding implicating β-arrestin as the pathway responsible for opioid-induced respiratory depression.

One may argue that although the mechanism of action remains unclear, the clinical data are clear about increased safety regarding respiratory depression with tramadol.

Here, the idea of increased safety in the context of opioids must be weighed carefully. Initially, tramadol was thought to be less addictive and less likely to be abused than other opioids. However, despite those early assumptions, years of clinical use have borne that tramadol produces stimulant and euphoric effects and is a drug of abuse.[42] Tramadol's story raises interesting questions. Although the concept that it might be less addictive (or not at all) have not borne out, and the pharmacodynamic effect of desmetramadol have come into question due to observations of decreased respiratory depression, its role as a potential biased opioid agonist remains unclear. If it is a biased opioid agonist, it raises the question of understanding these agents as safe. Although potentially leading to less respiratory depression, addiction remains problematic. Further, tramadol is confounded by its additional serotonergic and noradrenergic properties. Tramadol raises potentially more questions than answers and begs the question of biased opioid agonists and the potential for abuse and misuse and opens the discussion of truly answering questions around safety.

Abuse Potential of Biased Opioid Agonists

Although the earlier discussion raises questions in how to view and interpret the emerging field of biased opioid agonists, the question regarding abuse potential is perhaps more complicated and yet perhaps the most urgent. One of the premises of the commercial development of biased μ-opioid agonists was their increased safety regarding respiratory depression and gastrointestinal effects. The discussion has shown so far why this picture and presumption is likely more complicated than initially thought, and the more complete picture should be considered when developing, designing, and interpreting clinical studies and data of these new agents. In addition to reducing respiratory depression and gastrointestinal side effects, it has been suggested that biased opioid agonists may have lower abuse potential compared with full agonists.

Initial animal data from β-arrestin knockout mice suggested enhanced analgesia with decreased adverse effects, including the development of tolerance.[14] However, the same studies suggested that the rewarding effects of morphine were not mediated by the β-arrestin pathway implicating the G-protein pathway as the molecular actor for opioid reward in the mice.[14,43] Further studies done with oliceridine have shown that oliceridine retains abuse potential like that of other opioid analgesics such as morphine and oxycodone in animal models.[44] In a single human study, intravenous oliceridine and morphine produced similar results when looking at the endpoints of "liking" and "high," which are often predictive of abuse potential, thus agreeing with animal data regarding abuse potential of oliceridine.[44] As such, the understanding and discussion around safety should consider that biased opioid agonists seem to retain similar abuse potential as other opioid agonists. Interpreting animal data, once again, must be made with the understanding the knockout models affect multiple systems independent of opioid signaling, and should be given additional attention to interpreting and making conclusions regarding complicated phenotypes such as abuse potential.

Oliceridine is notable because it is easily the most-studied biased opioid agonist to date, developed under the framework that G-protein signaling produces desired analgesia while reducing adverse effects, including gastrointestinal effects, respiratory depression, tolerance, and abuse potential. The accuracy and completeness of this framework remain areas of active investigation, as the animal and clinical data have shown certain issues in translating the theoretical promise shown of biased opioid agonists in initial mice models. Notably, oliceridine seems to retain abuse potential though does show evidence of reduced adverse events related to gastrointestinal

Table 1
Representative opioids and candidate biased opioid agonists

Drug/ Candidate Agent	Biased at μ-Receptor?	Pharmacodynamics	Use
Morphine	No	Full μ-opioid agonist	Analgesic
Fentanyl	No	Full μ-opioid agonist (high efficacy)	Analgesic
Tramadol	Possible G-protein bias but disputed	Low-efficacy μ-opioid agonist, SNRI	Analgesic
Oliceridine	Possible G-protein bias but disputed	Low-efficacy μ-opioid agonist (data seem to suggest partial agonist)	Analgesic
PXM21	Possible G-protein bias but disputed	Low-efficacy μ-opioid agonist (data seem to suggest partial agonist)	Experimental
SR-17018	Possible G-protein bias but disputed	Low-efficacy μ-opioid agonist (data seem to suggest partial agonist)	Experimental
Mitragynine	Possible G-protein bias but disputed	Low-to-medium efficacy μ-opioid agonist	Experimental

and respiratory effects. However, this too is complicated considering oliceridine's potential pharmacodynamic profile as a partial μ-agonist in vitro, raising the question how much of the improved adverse effect profile is secondary to a preference for recruiting G-protein-coupled signaling rather than its effects as a partial agonist effect at the μ-opioid receptor, like buprenorphine.

Experimental Biased μ-Opioid Receptor Agonists

There are other candidate biased μ-opioid agonists in development, notably PZM21, mitragynine pseudoindoxyl, and SR-17018 (**Table 1**), all of which are currently still in the experimental stage.[45,46] Limited data from PZM21 and mitragynine pseudoindoxyl have shown that these compounds may have less abuse potential, and in general, these newer compounds seem to show a greater degree of G-protein recruitment when compared with β-arrestin than oliceridine in vitro.[44–46] Mitragynine is notable because it is an alkaloid found in *Mitragyna speciosa*, more commonly known as kratom.[47] Although biased agonism has been suggested as an explanation for its potential decreased abuse potential, other studies have again shown suggested it to be a partial agonist, with others suggesting it to be a full agonist.[47] Understanding some of its observed effects is complicated by known interactions with other receptors including adenosine, serotonin, and dopamine receptors, although the significance of these is not known. Although agents may be classified as biased μ-opioid receptors, our understanding is ever evolving and the data less clear.

A look at PZM21's data and story shows similarities to oliceridine. Initial data suggested PZM21 to have effective analgesic properties without respiratory depression or drug-seeking behavior, although subsequent studies again showed respiratory depression similar to that of morphine, although limited data continues to suggest that it may have less abuse potential compared with other oliceridine.[48] Studies looking at the pharmacodynamic mechanism have suggested that initial thoughts of PZM21 as a biased agonist may not be correct but rather its observed effects may be due to its pharmacodynamics meditated through weak partial agonism.[49] Interestingly, studies have demonstrated the ability of PZM21 to antagonize morphine in drug-seeking studies, raising the prospect that it could be used in the treatment of opioid use disorder not unlike buprenorphine's current role and use due to its properties as a partial opioid agonist.[50]

SR-17018 is notable as initial data showed a 100-fold bias for G-protein signaling over β-arresting signaling, although later studies demonstrated that there may be no bias at all.[32] Reasons for this may be related to issues with methodology and interpreting assays as previously discussed, again noting the importance of understanding the complex picture surrounding the development of potential biased opioid agonists. Despite this, SR-17018 demonstrates interesting pharmacokinetic and pharmacodynamic effects. It promises to be an interesting ligand, demonstrating the potential of the pursuit of biased opioid agonists to reveal and deepen our understanding of opioid pharmacology and perhaps, discover new avenues for exploration and drug development. Future studies and data will help clarify and further the field of biased opioid agonists, as will the data that will come from real-world use of oliceridine. Regardless, it is clear the concept has opened avenues for development and is expanding the understanding of opioid pharmacology.

SUMMARY

In its role as a first in-class drug, there is no doubt that further data from clinical use of oliceridine will help scientists and clinicians better understand this emerging field of potential biased opioid ligands. However, the data so far has shown that despite early animal data showing promise of selective G-protein recruitment in potential physiological effects, we need to scrutinize both the safety and abuse potential of these new agents, with oliceridine showing similar abuse potential to currently available opioid analgesics. It is also a cautionary tale that echoes the development of heroin in the late nineteenth century, the marketing of oxycontin as having an extremely small risk of addiction, and the experience of many abuse-deterrent opioid formulations the failed once brought to market.[51,52]

The story of the development of biased opioid agonists at every stage shows an ever-changing story. From initial promise of differential physiological effects from G protein compared with β-arrestin signaling, which was then disputed in subsequent studies, to issues with methodology classifying agents as biased opioid agonists with subsequent data suggestion potentially weak partial agonism to explain the observed phenotypic effects, the central thesis and guiding principle in the pursuit of biased opioid ligands has been the promise of safety. The changing science has challenged the notion of safety, and although skepticism should not translate into fatalism, prudent scrutiny and caution continue to be warranted, a lesson that the history of opioid development and introduction have painfully rendered.

The advent of new molecular tools and a greater understanding of the mechanism of the opioid receptor and its effect on human physiology puts the possibility of the development of an opioid with retained analgesic efficacy without it its significant adverse effects closer than before. Pursuing such a drug or class of drugs is warranted; to the author's knowledge, there are no preclinical or clinical development drugs that are as effective for acute pain as opioids. This is made clear by the fact that opioids are the mainstay even today for perioperative pain management despite their adverse effects including pruritis, nausea, vomiting, sedation, respiratory depression, addiction, and death.

A healthy scrutiny of the data and a call for more studies of opioid compounds is warranted. Biased opioid agonists in the lineage of oliceridine are not the only new opioids that may enter the market in the coming years. Data and experiments involving salvinorin A derivatives, piperidine benzimidazoles, carfentanil amides, biased κ-opioid receptors agonists, biased δ-opioid receptor agonists, strategies to decrease central nervous system entry of opioids to minimize the "rush" with abused drugs, mixing opioid agonism with other targets, as well as work in selectivity for μ-opioid receptor variants represent the continued efforts of scientists, industry, and clinicians to develop opioid analgesics with decreased adverse effects.[45,53–55] However, early periods of excitement have been tempered with the reality of drug development, and it remains clear that there is still much to elucidate in the molecular mechanism of opioid receptors and their observed physiological and behavioral phenotypes. Will pharmacological manipulation result in an opioid that separates the adverse effects and reward from analgesia? The answer remains unknown. Oliceridine represents possibly the start of a new direction but also highlights the need for scrutiny and careful inquiry because new drugs are developed and brought to clinical use given the varied results seen between animal models and human clinical trials. Notably, this healthy scrutiny was recently advocated by the lead researcher whose initial work in 1999 in β-arrestin knockout mice sparked interest in biased opioid agonists.[56] Physicians, scientists, and policy makers will need to work in parallel to ensure safe, timely, and appropriate access for opioids for pain relief, balancing innovation and safety.

CLINICS CARE POINTS

- Twenty-one years after first demonstration of differential effects between β-arrestin and G-protein pathways of the μ-opioid receptor, oliceridine became the first FDA-approved biased opioid agonist
- Preclinical data suggested marked differences in respiratory depression, addiction potential, gastrointestinal effects, and other adverse effects to potential agonists favoring G-protein signaling
- Clinical data have not borne out the degree and, in some cases, the phenotype, of safety, suggested by preclinical data, suggesting increased scrutiny, including potential other mechanisms of action, to ensure patient safety of future biased opioid agonists

DISCLOSURE

None.

REFERENCES

1. Bruchas MR, Roth BL. New technologies for elucidating opioid receptor function. Trends Pharmacol Sci 2016;37(4):279–89.
2. DeWeerdt S. Tracing the US opioid crisis to its roots. Nature 2019;573(7773):S10–2.
3. Michel MC, Charlton SJ. Biased agonism in drug discovery-is it too soon to choose a path? Mol Pharmacol 2018;93(4):259–65.
4. Smith JS, Lefkowitz RJ, Rajagopal S. Biased signaling: from simple switches to allosteric microprocessors. Nat Rev Drug Discov 2018;17(4):243–60.

5. Wingler LM, Lefkowitz RJ. Conformational basis of g protein-coupled receptor signaling versatility. Trends Cell Biol 2020;30(9):736–47.
6. Kenakin T. Biased receptor signaling in drug discovery. Pharmacol Rev 2019; 71(2):267–315.
7. Onfroy L, Galandrin S, Pontier SM, et al. G protein stoichiometry dictates biased agonism through distinct receptor-G protein partitioning. Sci Rep 2017;7(1):7885.
8. Goodman LS, Gilman A. The pharmacological basis of therapeutics: a textbook of pharmacology, toxicology, and therapeutics for physicians and medical students. 1st ed. New York: Macmillan Publishing; 1941.
9. Pert CB, Snyder SH. Opiate receptor: demonstration in nervous tissue. Science 1973;179(4077):1011–4.
10. Gillis A, Kliewer A, Kelly E, et al. Critical assessment of g protein-biased agonism at the μ-opioid receptor. Trends Pharmacol Sci 2020;41(12):947–59.
11. Siuda ER, Carr R, Rominger DH, et al. Biased mu-opioid receptor ligands: a promising new generation of pain therapeutics. Curr Opin Pharmacol 2017;32: 77–84.
12. Che T, Dwivedi-Agnihotri H, Shukla AK, et al. Biased ligands at opioid receptors: Current status and future directions. Sci Signal 2021;14(677):eaav0320.
13. Porter-Stransky KA, Weinshenker D. Arresting the development of addiction: the role of β -arrestin 2 in drug abuse. J Pharmacol Exp Ther 2017;361(3):341–8.
14. Bohn LM, Lefkowitz RJ, Gainetdinov RR, et al. Enhanced morphine analgesia in mice lacking beta-arrestin 2. Science 1999;286(5449):2495–8.
15. Bohn LM, Gainetdinov RR, Lin FT, et al. Mu-opioid receptor desensitization by beta-arrestin-2 determines morphine tolerance but not dependence. Nature 2000;408(6813):720–3.
16. Raehal KM, Walker JKL, Bohn LM. Morphine side effects in beta-arrestin 2 knockout mice. J Pharmacol Exp Ther 2005;314(3):1195–201.
17. Matthes HW, Smadja C, Valverde O, et al. Activity of the delta-opioid receptor is partially reduced, whereas activity of the kappa-receptor is maintained in mice lacking the mu-receptor. J Neurosci 1998;18(18):7285–95.
18. Montandon G, Slutsky AS. Solving the opioid crisis: respiratory depression by opioids as critical end point. Chest 2019;156(4):653–8.
19. Varga AG, Reid BT, Kieffer BL, et al. Differential impact of two critical respiratory centres in opioid-induced respiratory depression in awake mice. J Physiol 2020; 598(1):189–205.
20. Bachmutsky I, Wei XP, Kish E, et al. Opioids depress breathing through two small brainstem sites. Elife 2020;9:e52694.
21. Levitt ES, Abdala AP, Paton JFR, et al. M opioid receptor activation hyperpolarizes respiratory-controlling kölliker-fuse neurons and suppresses post-inspiratory drive. J Physiol 2015;593(19):4453–69.
22. Kliewer A, Gillis A, Hill R, et al. Morphine-induced respiratory depression is independent of β-arrestin2 signalling. Br J Pharmacol 2020;177(13):2923–31.
23. Tan HS, Habib AS. Oliceridine: a novel drug for the management of moderate to severe acute pain - a review of current evidence. J Pain Res 2021;14:969–79.
24. Chen XT, Pitis P, Liu G, et al. Structure-activity relationships and discovery of a G protein biased μ opioid receptor ligand, [(3-methoxythiophen-2-yl)methyl]({2-[(9R)-9-(pyridin-2-yl)-6-oxaspiro-[4.5]decan-9-yl]ethyl})amine (Trv130), for the treatment of acute severe pain. J Med Chem 2013;56(20):8019–31.
25. Commissioner, O. FDA Approves New Opioid for Intravenous Use in Hospitals, Other Controlled Clinical Settings. Available at: https://www.fda.gov/news-events/

press-announcements/fda-approves-newopioid- intravenous-use-hospitals-other-controlled-clinical-settings. Accessed 1 October 2022.
26. Pedersen MF, Wróbel TM, Märcher-Rørsted E, et al. Biased agonism of clinically approved μ-opioid receptor agonists and TRV130 is not controlled by binding and signaling kinetics. Neuropharmacology 2020;166:107718.
27. Liang DY, Li WW, Nwaneshiudu C, et al. Pharmacological characters of oliceridine, a μ-opioid receptor g-protein–biased ligand in mice. Anesth Analg 2019; 129(5):1414–21.
28. Altarifi AA, David B, Muchhala KH, et al. Effects of acute and repeated treatment with the biased mu opioid receptor agonist TRV130 (Oliceridine) on measures of antinociception, gastrointestinal function, and abuse liability in rodents. J Psychopharmacol 2017;31(6):730–9.
29. Viscusi ER, Skobieranda F, Soergel DG, et al. APOLLO-1: a randomized placebo and active-controlled phase III study investigating oliceridine (Trv130), a G protein-biased ligand at the μ-opioid receptor, for management of moderate-to-severe acute pain following bunionectomy. J Pain Res 2019;12:927–43.
30. Singla NK, Skobieranda F, Soergel DG, et al. Apollo-2: a randomized, placebo and active-controlled phase iii study investigating oliceridine (Trv130), a g protein-biased ligand at the μ-opioid receptor, for management of moderate to severe acute pain following abdominoplasty. Pain Pract 2019;19(7):715–31.
31. Singla N, Minkowitz HS, Soergel DG, et al. A randomized, Phase IIb study investigating oliceridine (Trv130), a novel μ-receptor G-protein pathway selective (M-gps) modulator, for the management of moderate to severe acute pain following abdominoplasty. J Pain Res 2017;10:2413–24.
32. Gillis A, Gondin AB, Kliewer A, et al. Low intrinsic efficacy for G protein activation can explain the improved side effect profiles of new opioid agonists. Sci Signal 2020;13(625):eaaz3140.
33. Aiyer R, Gulati A, Gungor S, et al. Treatment of chronic pain with various buprenorphine formulations: a systematic review of clinical studies. Anesth Analg 2018; 127(2):529–38.
34. Gudin J, Fudin J. A narrative pharmacological review of buprenorphine: a unique opioid for the treatment of chronic pain. Pain Ther 2020;9(1):41–54.
35. Olinvyk [package insert]. Chesterbrook, PA: Trevena Inc; 2020.
36. Li AH, Schmiesing C, Aggarwal AK. Evidence for continuing buprenorphine in the perioperative period. Clin J Pain 2020;36(10):764–74.
37. DeWire SM, Yamashita DS, Rominger DH, et al. A G protein-biased ligand at the μ-opioid receptor is potently analgesic with reduced gastrointestinal and respiratory dysfunction compared with morphine. J Pharmacol Exp Ther 2013;344(3): 708–17.
38. Nickolls SA, Waterfield A, Williams RE, et al. Understanding the effect of different assay formats on agonist parameters: a study using the μ-opioid receptor. J Biomol Screen 2011;16(7):706–16.
39. Kelly E. Efficacy and ligand bias at the μ-opioid receptor. Br J Pharmacol 2013; 169(7):1430–46.
40. Vasudevan L, Vandeputte M, Deventer M, et al. Assessment of structure-activity relationships and biased agonism at the Mu opioid receptor of novel synthetic opioids using a novel, stable bio-assay platform. Biochem Pharmacol 2020; 177:113910.
41. Zebala JA, Schuler AD, Kahn SJ, et al. Desmetramadol is identified as a g-protein biased μ opioid receptor agonist. Front Pharmacol 2019;10:1680.

42. Miotto K, Cho AK, Khalil MA, et al. Trends in tramadol: pharmacology, metabolism, and misuse. Anesth Analg 2017;124(1):44–51.
43. Bohn LM, Gainetdinov RR, Sotnikova TD, et al. Enhanced rewarding properties of morphine, but not cocaine, in beta(Arrestin)-2 knock-out mice. J Neurosci 2003; 23(32):10265–73.
44. Negus SS, Freeman KB. Abuse potential of biased mu opioid receptor agonists. Trends Pharmacol Sci 2018;39(11):916–9.
45. Faouzi A, Varga BR, Majumdar S. Biased opioid ligands. Molecules 2020;25(18): 4257.
46. James IE, Skobieranda F, Soergel DG, et al. A first-in-human clinical study with trv734, an orally bioavailable g-protein-biased ligand at the μ-opioid receptor. Clin Pharmacol Drug Dev 2020;9(2):256–66.
47. Kruegel AC, Gassaway MM, Kapoor A, et al. Synthetic and receptor signaling explorations of the mitragyna alkaloids: mitragynine as an atypical molecular framework for opioid receptor modulators. J Am Chem Soc 2016;138(21):6754–64.
48. Kelly E, Conibear A, Henderson G. Biased agonism: lessons from studies of opioid receptor agonists. Annu Rev Pharmacol Toxicol 2023;63:491–515.
49. Yudin Y, Rohacs T. The G-protein-biased agents PZM21 and TRV130 are partial agonists of μ-opioid receptor-mediated signalling to ion channels. Br J Pharmacol 2019;176(17):3110–25.
50. Kudla L, Bugno R, Skupio U, et al. Functional characterization of a novel opioid, PZM21, and its effects on the behavioural responses to morphine. Br J Pharmacol 2019;176(23):4434–45.
51. Litman RS, Pagán OH, Cicero TJ. Abuse-deterrent opioid formulations. Anesthesiology 2018;128(5):1015–26.
52. Van Zee A. The promotion and marketing of oxycontin: commercial triumph, public health tragedy. Am J Public Health 2009;99(2):221–7.
53. Miyazaki T, Choi IY, Rubas W, et al. Nktr-181: a novel mu-opioid analgesic with inherently low abuse potential. J Pharmacol Exp Ther 2017;363(1):104–13.
54. Ding H, Czoty PW, Kiguchi N, et al. A novel orvinol analog, BU08028, as a safe opioid analgesic without abuse liability in primates. Proc Natl Acad Sci U S A 2016;113(37):E5511–8.
55. Pasternak GW. Mu opioid pharmacology: 40 years to the promised land. Adv Pharmacol 2018;82:261–91.
56. Servick K. Safety benefits of 'biased' opioids scrutinized. Science 2020; 367(6481):966.

Pain Medicine Education in the United States

Success, Threats, and Opportunities

Anuj K. Aggarwal, MD[a,*,1], Lynn Kohan, MD[b], Susan Moeschler, MD[c], James Rathmell, MD[d], Jane S. Moon, MD[e], Meredith Barad, MD[a,1]

KEYWORDS

• Pain medicine • Graduate medical education • Multidisciplinary • Chronic pain

KEY POINTS

- Training of pain medicine practitioners has quickly transitioned from an apprenticeship model to a structured educational model under the auspices of the ACGME and national leadership.
- Pain medicine education continues to adapt to evolving educational pedagogy.
- Challenges due to the explosive growth in pain knowledge and lack of national standardization offer opportunities for pain medicine educators to shape the future of the specialty.

The year 2022 marked the 30th anniversary of the Accreditation Council for Graduate Medical Education's (ACGME) first accreditation of training programs in the specialty of pain medicine. It offers a time to reflect on the past, present, and future of pain medicine education in the United States through the lens of successes, threats, and opportunities. The training of future pain practitioners is key to shaping and maintaining the growth of the field, as well as addressing emerging challenges.

HISTORICAL BACKGROUND

The treatment of pain, the oldest medical problem, and the training of practitioners to treat it have been central themes in the history of medicine, with rich stories spanning

[a] Department of Anesthesiology, Perioperative and Pain Medicine, Stanford University School of Medicine, Stanford, CA 94305, USA; [b] Department of Anesthesiology, University of Virginia, 545 Ray C Hunt Drive, Suite 3168, Charlottesville, VA 22903, USA; [c] Department of Anesthesiology, Mayo Clinic, 200 First Street Southwest, Rochester, MN 55905, USA; [d] Department of Anesthesiology, Perioperative, and Pain Medicine, Brigham and Women's Health Care, 75 Francis Street, Boston, MA 0215, USA; [e] Department of Anesthesiology and Perioperative Medicine, University of California, Los Angeles, 757 Westwood Plaza, Suite 3325, Los Angeles, CA 90095-7403, USA

[1] Present address: 450 Broadway Street, Pavilion A, 1st Floor MC 5340, Redwood City, CA 94063.

* Corresponding author.

E-mail address: akaggarw@stanford.edu

Anesthesiology Clin 41 (2023) 329–339

https://doi.org/10.1016/j.anclin.2023.03.004

anesthesiology.theclinics.com

1932-2275/23/

the spectrum of human cultures and civilizations. Long viewed as a fundamental human experience with philosophical and religious meaning, pain would not be explored scientifically until the 1800s. By the end of the 19th century, the world had witnessed the first public demonstration of surgical anesthesia and the first synthesis of potent analgesics like morphine and aspirin. Physicians had also begun to see the multifaceted nature of pain not only as an acute phenomenon but also as a chronic illness, as well as a severe affliction in progressive diseases like cancer.[1]

It was only in the second half of the 20th century that the notion of chronic pain as a disease entity in and of itself came into the mainstream.[1] World War II provided a unique opportunity for physicians to treat complex injuries, and two anesthesiologists—Henry K. Beecher, MD, the first Anesthetist-in-Chief at the Massachusetts General Hospital (Boston, MA), and John J. Bonica, MD, future founding Chair of the Department of Anesthesiology at the University of Washington (Seattle, WA)—separately pioneered an understanding of pain as a multidisciplinary problem.

During his two-year stint in the Mediterranean Theater, Henry Beecher provided anesthesia for severely wounded soldiers and marveled at the highly subjective experience of pain. His observation that many soldiers experienced far less pain than civilians with similar injuries led him to conclude that "strong emotions can block pain."[2] His battlefield observations during the war followed by his extensive research after the war resulted in a new analgesic testing method using double-blinded crossover trials, simple numerical scales to quantify pain, and clear demonstration of the power of the placebo effect.[2–4]

John Bonica, a professional wrestler-turned-anesthesiologist, is widely recognized to be the founder of the discipline of pain medicine. As Chief of Anesthesia at Madigan Army Hospital (Tacoma, Washington) during the war, he championed the use of regional anesthesia and pioneered the concept of multidisciplinary pain management by holding informal lunch meetings to discuss complex patients with a neurologist, psychiatrist, internist, and orthopedic surgeon. In 1973, his efforts led to the formation of the International Association for the Study of Pain (IASP), signifying the formal start of the discipline of pain medicine. [5] Just a few years later, Bonica emphasized the need for "education and training of students, house officers, physicians, and other health professionals to improve the care of patients suffering from pain."[6] Highly conscious of the societal burden of chronic pain, Bonica understood that strong education in pain management would be essential to addressing this public health dilemma.

THE ADVENT OF MULTIDISCIPLINARY PAIN MEDICINE FELLOWSHIPS

Little literature or documentation about academic pain programs existed prior to the late 1980s. William Brose, MD, the founder of the pain medicine division at Stanford University, in personal correspondence with the authors, recalls much of pain education training as using an apprenticeship model without a formal curriculum or integrated educational experiences before the late 1980s. The University of Washington was a notable exception under the leadership of John Loeser, MD, after Bonica's retirement.

In 1989, Stephen Abrams, then Chair of the American Society of Anesthesiologists Committee on Pain Therapy and Chair of the American Society of Regional Anesthesia and Pain Medicine (ASRA) Committee on Pain Standards, wrote a letter to the American Board of Anesthesiology (ABA) that called for a certification process for anesthesiologists who had "demonstrated competence in the management of pain."[7] Concurrently, Abrams advocated for the ACGME and its Residency Review

Committee (RRC) to start the process of accreditation of subspecialty-training programs in pain medicine within anesthesiology programs. Notably, the backdrop to this effort was an emerging framework for pain certification that was fragmented.[8] For example, in the 1980s, the American Academy of Pain Management offered certification without an examination, the American Academy of Pain Medicine had plans for a certification examination, and the American Board of Medical Specialties (ABMS) had declined an application by the American Academy of Pain Medicine to formalize pain medicine as a new primary medical specialty.[8] It was notable that the ABMS had received multiple inquiries regarding the establishment of pain medicine as a subspecialty, sparking fears that pain medicine would be fragmented as a subspecialty among numerous primary specialties.[8]

In 1989, recognizing the issue facing pain medicine and other medical specialties, the ACGME convened a conference to address the issue of medical specialties that did not yet have certification.[9] Following that meeting, under the leadership of Bill Owens who was then a member of both the ABA Board of Directors and the ACGME RRC for Anesthesiology, the ABA applied to the ABMS for recognition of pain management as a subspecialty within anesthesiology in January 1991. The ABMS approval in March 1991 made pain management only the second subspecialty within anesthesiology to receive recognition—the first being critical care medicine in 1985.[8] The ABMS approval paved the way for the ACGME to develop program requirements for accreditation of programs in pain management at the same time that the ABA was developing the examination that would lead to a certificate of added qualifications in pain management (later renamed as subspecialty certification in pain medicine), which was first administered in September 1993.[10]

Since then, the number of ACGME-accredited fellowships has grown. In 1994, the second year that the ACGME included pain medicine fellowships in its list of accredited programs, there were 55 fellowships, reflecting the rapid growth from the mid-1980s to the 1990s in formalized pain education. Most recently, as of September 2022, there were 113 ACGME-accredited pain fellowships.[11,12]

With the establishment of pain management with subspecialty board certification through the ABA and formal accreditation of training programs by the ACGME, pain management education began to grow and become more streamlined in the larger context of graduate medical education. Dr Bonica's original push to develop multidisciplinary pain care evolved into collaboration between four specialties who agreed to a single and unified set of program requirements for all ACGME-accredited pain fellowships regardless of sponsoring specialty. In 1999, the ABA invited representatives of the American Board of Psychiatry and Neurology (ABPN) and the American Board of Physical Medicine & Rehabilitation (ABPMR) to join the ABA's Pain Management Examination Committee to broaden the examination beyond its prior focus on regional anesthesia, and in 2000, the ABPN and ABPMR began issuing certificates of subspecialty certification in pain management to those diplomates who passed the expanded ABA examination. Between 2002 and 2006, the ACGME working in collaboration with the ABA, ABPN, and ABPMR developed new program requirements for pain fellowship training programs aimed at improving the quality of education in pain medicine and promoting a multidisciplinary approach to care. The new program requirements were adopted in 2006. In 1999, the ABMS introduced 6 core competencies for all specialties, and the ACGME, as part of the ACGME educational milestones project, asked each specialty to develop subcompetencies and milestones within each of the 6 core competencies. The first version for pain medicine was released in 2013.[13,14] With the evolution of the field and iterative processes at the ACGME, the second version of the milestones for pain medicine was released in 2022, reflecting the incorporation and standardization of pain education under a comprehensive medical education pedagogy since the 1980s.[15] The specialty was given the title pain medicine to reflect the more comprehensive role of diagnosis, treatment, management, consultation, and interdisciplinary collaboration recognizing chronic pain as a disease state rather than pain management, implying a focus solely on treating of a symptom.

The involvement of multiple disciplines has posed unique challenges for pain medicine training programs, and efforts at the start of the 21st century by program directors at various pain fellowships culminated in the formal incorporation of the Association of Pain Program Directors (APPD) in 2013, with formal affiliations with the American Academy of Pain Medicine and ASRA. The APPD helped initiate the first pain medicine fellowship match in 2013 and the first common application via the Electronic Residency Application Service (ERAS) in 2014.[16] The recent history of pain medicine education has been dominated by efforts to craft pain medicine into a distinct specialty, with certification and standardization of training programs to aid in the growth of the specialty under the guidance of the ACGME.

Since their inception in 1982, every version of the ACGME Program Requirements for Pain Medicine Training Programs contained the requirement that allowed only 1 training program per institution. This requirement was the deliberate work of Bill Owens and the team that originally crafted the first program requirements and was aimed at preventing the fragmentation of pain care among multiple programs within a single institution. In 2019, the ACGME removed this provision from the program requirements, paving the way for physical medicine and rehabilitation (PM&R), neurology, psychiatry, and other disciplines to be granted ACGME accreditation using the same accreditation requirements as pain medicine fellowships within anesthesiology. This echoed the concern for fragmentation of the field during the 1980s; however, as of February 2023, all pain medicine programs listed by the ACGME are accredited within anesthesiology, including those with core programs in PM&R and neurology.[12] While other non-ACGME fellowships do exist, such as interventional spine and musculoskeletal medicine fellowships, ACGME-accredited fellowships continue to emphasize and standardize the multidisciplinary nature of chronic pain management.[17] The threat of training fragmentation, however, is ever present given the multidisciplinary nature of the specialty.

As of February 2023, there are 114 accredited pain fellowship programs. The most recent year for which the ACGME published data, 2019-2020, noted 108 programs with 386 fellows. The mean age of pain fellows was 33.8 years, 22.8% were female, and 42 identified as underrepresented minorities in medicine.[18] Of the 386 fellows, 252 were from US allopathic medical schools, 70 from international medical schools, and 64 from US osteopathic medical schools.[18] Pain fellowships reported a total of 993 faculty, with a mean of 9.2 faculty per fellowship with a range from 2 to 31 faculty.[18] Data from the ERAS, most recently from 2021, showed 540 applicants, relatively unchanged from 2017 when there were 538 applicants; it should be noted that in 2021, only 428 of the 540 applicants went on to participate in the match.[19] However from 2017 to 2021, the average number of programs applied to per applicant increased from 33.4 to 49.3, placing pain medicine third among all fellowships using ERAS for this ratio, behind cardiology and gastroenterology.[20]

Notably, almost all ACGME-accredited pain fellowships use the National Resident Matching Program. In 2018, 98 of 104 programs used the match; the number had increased to 109 of 113 programs by 2022.[19] The rapid increase in the number of programs applied to per applicant, coinciding with the COVID-19 pandemic and the transition to virtual interviews, poses questions and challenges for future pain applicants. The demographics of pain medicine fellows reflect the continued underrepresentation of women and certain racial minorities in relation to not only the general American population but also to pipeline trainees and the field of medicine as a whole.[21,22] It has been repeatedly recognized that diversity and equity play a role in the delivery of care, and this represents an area within pain education that requires focus and improvement. Greater efforts should be made within the field to recruit and retain women and minorities who are traditionally underrepresented in medicine.[21,22] Future areas of research should include the recruitment of LGBTQ + trainees, trainees with military backgrounds, and trainees representing populations with other unique needs with respect to pain medicine, including geographic regions and socioeconomic status.

DEVELOPMENT OF A CURRICULUM

The growth of the sheer volume of treatment strategies and research in pain management, the recognition of the burden of pain on health and chronic pain being viewed as a disease in its own right, the need for team-based care, the devastating and ongoing effects of opioid addiction in the United States, and the growth of neuromodulation technologies are just some of the defining features of the specialty today.[23,24] This explosive growth in knowledge stands in contrast to the lack of a national shared curriculum for pain fellowship education and poses unique challenges. While the ACGME highlights core competencies to be achieved by graduating fellows, granular knowledge (eg, specific procedures or specific medications) is not a part of the ACGME milestone framework.

This gap between the vast range of knowledge required by the field and the lack of a standardized training curriculum was recognized early by the IASP and was reinforced when an interprofessional group reported to the IASP that a curriculum was essential to develop pain education initiatives. This report led to the publication of the first edition of the IASP's core curriculum in 1991.[25,26] The original ABA Pain Medicine Examination purposefully adopted a condensed version of the IASP core curriculum, and the multidisciplinary members of the ABA Pain Medicine Examination have periodically revised the content outline, with the most recent revision published in April 2022.

Today, reliance on the ABA Pain Medicine Examination outline, and by extension, the ABA guides for the In-Training Exam for Pain Medicine for curriculum design leaves both knowledge and skill gaps among many graduating trainees. Despite the ABAs periodic reassessment of the pain medicine examination content outline, it has not kept pace with the knowledge goals that many pain education leaders feel are most important. While the ABA Pain Medicine Examination content outline helps to establish a curriculum for pain management fellowships and the ACGME Pain Milestones establish principles for the skills and competencies that pain medicine physicians should have by the end of training, many challenges and opportunities remain. Among the most important gaps in training are uniform agreement on which procedures should be taught in all training programs and how should a trainees' skills in performing those procedures be assessed.

This challenge is highlighted most acutely by the growing push for mastery-based learning and its application to interventions and procedures for pain management. Mastery-based learning has steadily made its way into medical education over the last 10 years. It is a framework for actively developing expertise rather than passively absorbing information.[27,28] The basic principles are as follows:

1. Baseline, or diagnostic testing;
2. Clear learning objectives, sequenced as units, usually in increasing difficulty;
3. Engagement in educational activities (eg, deliberate skills practice, calculations, data interpretation, reading) focused on reaching the objectives;

4. A set minimum passing standard (eg, test score) for each educational unit;
5. Formative testing to gauge unit completion at a preset minimum passing standard for mastery;
6. Advancement to the next educational unit given measured achievement at or above the mastery standard; and
7. Continued practice or study on an educational unit until the mastery standard is reached.[28]

In practice, the ACGME milestones 2.0 help describe the knowledge and skills required of the pain medicine graduate. However, as described above, these milestones are not specific or granular. To address this deficiency, Entrustable Professional Activities (EPAs) have emerged to translate competencies into measurable or observable outcomes, using a mastery education checklist to measure and observe progress.[29] While many specialties and fellowships have developed EPAs for their respective fields, this has yet to occur for pain medicine, likely due to the specialty's unique challenges. The diversity of core programs, the diversity of training backgrounds of pain fellows, and the sheer breadth of the field will pose challenges to arriving at a unified set of EPAs.

This difficulty is highlighted by looking at interventions and procedures for pain medicine. While the APPD has begun efforts to understand the landscape of which procedures pain fellows are currently being trained to perform, there continues to be an absence of consensus on familiarity with which procedures, imaging modalities, and techniques should be expected of a pain fellowship graduate. The rapid and early adoption based on limited clinical data of many interventional pain procedures and then abrupt abandonment as additional clinical trials appear have made it all but impossible to establish which procedures should be part of the core training of every pain medicine specialist. This makes it challenging to develop a standardized curriculum, as well as EPAs.

While organizations such as the North American Neuromodulation Society have led specific efforts (eg, development of an educational curriculum for spinal cord stimulation), pain medicine is still in the formative stages of establishing a structured curriculum akin to that found in other interventional specialties.[30] Without a structured curriculum, pain medicine education is threatened with fragmentation, which poses further challenges for all parties, including trainees, hiring institutions, health care payors, and patients. Shared standards of training—made challenging with continued innovation in technologies, imaging, techniques, and modalities—are necessary for the success and growth of the field.

This rapid growth of innovation has created a role for industry in training pain medicine fellows. From 2009 to 2012, several articles were published discussing the "business of pain" and outlining ethical elements of professionalism in the shifting business of pain medicine. The AAPM's Ethics Council Statement on conflict of interest was the most notable example.[31] In its statement, the AAPM addressed the potential consequences of entanglement between pharmaceutical and device companies and individuals. This was seen with the closure of the American Pain Society due, in part, to numerous lawsuits tying the organization to the opioid epidemic.

Today, we are yet at another inflection point, with numerous advances in neuromodulation that pose challenges in teaching advanced skill sets within an already compressed 1-year pain fellowship. This gap is currently being filled with industry-sponsored workshops, many of which occur at meetings of various organizations and offer attractive benefits. Given the sheer number of pain fellowships, along with their generally small size, these workshops offer economies of scale in concentrating both teaching talent and a wealth of resources within the training sessions. However, while pain medicine, as in other specialties, will have to work alongside industry partners, the question of who is in control of educating future pain physicians remains as relevant as ever. This is especially salient in the context of the past 30 years when we examine the role of pharmaceutical companies in educating pain physicians and the subsequent fallout from these relationships. Understanding this history and building on the lessons learned from the problems that have historically befallen the field of pain medicine should guide future steps.

We cannot overstate how real these issues are. How do we ensure that our fellows achieve mastery of a given skill set? What is the skill set? As the number of interventions performed under the umbrella of pain medicine far exceeds what one can learn in a brief fellowship, who should be teaching procedures? Industry? Academic pain physicians? Are these borders too blurry to distinguish? These are questions that the field will need to grapple with and eventually answer and that, for now, offer avenues for future research in pain education and collaboration opportunities.

FUTURE CHALLENGES

So far, we have looked at the evolution of pain medicine from an apprentice-based model to a formal ACGME-accredited multidisciplinary specialty, with national leadership through multiple societies (AAPM, ASRA, APPD). Pain medicine has recently published updated milestones and is likely headed toward development of EPAs. However, pain medicine still faces numerous challenges: (1) the recruitment and training of pain fellows who better reflect our patient population, (2) continued threats of fragmentation of the field, (3) the development of a standardized curriculum, and (4) the training of pain physicians for an ever-growing body of interventions and modalities, which raises questions regarding the role of industry. More research and data are needed to address each challenge accurately.

Some of the issues above highlight perennial discussions within pain medicine education from the past three decades. Should pain fellowships be lengthened to address the growing body of knowledge and interventions? Should training in other subspecialities (eg, radiology) be formalized? What is the balance between skill acquisition for pain interventions and training pain physicians within a biopsychosocial paradigm? How do we address the tension between the two in pain medicine education, and how do we mentor and guide pain medicine trainees? Time and again, data have shown that interdisciplinary pain medicine is efficacious, cost-effective, and safe, and yet trends within pain medicine continue to threaten this training model.[32]

There have been calls by leaders in the field for extension of the current pain medicine fellowship model from 1-year to a 2-year fellowship to address the explosive growth in technology, medications, mind-body/psychological therapies, physical rehabilitative approaches, and integrative approaches that have been shown to be effective as part of an interdisciplinary care model. While not a topic that has been published on, it merits discussion given its endurance in discussions at national societies and among educational leaders in pain medicine. Practical or not, the decisions of length of training have been constrained by numerous factors including financial barriers, potential concerns of attracting talent into the field, and support from health care systems. Few argue that there is no need for lengthening of training from an educational perspective. There are opportunities for the field of pain medicine to closely study current training paradigms and understand how other specialties have adapted and changed training length to meet the demands of expanding diagnostics and treatment options.

Despite the focus on challenges, we would be remiss if we did not note that pain medicine has shown an ability to adapt to and respond to society's needs as well. Just as the opioid epidemic challenged and changed pain education, COVID-19 also transformed the field. The pandemic accelerated the adoption of telehealth, raising new concerns about teaching physical examination skills (both virtual and in person) and showing pain educators the continued need for flexibility to adapt to societal forces that influence the field.

While we have highlighted various successes, threats, and opportunities within pain medicine education at the fellowship level, the leadership of educational efforts in pain medicine at the undergraduate medical education level and other specialties remains an untapped opportunity. The 2011 Institute of Medicine (IOM) report, "Relieving pain in America: a blueprint for transforming prevention, care, education, and research", emphasized that chronic pain continues to be a widespread and costly problem in the United States.[23] The IOM report echoed an American Academy of Pain Medicine position statement (2000) and a National Pain Summit report (2010) in calling for improved pain management education in medical schools as an essential component of addressing the public health crisis. Given the sheer number of chronic pain sufferers, many of whom seek initial care from primary health care providers and other specialists, it has been suggested that basic education for both acute and chronic pain management should start early in medical school, be emphasized in primary care residency programs (ie, family medicine, internal medicine, obstetrics and gynecology, general surgery, pediatrics, psychiatry), and be expanded beyond the purview of anesthesiology and PM&R departments.[33] Evidence suggests that few physicians feel comfortable managing chronic pain patients and that most primary care residents view their pain management education in both medical school and residency as inadequate.[34–38]

In response to the 2011 IOM report, the Department of Health and Human Services tasked the Interagency Pain Research Coordinating Committee to oversee the creation of a National Pain Strategy (NPS). Released in 2016, the NPS addressed professional education and training, particularly to address competencies in pain management across undergraduate and graduate medical education levels, called for the development of a Web-based pain education portal, and recommended that we ensure that pain medicine specialists are trained to lead teams to manage acute and chronic pain patients.[39] Since 2016, steps have been taken in these areas, including the updated Pain Medicine Milestones 2.0 released in 2022 with an increased emphasis on the latter for pain medicine fellowships and increased tracking by the Association of American of Medical Colleges (AAMC) regarding pain management for medical schools.[40] For 2019-2020, the last year for which data are publicly available, 150 of 153 schools reported pain management curriculum in required or elective courses.[41] A more in-depth analysis of curriculum for pain management at the medical school level has focused on substance use disorder domains and pain management in response to the opioid epidemic as discussed in a report published in 2018 by the AAMC; however, this in itself represents opportunities for pain medicine as a field to lead in education.[42] While steps have been taken as called upon in the NPS to expand pain management competency across graduate and undergraduate education, opportunity exists to study the nature of the content. Furthermore, opportunity exists to expand the focus of pain management centering on the opioid epidemic to pain medicine as a chronic disease state, with its unique diagnostic and treatment challenges. It is in this space that pain medicine as a field can and needs to lead.

As the specialty to which other health care providers will refer their most complex patients, the involvement of pain medicine physicians in pain education throughout the continuum of medicine, from medical school to various graduate medical education training programs, and into continuing medical education, is essential to address the immense burden of pain in our society. Within pain education, we must address the challenges in training future pain physicians, seize the opportunities afforded by technology and the growing integration of our field into a national graduate medical education system, and train future pain physicians to be educators. We should lead efforts to ensure the future of the specialty by teaching the principles of interdisciplinary pain management across the spectrum of medicine in hopes of achieving the ultimate goal of pain management: the alleviation of human suffering.

DISCLOSURE

The authors have nothing to disclose.

REFERENCES

1. Meldrum ML. A capsule history of pain management. JAMA 2003;290(18):2470–5.
2. Beecher HK. Pain in men wounded in battle. Ann Surg 1948;123:96–105.
3. Beecher HK. Measurement of subjective responses: quantitative effects of drugs. New York, NY: Oxford University Press; 1959.
4. Beecher HK. The powerful placebo. J Am Med Assoc 1955;159(17):1602–6.
5. Liebeskind JC, Meldrum ML, John J. Bonica, world champion of pain. In: Jensen TS, Turner JA, Wiesenfeld-Hallin Z, editors. Proceedings of the eighth world congress on pain: progress in pain research and management, vol. 8. Seattle, Wash: International Association for the Study of Pain Press; 1997. p. 19–32.
6. Bonica JJ. Introduction to the first World Congress on Pain. Goals of the IASP and the World Congress. In: Bonica JJ, Albe-Fessard D, editors. Advances in pain research and therapy, vol. 1. New York: Raven Press; 1976. p. xxvii–xxxix, proceedings of the First World Congress on Pain.
7. Abram SE. Letter to the American board of anesthesiology. Archives of the American Board of Anesthesiology; 1989.
8. Owens WD, Abram SE. The genesis of Pain Medicine as a subspecialty in anesthesiology. J Anesth Hist 2020;6(1):13–6.
9. The American Board of Anesthesiology. Minutes of Fall Meeting. Archives of the American Board of Anesthesiology. September 10-15, 1989, San Francisco, CA.
10. American Council of Graduate Medical Education: 1993–1994 Directory of Graduate Medical Education: Special Requirements for Residency Training in Pain Management, pages 23–25. Available at: https://www.acgme.org/Portals/0/PDFs/1993-94.pdf. Accessed 5 September, 2022.
11. American Council of Graduate Medical Education: 1995-1996 Directory of Graduate Medical Education. Available at: https://www.acgme.org/globalassets/PDFs/1995-96.pdf. Accessed 25 September, 2022.
12. American Council of Graduate Medical Education: Accreditation Data System (AD). Available at: https://apps.acgme-i.org/ads/Public/. Accessed 30 September, 2022.
13. Nasca TJ, Philibert I, Brigham T, et al. The next GME accreditation system–rationale and benefits. N Engl J Med 2012;366(11):1051–6.
14. Swing SR. The ACGME outcome project: retrospective and prospective. Med Teach 2007;29(7):648–54.
15. Edgar L, Roberts S, Holmboe E. Milestones 2. 0: a step forward. J Grad Med Educ 2018;10(3):367–9.

16. The Association of Pain Program Directors. About Us. Accessed 30 September, 2022. Available at: https://appdhq.org/about/
17. North American Spine Society. 2022-2023 Interventional Spine and Musculoskeletal Medicine (ISMM) Fellowships. Accessed 30 September, 2022. Available at: https://www.spine.org/Portals/0/assets/downloads/Education/Match-Opportunities.pdf
18. Data resource book academic year 2020-2021. Accreditation Council for Graduate Medical Education; 2021.
19. National Resident Matching Program: Match Data Analytics. Available at: https://www.nrmp.org/match-data-analytics/fellowship-data-reports/. Accessed 30 September, 2022
20. American Association of Medical Colleges: Electronic Residency Application Service Statistics. Available at: https://www.aamc.org/data-reports/interactive-data/eras-statistics-data. Accessed 30 September, 2022
21. Odonkor CA, Leitner B, Taraben S, et al. Diversity of Pain Medicine trainees and faculty in the United States: a cross-sectional analysis of fellowship training from 2009–2019. Pain Med 2021;22(4):819–28.
22. Doshi TL, Bicket MC. Why aren't there more female Pain Medicine physicians? Reg Anesth Pain Med 2018;43(5):516–20.
23. Institute of Medicine (US). Committee on advancing pain research, care, and education. Relieving pain in America: a blueprint for transforming prevention, care, education, and research. National Academies Press (US); 2011.
24. Cohen SP, Vase L, Hooten WM. Chronic pain: an update on burden, best practices, and new advances. Lancet 2021;397(10289):2082–97.
25. Watt-Watson J, Hunter J, Pennefather P, et al. An integrated undergraduate pain curriculum, based on IASP curricula, for six health science faculties. Pain 2004;110(1–2):140–8.
26. Fields HL. Core curriculum for professional education in pain. Seattle: IASP Publications; 1991.
27. McGaghie WC, Siddall VJ, Mazmanian PE, et al. Lessons for continuing medical education from simulation research in undergraduate and graduate medical education: effectiveness of continuing medical education: American College of Chest Physicians Evidence-Based Educational Guidelines. Chest 2009;135(3 Suppl):62S–8S.
28. McGaghie WC. Mastery learning: it is time for medical education to join the 21st century. Acad Med 2015;90(11):1438–41.
29. Cate OT, Carraccio C. Envisioning a true continuum of competency-based medical education, training, and practice. Acad Med 2019;94(9):1283–8.
30. Abd-Elsayed A, Abdallah R, Falowski S, et al. Development of an educational curriculum for spinal cord stimulation. Neuromodulation: Technology at the Neural Interface 2020;23(5):555–61.
31. Dubois MY. American academy of Pain Medicine ethics council statement on conflicts of interest: interaction between physicians and industry in Pain Medicine. Pain Med 2010;11(2):257–61.
32. Turk DC, Swanson K. Efficacy and cost-effectiveness treatment of chronic pain; an analysis and evidence-based synthesis. In: Schatman ME, Campbell A, editors. Chronic pain management: guidelines for multidisciplinary program development. New York: Informa Healthcare; 2007. p. 15–38.
33. Loeser JD. The education of pain physicians. Pain Med 2015;16(2):225–9.
34. Upshur CC, Luckman RS, Savageau JA. Primary care provider concerns about management of chronic pain in community clinic populations. J Gen Intern Med 2006;21:652–5.

35. Breuer B, Cruciani R, Portenoy RK. Pain management by primary care physicians, pain physicians, chiropractors, and acupuncturists: a national survey. Southampt Med J 2010;103:738–47.
36. Yanni LM, McKinney-Ketchum JL, Harrington SB, et al. Preparation, confidence, and attitudes about chronic noncancer pain in graduate medical education. J Grad Med Educ 2010;2:260–8.
37. Regunath H, Cochran K, Cornell K, et al. Is it painful to manage chronic pain? A cross-sectional study of physicians in-training in a university program. Mo Med 2016 Jan-Feb;113(1):72–8.
38. Shipton EE, Bate F, Garrick R, et al. Systematic review of Pain Medicine content, teaching, and assessment in medical school curricula internationally. Pain Ther 2018;7:139–61.
39. Department of Health and Human Services. National Pain Strategy: a comprehensive population health strategy for pain. 2016. Available at: https://www.iprcc.nih.gov/sites/default/files/documents/IOM_Pain_Report_508C.pdf. Accessed 27 November, 2022
40. Aggarwal A, Barad M, Braza DW, et al. Pain Medicine Milestones 2/0: A Step into the Future. Pain Med. Published online February 14, 2023.
41. Association of American Medical Colleges. Curriculum Topics in Required and Elective Courses at Medical School Programs. Available at: https://www.aamc.org/data-reports/curriculum-reports/interactive-data/curriculum-topics-required-and-elective-courses-medical-school-programs. Accessed 27 November, 2022
42. Howley L, Whelan A, Rasouli T. Addressing the Opioid Epidemic: U.S. Medical School Curricular Approaches. AAMC Analysis in Brief 2018;18(1):1–3. Available at: https://www.aamc.org/media/8841/download?attachment.

Psychological Approaches for Migraine Management

John A. Sturgeon, PhD[a,*], Dawn M. Ehde, PhD[b], Beth D. Darnall, PhD[c], Meredith J. Barad, MD[d], Daniel J. Clauw, MD[a,e,f], Mark P. Jensen, PhD[b]

KEYWORDS

• Migraine • Psychological treatment • Cognitive-behavioral therapy • Biofeedback • Relaxation therapy • Telehealth

KEY POINTS

- Psychological therapies are a central aspect of best-practice migraine management.
- The best-supported interventions are relaxation strategies, cognitive-behavioral therapy, and biofeedback, with less robust evidence for mindfulness meditation, hypnosis, acceptance and commitment therapy, and trigger management interventions.
- Areas of continued need in psychological intervention research for migraine include high-quality clinical trials, brief and telehealth-based treatment delivery, incorporation of trauma and life stress approaches, and identification of treatment outcome moderators.

INTRODUCTION

Migraine headaches are among the most common and costly medical symptoms in the world; migraine affects more than 1 billion people worldwide.[1] Migraine was identified as the seventh most common cause of years lost to disability across all medical conditions in both 1990 and 2010[2] and accounts for more than 50% of years lost to disability for people with a neurological condition.[3] Direct costs from migraine-related medical care have been estimated to be $9.2 billion annually over the past 15 years.[4]

[a] Department of Anesthesiology, University of Michigan Medical School, 24 Frank Lloyd Wright Drive, Ann Arbor, MI 48105, USA; [b] Department of Rehabilitation Medicine, University of Washington School of Medicine, 325 Ninth Avenue, Box 359612, Seattle, WA 98104, USA; [c] Department of Anesthesiology, Perioperative and Pain Medicine, Stanford University School of Medicine, 430 Broadway Street, Pavilion C, 3rd Floor MC6343, Redwood City, CA 94063, USA; [d] Department of Anesthesiology, Perioperative and Pain Medicine, Stanford University School of Medicine, 1070 Arastradero, Suite 200, MC 5596, Palo Alto, CA 94304, USA; [e] Department of Psychiatry, University of Michigan Medical School, 24 Frank Lloyd Wright Drive, Ann Arbor, MI 48105, USA; [f] Department of Internal Medicine-Rheumatology, University of Michigan Medical School, 24 Frank Lloyd Wright Drive, Ann Arbor, MI 48105, USA

* Corresponding author. 24 Frank Lloyd Wright Drive, Lobby M, Suite 3100, Ann Arbor, MI 48105.

E-mail address: jsturgeo@med.umich.edu

Anesthesiology Clin 41 (2023) 341–355

https://doi.org/10.1016/j.anclin.2023.02.002

Migraine headaches are defined as a neurovascular condition, associated with vascular activity abnormality, altered connectivity between brain regions, circulating neuropeptides, and cervical and cranial nerve dysfunction.[5] However, there is considerable variability in the intensity, frequency, and functional impact of migraine-related pain between individuals and across time.[3,5,6] As with other chronic pain conditions, it is useful to consider not only the objective pathophysiology but also the coping responses and social environment of the individual to fully understand the factors contributing to disease activity and resulting function.

Modern biopsychosocial conceptualizations of chronic pain recognize the significant contributions of psychological and social factors alongside biological factors to the experience and impact of pain; this model provides a strong conceptual fit for migraine pain and migraine-related disability.[6] A key benefit of applying a biopsychosocial lens is the ability to identify psychosocial risk factors that can be modified by psychological interventions and complementary biomedical interventions to reduce migraine pain and associated disability.

PSYCHOSOCIAL RISK FACTORS IN MIGRAINE

Several psychosocial risk factors warrant mention as potential targets of psychological interventions in migraine: maladaptive cognitive appraisals, behavioral avoidance, emotional distress, and sleep disturbance. Importantly, as these risk factors develop, they can interact and contribute to even greater migraine severity and disability over time (**Fig. 1**).

Cognitive appraisals: Cognitive appraisals are interpretations individuals make about the meaning of their medical condition and the degree to which they can manage their symptoms. The appraisal pattern most often studied in migraine and other chronic pain conditions is pain catastrophizing.[7] It is a multidomain construct

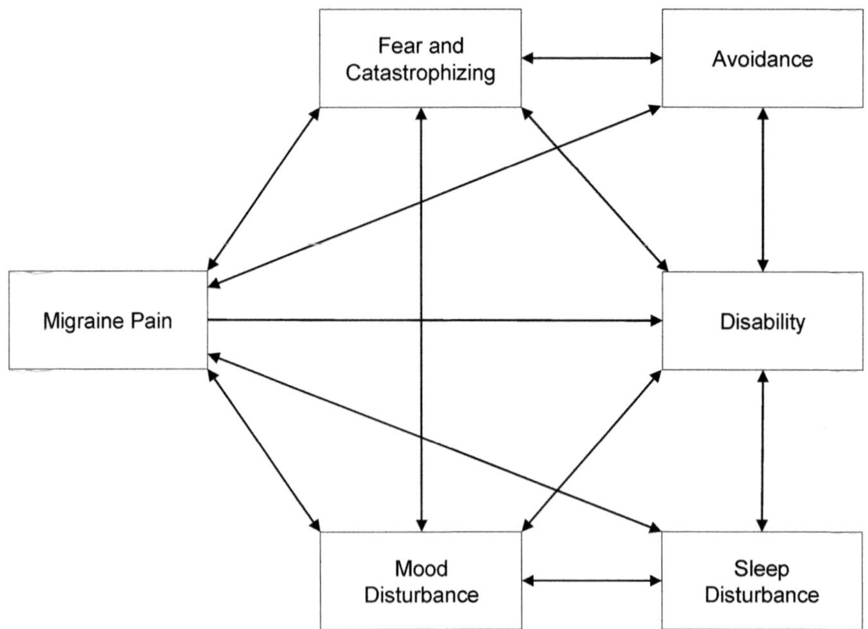

Fig. 1. Biopsychosocial model of vulnerability factors in migraine.

related to feeling helplessness about pain, magnifying negative aspects of pain, and an inability to disengage from negative thoughts about pain.[8] Among individuals with migraine, greater catastrophizing is associated with greater long-term disability[9] and emotional distress.[7] Importantly, catastrophic or fearful appraisals of migraine symptoms can fuel maladaptive behavioral patterns that compound the negative impacts of migraine on function and well-being.[10,11]

Behavioral avoidance: Individuals with migraine can engage in progressively greater avoidance of activities associated with headaches. Although effective management may involve some adaptive avoidance (eg, of particularly potent migraine triggers), consistent and indiscriminate avoidance can increase migraine severity and disability by worsening sensitivity to migraine triggers and undermining meaningful goal pursuits.[11] As noted previously, individuals with high levels of catastrophizing and fear associated with migraine report greater avoidance of activity even during interictal periods.[9] Unfortunately, extreme avoidance of activities commonly associated with a healthy lifestyle (eg, physical exercise, pleasurable activities) can reinforce existing catastrophic appraisals of migraine, making them even more difficult to change.[10,11]

Emotional distress: Strong evidence links migraine with emotional distress; several psychiatric conditions including major depressive disorder, panic disorder, social phobia, and bipolar disorder are more common in individuals with migraine compared with those with no history of migraine.[12] Further, emotional distress, including both immediate negative emotional states[13] and psychosocial stress,[14] is commonly identified causes of migraine. Similarly, depressive and anxious symptom severity shows significant bidirectional relationships with migraine intensity and frequency in cross-sectional and longitudinal research.[15]

Sleep disturbance: Insomnia is more common in individuals with migraine than those with no history of migraine,[16] and there is a significant bidirectional longitudinal relationship between migraine severity and insomnia symptoms. The role of insomnia in migraine is intertwined with other risk factors; there is a well-established bidirectional link between mood disturbance and insomnia in migraine,[17] and insomnia and emotional distress independently predict migraine severity and disability in longitudinal research.[18] Individuals with migraine and comorbid insomnia may be vulnerable to behavioral patterns that worsen both. Avoidance coping responses to migraine (eg, lying in bed in a dark room during the day) can precipitate and perpetuate sleep disturbance, with subsequent disruption in sleep physiology and then increasing the propensity for headaches; over time, these cycles may interact and transform or perpetuate episodic migraine into patterns of chronic migraine.[19]

Social and environmental factors: When considering psychological treatments for migraine, it is important to keep in mind that the pain experience is also influenced by social and environmental factors.[20] For example, perceived lack of social support, increased isolation, and lack of time for self-care have been associated with increased migraine severity.[21] Structural and enacted stigma have also been associated with increased disability in people with migraine.[22]

Given the clear contributions of psychosocial factors to migraine, it follows that its severity and impact could be effectively managed from a biopsychosocially informed multidisciplinary approach that targets these factors for change.[1] A prevailing goal of psychological approaches for migraine is to position individuals with migraine as active managers of their condition. Importantly, psychological interventions tend to show the greatest benefit when used in concert with pharmacological and other medical approaches; best practices therefore emphasize the integrative approaches involving biomedical, psychological, and other approaches (eg, lifestyle management).[1]

What follows is a narrative review of evidence-based psychological interventions and the base of current evidence supporting their use, followed by a discussion of future directions in psychological treatments for migraine. The interventions with the largest base of research supporting their efficacy are relaxation strategies, biofeedback, and cognitive-behavioral therapy (CBT).[23] A second set of interventions (acceptance and commitment therapy, mindfulness meditation interventions, trigger-focused coping interventions, and hypnosis) have also been studied, but to a more limited extent.

Interventions with the Strongest Supporting Evidence for Migraine

Relaxation strategies: Relaxation strategies are a common component of psychological management of migraine. These approaches are intended to elicit a relaxation response through increased parasympathetic nervous system activity[24] and/or a reduction in sympathetic nervous system activity.[25] These interventions are most effective when used prophylactically (eg, as routine parts of daily life, in response to migraine-related risk factors such as stress); there is less evidence supporting analgesic benefits during the ictal period.[26]

This pattern of practice is based on a model that proposes that stress may elicit or potentiate pathophysiological processes that can contribute to migraine onset and greater migraine severity, including premonitory activation of brain regions associated with pain processing, sensitization of central and peripheral nervous system processes, and activation of interactive processes involving the autonomic nervous system and hypothalamic–pituitary–adrenal axis.[14] Consequently, relaxation techniques may dampen some neurophysiological responses and reduce the risk of a migraine attack.

The most common relaxation strategies are diaphragmatic breathing, progressive muscle relaxation (PMR), guided imagery, and autogenic training. Diaphragmatic breathing teaches individuals to expand their lungs into the diaphragm by taking slow, deep, and smooth breaths, often while in a relaxed or supine position.[27] Diaphragmatic breathing practices seem to lower pulse rate and reduce sympathetic nervous system responses.[28] Diaphragmatic breathing practices do not require equipment, can be taught quickly, and can be readily used in most situations; even brief practices of a few minutes at a time can be beneficial, though longer breathing practices (20–30 minutes at a time) are typical.[29] Of note, diaphragmatic breathing can be used in conjunction with other relaxation-focused strategies such as guided imagery, hypnosis, and biofeedback.[25,30]

PMR emphasizes purposeful relaxation of specific muscle groups.[31] PMR typically requires upwards of 20 minutes per day focused on gentle tensing and relaxing of one muscle group at a time and moving through large muscle groups in the body.[32] In more advanced practice, patients may be able to elicit relaxation of muscle groups through awareness of tension without needing to tense of the muscle group.[32] There is evidence that PMR alters autonomic nervous system responses that underlie or exacerbate migraine, including activation for neural circuits related to modulation of attention and emotion[33] and central information processing.[34]

Guided imagery techniques involve purposeful direction of attention away from distressing experiences like pain and toward typically pleasurable or positive images.[35] Guided imagery is often conducted in combination with diaphragmatic breathing or autogenic training when treating migraine[36] and demonstrates promising efficacy in reducing pain, although there are methodological problems with the research in this area.[37] The therapeutic benefit of guided imagery seems to be due in part to distraction from the distressing aspects of pain.[38]

Autogenic training is intended to reduce states of high sympathetic arousal by teaching patients to observe and (if possible) shift toward feelings of relaxation through self-suggestion (eg, eliciting feelings of warmth/heaviness in the hands, arms, or abdomen, regulation of breathing, internal organs, and heartbeat).[39] This approach shares some features with hypnosis,[39] such as the utilization of suggestions (and later self-suggestions) toward feelings of calm and beliefs in control over interoceptive signals. Autogenic training yields measurable changes in physiological stress indices such as increased heart rate variability and reduced heart rate, muscle tension, and blood pressure.[39] Autogenic training has demonstrated efficacy in reducing migraine intensity and frequency[39,40] as well as broader effects on improving mood and quality of life.[41]

Biofeedback: Biofeedback uses measurements of physiologic processes that are usually outside of conscious awareness, which are then fed back to patients in real time (eg, through a visual display or auditory feedback) with the goal of teaching them to recognize and modulate indices of stress. Biofeedback uses multiple modalities including respiratory rate, skin conductance response, electromyographic muscle group activity measurement, extremity temperature modulation, blood volume pulse, heart rate variability, and electroencephalography-assessed neuronal activity.[42] Although biofeedback in migraine is intended to improve control over physiologic stress responses,[43] a significant degree of benefit from biofeedback may be attributable to changes in cognitive factors such as perceived self-efficacy for managing headaches.[44] Meta-analytic studies conclude moderate impact of biofeedback on migraine frequency, intensity, duration, and impact, with comparable levels of effect across biofeedback modalities.[45]

Cognitive-behavioral therapy: CBT is considered the "gold standard" for treatment of chronic pain conditions,[46] and there is a large evidence base supporting the efficacy of CBT for reducing migraine pain and disability.[47] CBT is also useful for patients with comorbid migraine and mood disorders, as CBT also demonstrates efficacy for improving most mood disorders.[25] Similarly, CBT-based interventions for insomnia improve both migraine severity and sleep quality.[48]

The CBT approach for migraine emphasizes developing a "coping skills toolbox"[49] that addresses migraine triggers and unhelpful cognitive or behavioral responses to headaches through cognitive and behavioral strategies to reduce the frequency and impact of migraine headaches.[50] CBT sessions often include training in relaxation strategies like those described above, more regular engagement in healthy behaviors such as drinking water and tolerable levels of exercise, graded activity approaches focused on teaching patients to build in periods of rest and gradually build up tolerable levels of valued activity throughout the day despite pain, behavioral activation approaches (eg, scheduling of pleasurable events to improve motivation and mood), and use of cognitive and behavioral strategies for improving sleep and decreasing avoidance behaviors.[50] With CBT, patients also learn to recognize automatic thoughts associated with migraine symptoms and related stressors (eg, missing valued activities due to a headache), to understand the impact of these thoughts on pain, mood, and behavior, and to develop strategies for reappraising or replacing maladaptive thoughts with more adaptive ones. Some CBT programs also include training in assertive communication to address interpersonal issues that may contribute to stress or interfere with self-care (eg, communicating about the need to exercise or practice relaxation).[25]

Emerging Therapies

Mindfulness-based therapies: The most common therapeutic application of mindfulness is mindfulness-based stress reduction (MBSR), which has demonstrated efficacy across multiple chronic pain conditions.[51] More recent adaptations have examined mindfulness-based cognitive therapy, which integrates principles of mindfulness and CBT.[52] Mindfulness meditation typically emphasizes regular (ie, daily) meditation practice.[51] Mindfulness approaches teach patients to attend to the interoceptive and external events (eg, breathing, eating, thoughts, emotions, pain, interpersonal communication) in a calm and nonjudgmental fashion, allowing the patient to free themselves from automatic patterns of cognitive, behavioral, and emotional reactions that may worsen distress or disability.[53] The base of evidence for mindfulness interventions for migraine is smaller and more heterogeneous in terms of study quality than that for the interventions described above. However, recent reviews have concluded that they are more reliably effective in reducing migraine-related distress and disability, but show equivocal effects on migraine frequency or intensity.[53]

Acceptance and commitment therapy: Acceptance and commitment therapy (ACT) integrates CBT with mindfulness principles.[26] Like mindfulness, ACT teaches patients to adopt a nonjudgmental (accepting) view of their internal experience, including pain, thoughts, and emotions.[54] Subsequent sessions are spent teaching patients to orient their behavioral efforts toward valued goals derived from their personal values (committed action) rather than ineffective efforts to diminish pain symptoms.[55] Unlike CBT, ACT emphasizes promotion of flexible psychological processes rather than changing the content of thoughts or reduction of symptoms or stress; patients are encouraged to pursue personally meaningful goals even in the presence of pain, distress, or negative thoughts.[56] The base of research for ACT in migraine is small. The evidence that exists suggests that ACT may improve function and reduce distress, but have equivocal effects on migraine pain.[57]

Learning to cope with triggers: As noted previously, a central contention in behavioral migraine management addresses how patients manage migraine triggers. Martin and colleagues[58] have developed a hybrid behavioral intervention (Learning to Cope with Triggers [LCT]) that emphasizes recognition of migraine triggers and learning to make mindful and deliberate decisions about avoidance versus “living alongside” triggers as a means of bolstering function and reducing the risk of sensitization to triggers. A few randomized clinical trials have indicated preliminary evidence of reductions in migraine frequency and intensity and associated disability with LCT treatment[58,59] and LCT principles have been integrated with CBT,[59] suggesting that this approach may be a useful complement to other evidence-based interventions. However, there is considerable debate on the topic of desensitization approaches in migraine, as it may be impossible or counterproductive to increase exposure to or otherwise change the frequency of major triggers.[60] At this stage, it seems sufficient to state that there is potential benefit in psychological approaches that promote flexible responding to migraine triggers that is worthy of additional study.

Hypnosis: Clinical hypnosis approaches have demonstrated efficacy across a variety of chronic pain conditions.[61] A clinical hypnosis session typically involves two steps: an induction that encourages the patient to experience a state of focused attention followed by a clinical suggestion or series of suggestions (eg, greater comfort, changing location of uncomfortable sensations, increased feelings of calm or control, or increased frequency of adaptive pain-related thoughts).[62] For many patients, hypnosis training can be transitioned into a self-guided hypnosis practice to be used outside of therapy.[63] In the area of migraine management, there is a relatively small base of research suggesting that hypnosis can reduce migraine frequency and intensity.[64] However, the efficacy of hypnosis as a monotherapy is unclear as it is often used in concert with CBT or relaxation techniques.[64]

DISCUSSION

Although the literature base examining psychological interventions for migraine is large, one key issue concerns research quality; recent reviews have concluded that most of the clinical trials involving psychological interventions for migraine yield only low-quality evidence due to methodological flaws, inconsistent reporting of important methodological details, variability in sampling, or variability in the use of control or comparator conditions.[65,66] Although a reasonable consensus exists that psychological interventions yield some degree of benefit for migraine pain, disability, and distress,[23,65] there is nevertheless a strong need for high-quality clinical trials testing all of the aforementioned interventions to determine the scope and magnitude of their effectiveness with more confidence. At present, although CBT, relaxation therapy, and biofeedback show the strongest empirical base of support, many of the published studies yield only very low-quality evidence. As noted previously, psychological interventions are most efficacious in the context of multidisciplinary management plan. However, we wish to highlight that more rigorous clinical trials would be invaluable both for examining psychological interventions as monotherapies and in concert with medical and other non-pharmacological interventions. We discuss other future directions for research below.

Improving patient access: Improving patient access is another key consideration for future research. This includes the need to evaluate the feasibility and efficacy of brief and telehealth-based interventions for migraine. Specialty-trained mental health providers often deliver psychological interventions for migraine (eg, health or rehabilitation psychologists); however, access to specialty-trained mental health is limited and quite rare outside tertiary care settings.[67] Further, interventions such as CBT, MBSR, or relaxation therapy typically require weekly sessions over a span of 8 to 12 weeks. Thus, even among patients who are able to find these services through a specialty clinic, significant time, cost, and associated patient burden pose a major barrier to patient access.[67] Thus, brief and scalable interventions are needed to improve access to psychological treatment for migraine. Brief psychological interventions show preliminary evidence of feasibility in pilot studies with individuals with headache, but larger and more rigorous studies are needed to determine their efficacy.[55,68]

Telehealth interventions: Another key aspect to improving patient access to psychological interventions for migraine is telehealth. Behavioral interventions demonstrate comparable effects to in-person treatment when delivered via telehealth modalities (eg, telephone, Internet), suggesting that these services can be valuable options for individuals not regularly seen in specialty clinics.[69] However, response to telehealth or mHealth (mobile health) interventions may vary between contemporaneous and asynchronous delivery systems; the availability of a live therapeutic provider may improve patient ratings of treatment acceptability[70] and patient engagement[71] and reduce rates of treatment attrition compared with strictly self-guided Internet-based interventions.[72] Consequently, additional research is needed to determine whether specific interventions may be better suited for minimal-contact interventions and which may require more active, contemporaneous engagement with a provider. We speculate that, particularly for patients uninitiated with or ambivalent about psychologically based management strategies, initial contact with a live therapist may be indicated to build competence and self-efficacy regarding the use of migraine management strategies.

Life stress/trauma-informed approaches: Major life stressors are a significant risk factor for the presence of a migraine disorder,[73] transition from episodic to chronic migraine,[14] and for overlapping non-headache pain conditions, which exacerbate patterns of migraine-related distress and disability.[74] Similarly, individuals with a history of trauma and ongoing symptoms of post-traumatic stress disorder show greater severity and burden of migraine symptoms compared with those without a history of trauma.[75]

Although the mechanisms connecting trauma/life stress and migraine are likely multifactorial,[73] one potential mechanism concerns patterns of emotional avoidance or suppression that can arise when individuals face highly threatening or invalidating environments. Of note, patterns of emotional avoidance or suppression seem to be more common in individuals with migraine, particularly among those with a history of trauma or adverse life experiences,[76,77] and these avoidance/suppression patterns demonstrate a direct relationship with severity of migraine symptoms.[78] Novel psychotherapies (eg, Emotional Awareness and Expression Therapy) that teach patients to recognize, express, or otherwise act on their own emotions in new and more productive ways show at least comparable benefit to CBT and in some cases superior efficacy in reducing pain intensity in conditions that may have a nociplastic pain component like fibromyalgia.[79] Although there is preliminary efficacy for emotional expression-focused approaches in headache,[80] large-scale randomized trials in migraine have not yet been conducted and remain as a viable future direction for research, particularly for patients with migraine and identifiable histories of major life stress or trauma.

Precision medicine: As in other chronic pain conditions,[46] there is a pressing need to move beyond determining *if* psychological interventions for migraine improve outcomes, to *for whom* and *how* the interventions work. The current literature suggests that as many as 50% who receive a psychological intervention for migraine do not achieve a clinically significant (ie, 50% or greater) degree of pain relief.[65] This may be due to a mismatch between a specific treatment and a specific individual; for example, CBT may not benefit those who do not have problematic levels of maladaptive thinking (eg, pain catastrophizing) or behavior (eg, inactivity) before entering treatment.[81] A better understanding of the patient characteristics associated with response to specific interventions (ie, treatment effect moderators) may improve migraine care by matching patients to the treatment that they are most likely to benefit from and to tailor specific interventions to the moderating patient characteristics. Research examining moderators is underway in several pain populations, including low back pain[82] and multiple sclerosis[83]; despite long-standing calls for moderation research,[28] this area of research in migraine has remained very limited.

Practical and clinical considerations: There is an unfortunate shortfall of mental health providers with specialized training in management of chronic pain and headache conditions. Indeed, many medical systems do not have consistent access to headache- or chronic pain-trained mental health providers, which can complicate efforts to promote multidisciplinary migraine management. We would like to acknowledge ongoing efforts to expand pain management approaches as a more common aspect of mental health training curricula.[84,85]

However, it is likely that this scarcity of appropriately trained mental health providers will continue for the foreseeable future; consequently, there may be alternative pathways that providers may pursue to access the psychological treatments detailed above.

For medical providers who do not have co-located mental health services within their department or institution, a few options may be considered. Mental health providers who offer psychological services for pain or migraine management (eg, CBT, MBSR) may be identified through the Therapist Search function of the Psychology Today Web site, which allows for filtering by insurance type, therapy and condition type, among other factors. Some state-level psychological associations also offer similar listings but may include only doctoral-level psychological providers. In addition, there are public lists of providers trained in MBSR (https://www.mindfulleader.org/mbsr-certified-teacher-directory), ACT (https://contextualscience.org/), and biofeedback (https://www.bcia.org/consumers-find-a-practitioner). Therapists trained in Empowered Relief, an empirically supported brief cognitive-behavioral intervention for chronic pain, can be found at their training Web site through Stanford University (https://empoweredrelief.stanford.edu/find-provider). Further, Internet-based intervention classes may be available both locally and nationally; for example, Internet-based MBSR courses are offered through the University of Massachusetts Medical School (https://www.ummhealth.org/). However, it should be noted that these services are not uniformly available across insurance payors or across geographic regions.

In cases where patients are not able to find pain-trained mental health professionals, it may be possible to engage patients in the use of self-management techniques through referral to Web sites, phone apps, or books that outline how to use empirically supported therapeutic approaches. The University of Michigan's Pain Guide (https://painguide.com) is an evidence-based education and self-management resource that includes information about pain, self-management tools, and tracking tools as well as a section on migraine.[86] The University of California-Los Angeles Mindful Awareness Research Center offers free recordings of guided mindfulness meditations through their Web site and corresponding phone app (https://www.uclahealth.org/programs/marc/free-guided-meditations/guided-meditations). For patients with co-occurring insomnia or post-traumatic stress disorder (PTSD), there are free self-guided programs based in CBT for insomnia and PTSD through the Veterans Affairs Web site (CBT-I Coach and PTSD Coach, respectively; https://www.ptsd.va.gov). Proprietary phone apps also review the principles of relaxation therapy (eg, Calm, Breathe2Relax) and mindfulness meditation (eg, Headspace, Insight Timer). However, it is likely that the degree of efficacy from these applications will vary across patients, as noted previously interventions that rely on asynchronous delivery of psychological treatment for migraine are vulnerable to reduced patient engagement and adherence compared with engagement with a live therapist.[70–72]

Similarly, there may be books that describe CBT, mindfulness meditation, and ACT principles in actionable ways; though the research on bibliotherapy is quite limited in the area of chronic pain or migraine management, there is preliminary evidence of efficacy when these materials are rigorously developed.[87,88]

Particularly for patients with high levels of migraine-related symptom burden, significant psychiatric comorbidities, or ambivalence about engagement with mental health treatments, it may be necessary to reinforce the importance of patient engagement with the material presented in self-help books regularly during medical visits and to refer them for psychiatric or psychological care, even if the provider does not have expertise in pain management. In cases where patients may have an ongoing relationship with a mental health provider, it may also be feasible to encourage the patients to bring self-guided materials like those listed above and review them in future treatment sessions. Even in cases where mental health providers are not specifically trained in psychological approaches for chronic pain or migraine management, they may have had training in CBT, MBSR, or ACT for other conditions such as depression or anxiety and would be able to reinforce and support the use of psychological approaches such as relaxation, cognitive reappraisal, meditation, and behavioral or social activation. They should also be able to assess and treat common co-occurring conditions, including mood disorders and insomnia.

From the standpoint of communicating with patients about the role of psychological interventions, we encourage all health care providers to present a biopsychosocial conceptualization of migraine headaches (ie, brain-based neurophysiological processes that are reciprocally related to thoughts, emotions and behaviors as well as factors in the broader social environment) and to impress on their patients the importance of multidisciplinary approaches and self-management of migraine headaches. Explaining to patients that psychological techniques are intended to complement, rather than replace, biomedical management may assuage concerns about their headache condition being viewed as illegitimate, the possibility of having needed medical treatments withdrawn, or their symptoms being viewed as occurring "all in the head." In cases where patients or providers may be unsure about how to choose an appropriate psychological treatment, these decisions may be informed either by which treatments are immediately available (eg, through the current medical system, covered treatment services under insurance programs) or by patient preference. It may be useful to encourage patients to begin psychological treatment with an approach they feel might be most useful as a first step to fostering a more diverse set of coping responses to migraine.

SUMMARY

Psychological interventions are a central aspect of best-practice migraine management and can address major psychosocial contributors to the severity and impact of migraine. Despite some important limitations in methodological approaches and study design, the extant base of research supports the conclusion that psychological interventions can improve migraine symptoms and disability, both independently and in concert with medical and lifestyle interventions. However, several essential areas remain for future study, including improving the methodological quality of clinical trials, improving patient access, and incorporating of treatments for historically overlooked migraine-relevant factors such as trauma and emotional avoidance.

CLINICS CARE POINTS

- Psychological therapies are a central component of best-practice approaches for migraine management and are best used in conjunction with biomedical and other non-pharmacological interventions.
- Cognitive-behavioral therapy, relaxation strategies, and biofeedback have the strongest base of evidence for their effectiveness.
- Other interventions (mindfulness interventions, acceptance and commitment therapy, hypnosis, learning to cope with triggers) have shown preliminary efficacy but require more thorough evaluation through large-scale clinical trials.
- Greater consideration to patient-specific factors (eg, experiences of major life stress or trauma, treatment-relevant factors such as self-efficacy or motivation) and improving patient access through brief and telehealth interventions can potentially improve the quality and reach of psychological interventions.

- There is a strong need for additional rigorous clinical trials for all psychological approaches for migraine, as the quality of evidence from existing studies is low due to the methodological limitations of those studies.

DISCLOSURES

J.A. Sturgeon is funded under an award from NINDS K23NS125004. M.P. Jensen receives royalties from books and facilitation of clinical workshops on the use of hypnosis for chronic pain management. The authors have no conflicts of interest to disclose.

REFERENCES

1. Ashina M, Katsarava Z, Do TP, et al. Migraine: epidemiology and systems of care. Lancet 2021;397(10283):1485–95.
2. Vos T, Flaxman AD, Naghavi M, et al. Years lived with disability (YLDs) for 1160 sequelae of 289 diseases and injuries 1990–2010: a systematic analysis for the Global Burden of Disease Study 2010. Lancet 2012;380(9859):2163–96.
3. Steiner TJ, Stovner LJ, Birbeck GL. Migraine: the seventh disabler. London, England: Sage Publications Sage UK; 2013. p. 289–90.
4. Raval AD, Shah A. National trends in direct health care expenditures among US adults with migraine: 2004 to 2013. J Pain 2017;18(1):96–107.
5. Charles A. The pathophysiology of migraine: implications for clinical management. Lancet Neurol 2018;17(2):174–82.
6. Leonardi M, Raggi A, Grazzi L, et al. Disability, ICF biopsychosocial model and burden of migraine. J Headache Pain 2015;16(1):1–2.
7. Seng EK, Buse DC, Klepper JE, et al. Psychological factors associated with chronic migraine and severe migraine-related disability: An observational study in a tertiary headache center. Headache J Head Face Pain 2017;57(4):593–604.
8. Sullivan MJ, Bishop SR, Pivik J. The pain catastrophizing scale: development and validation. Psychol Assess 1995;7(4):524.
9. Black AK, Fulwiler JC, Smitherman TA. The role of fear of pain in headache. Headache J Head Face Pain 2015;55(5):669–79.
10. Farris SG, Thomas JG, Abrantes AM, et al. Intentional avoidance of physical activity in women with migraine. Cephalalgia Reports 2018;1. 2515816318788284.
11. Buse DC, Rupnow MF, and Lipton RB. Assessing and managing all aspects of migraine: migraine attacks, migraine-related functional impairment, common comorbidities, and quality of life, Mayo Clin Proc, 2009;84(5):422–435.
12. Jette N, Patten S, Williams J, et al. Comorbidity of migraine and psychiatric disorders—a national population-based study. Headache J Head Face Pain 2008; 48(4):501–16.
13. Mollaoğlu M. Trigger factors in migraine patients. J Health Psychol 2013;18(7): 984–94.
14. Stubberud A, Buse DC, Kristoffersen ES, et al. Is there a causal relationship between stress and migraine? Current evidence and implications for management. J Headache Pain 2021;22(1):1–11.
15. Antonaci F, Nappi G, Galli F, et al. Migraine and psychiatric comorbidity: a review of clinical findings. J Headache Pain 2011;12(2):115–25.
16. Uhlig B, Engstrøm M, Ødegård S, et al. Headache and insomnia in population-based epidemiological studies. Cephalalgia 2014;34(10):745–51.
17. Hertenstein E, Feige B, Gmeiner T, et al. Insomnia as a predictor of mental disorders: a systematic review and meta-analysis. Sleep Med Rev 2019;43:96–105.

18. Walters AB, Hamer JD, Smitherman TA. Sleep disturbance and affective comorbidity among episodic migraineurs. Headache J Head Face Pain 2014;54(1): 116–24.
19. Ong JC, Park M. Chronic headaches and insomnia: Working toward a biobehavioral model. Cephalalgia 2012;32(14):1059–70.
20. Fordyce W. Behavioral methods for chronic pain and illness. 1977, LWW, St. Louis, MO.
21. Griep RH, Toivanen S, Santos IS, et al. Work-family conflict, lack of time for personal care and leisure, and job strain in migraine: results of the Brazilian Longitudinal Study of adult Health (ELSA-Brasil). Am J Ind Med 2016;59(11):987–1000.
22. Parikh SK, Kempner J, Young WB. Stigma and migraine: developing effective interventions. Curr Pain Headache Rep 2021;25(11):1–10.
23. Sullivan A, Cousins S, Ridsdale L. Psychological interventions for migraine: a systematic review. J Neurol 2016;263(12):2369–77.
24. Benson H, Beary JF, Carol MP. The relaxation response. Psychiatry 1974;37(1): 37–46.
25. Singer AB, Buse DC, Seng EK. Behavioral treatments for migraine management: useful at each step of migraine care. Curr Neurol Neurosci Rep 2015;15(4):14.
26. Kropp P, Meyer B, Meyer W, et al. An update on behavioral treatments in migraine–current knowledge and future options. Expert Rev Neurother 2017; 17(11):1059–68.
27. Hazlett-Stevens H, Craske MG. Breathing retraining and diaphragmatic breathing techniques. In: O'Donohue W, Fisher JE, Hayes SC, editors. Cognitive Behavior Therapy: Applying in Empirically Supported Techniques in your Practice. Hoboken: John Wiley and Sons; 2003. p. 59–64.
28. Andrasik F. Behavioral treatment of migraine: current status and future directions. Expert Rev Neurother 2004;4(3):403–13.
29. Carlson CR. Psychological considerations for chronic orofacial pain. Oral Maxillofac Surg Clin 2008;20(2):185–95.
30. Fukui T, Williams W, Tan G, et al. Combining hypnosis and biofeedback to enhance chronic pain management. Aust J Clin Hypnother Hypn 2020; 41(1):3–15.
31. Jacobsen E. Progressive relaxation. Chicago: University of Chicago Press; 1929.
32. Bernstein DA, Borkovec TD. Progressive relaxation training: A manual for the helping professions. Champaign, IL: Research Press; 1973.
33. Bushnell MC, Čeko M, Low LA. Cognitive and emotional control of pain and its disruption in chronic pain. Nat Rev Neurosci 2013;14(7):502–11.
34. Meyer B, Keller A, Wöhlbier H-G, et al. Progressive muscle relaxation reduces migraine frequency and normalizes amplitudes of contingent negative variation (CNV). J Headache Pain 2016;17(1):1–9.
35. Pistoia F, Sacco S, Carolei A. Behavioral therapy for chronic migraine. Curr Pain Headache Rep 2013;17(1):1–8.
36. Pérez-Muñoz A, Buse DC, Andrasik F. Behavioral interventions for migraine. Neurol Clin 2019;37(4):789–813.
37. Posadzki P, Lewandowski W, Terry R, et al. Guided imagery for non-musculoskeletal pain: a systematic review of randomized clinical trials. J Pain Symptom Manage 2012;44(1):95–104.
38. Hart J. Guided imagery. Alternative Compl Ther 2008;14(6):295–9.
39. Seo E, Hong E, Choi J, et al. Effectiveness of autogenic training on headache: a systematic review. Complement Ther Med 2018;39:62–7.

40. Kohlert A, Wick K and Rosendahl J. Autogenic training for reducing chronic pain: a systematic review and meta-analysis of randomized controlled trials, Int J Behav Med, 2022;29(5):1–12.
41. Stetter F, Kupper S. Autogenic training: a meta-analysis of clinical outcome studies. Appl Psychophysiol Biofeedback 2002;27(1):45–98.
42. Nestoriuc Y, Martin A, Rief W, et al. Biofeedback treatment for headache disorders: a comprehensive efficacy review. Appl Psychophysiol Biofeedback 2008;33(3):125–40.
43. Andrasik F. Biofeedback in headache: an overview of approaches and evidence. Cleve Clin J Med 2010;77(Suppl 3):S72–6.
44. Seng EK, Holroyd KA. Dynamics of changes in self-efficacy and locus of control expectancies in the behavioral and drug treatment of severe migraine. Ann Behav Med 2010;40(3):235–47.
45. Nestoriuc Y, Martin A. Efficacy of biofeedback for migraine: a meta-analysis. Pain 2007;128(1–2):111–27.
46. Ehde DM, Dillworth TM, Turner JA. Cognitive-behavioral therapy for individuals with chronic pain: efficacy, innovations, and directions for research. Am Psychol 2014;69(2):153.
47. Bae J-y, Sung H-K, Kwon N-Y, et al. Cognitive behavioral therapy for migraine headache: a systematic review and meta-analysis. Medicina 2021;58(1):44.
48. Sullivan DP, Martin PR, Boschen MJ. Psychological sleep interventions for migraine and tension-type headache: a systematic review and meta-analysis. Sci Rep 2019;9(1):1–8.
49. Thorn BE. Ronald Melzack Award Lecture: putting the brain to work in cognitive behavioral therapy for chronic pain. Pain 2020;161:S27–35.
50. Seng EK. Using cognitive behavioral therapy techniques to treat migraine. J Health Soc Pol 2018;44(2):68–73.
51. Rosenzweig S, Greeson JM, Reibel DK, et al. Mindfulness-based stress reduction for chronic pain conditions: variation in treatment outcomes and role of home meditation practice. J Psychosom Res 2010;68(1):29–36.
52. Segal Z, Williams M, Teasdale J. Mindfulness-based cognitive therapy for depression. New York, USA: Guilford Publications; 2018.
53. Wells RE, Seng EK, Edwards RR, et al. Mindfulness in migraine: a narrative review. Expert Rev Neurother 2020;20(3):207–25.
54. Wetherell JL, Afari N, Rutledge T, et al. A randomized, controlled trial of acceptance and commitment therapy and cognitive-behavioral therapy for chronic pain. Pain 2011;152(9):2098–107.
55. Smitherman TA, Wells RE, Ford SG. Emerging behavioral treatments for migraine. Curr Pain Headache Rep 2015;19(4):13.
56. Vasiliou VS, Karademas EC, Christou Y, et al. Mechanisms of change in acceptance and commitment therapy for primary headaches. Eur J Pain 2022;26(1):167–80.
57. Galvez-Sánchez CM, Montoro CI, Moreno-Padilla M, et al. Effectiveness of acceptance and commitment therapy in central pain sensitization syndromes: a systematic review. J Clin Med 2021;10(12):2706.
58. Martin PR, Reece J, Callan M, et al. Behavioral management of the triggers of recurrent headache: a randomized controlled trial. Behav Res Ther 2014;61:1–11.
59. Martin PR, Reece J, MacKenzie S, et al. Integrating headache trigger management strategies into cognitive-behavioral therapy: A randomized controlled trial. Health Psychol 2021;40(10):674.

60. Martin PR. Triggers of primary headaches: issues and pathways forward. Headache J Head Face Pain 2020;60(10):2495–507.
61. Thompson T, Terhune DB, Oram C, et al. The effectiveness of hypnosis for pain relief: a systematic review and meta-analysis of 85 controlled experimental trials. Neurosci Biobehav Rev 2019;99:298–310.
62. Dillworth T, Jensen MP. The role of suggestions in hypnosis for chronic pain: a review of the literature. Open Pain J 2010;3(1):39.
63. Hammond DC. Review of the efficacy of clinical hypnosis with headaches and migraines. Int J Clin Exp Hypn 2007;55(2):207–19.
64. Flynn N. Systematic review of the effectiveness of hypnosis for the management of headache. IJCEH (Int J Clin Exp Hypn) 2018;66(4):343–52.
65. Dudeney J, Sharpe L, McDonald S, et al. Are psychological interventions efficacious for adults with migraine? A systematic review and meta-analysis. Headache J Head Face Pain 2022;62(4):405–19.
66. Sharpe L, Dudeney J, de C Williams AC, et al. Psychological therapies for the prevention of migraine in adults, Cochrane Database Syst Rev, 2019;7:CD012295.
67. Penzien DB, Irby MB, Smitherman TA, et al. Well-established and empirically supported behavioral treatments for migraine. Curr Pain Headache Rep 2015; 19(7):1–7.
68. Vekhter D, Robbins MS, Minen M, et al. Efficacy and feasibility of behavioral treatments for migraine, headache, and pain in the acute care setting. Curr Pain Headache Rep 2020;24(10):1–9.
69. McGeary DD, McGeary CA, Gatchel RJ, et al. Assessment of research quality of telehealth trials in pain management: a meta-analysis. Pain Pract 2013;13(5): 422–31.
70. Eccleston C, Fisher E, Brown R, et al. Psychological therapies (Internet-delivered) for the management of chronic pain in adults. Cochrane Database Syst Rev 2014; 2:CD010152.
71. Mehta S, Peynenburg VA, Hadjistavropoulos HD. Internet-delivered cognitive behaviour therapy for chronic health conditions: a systematic review and meta-analysis. J Behav Med 2019;42(2):169–87.
72. Buhrman M, Gordh T, Andersson G. Internet interventions for chronic pain including headache: a systematic review. Internet Interventions 2016;4:17–34.
73. Tietjen GE, Buse DC, Collins SA. Childhood maltreatment in the migraine patient. Curr Treat Options Neurol 2016;18(7):1–15.
74. Barad MJ, Sturgeon JA, Hong J, et al. Characterization of chronic overlapping pain conditions in patients with chronic migraine: A CHOIR study. Headache J Head Face Pain 2021;61(6):872–81.
75. Smitherman TA, Kolivas ED. Trauma exposure versus posttraumatic stress disorder: relative associations with migraine. Headache J Head Face Pain 2013;53(5): 775–86.
76. Bottiroli S, Galli F, Viana M, et al. Traumatic experiences, stressful events, and alexithymia in chronic migraine with medication overuse. Front Psychol 2018; 9:704.
77. Özsoy F, Taşcı İ. Defense mechanisms, dissociation, alexithymia and childhood traumas in chronic migraine patients. J Ration Emot Cogn Behav Ther 2021; 39(1):101–13.
78. Shim E-J, Park A, Park S-P. The relationship between alexithymia and headache impact: the role of somatization and pain catastrophizing. Qual Life Res 2018; 27(9):2283–94.

79. Lumley MA, Schubiner H, Lockhart NA, et al. Emotional awareness and expression therapy, cognitive-behavioral therapy, and education for fibromyalgia: a cluster-randomized controlled trial. Pain 2017;158(12):2354.
80. Slavin-Spenny O, Lumley MA, Thakur ER, et al. Effects of anger awareness and expression training versus relaxation training on headaches: A randomized trial. Ann Behav Med 2013;46(2):181–92.
81. Day MA, Ehde DM, Jensen MP. Psychosocial pain management moderation: the limit, activate, and enhance model. J Pain 2015;16(10):947–60.
82. Day MA, Ward LC, Thorn BE, et al. Mechanisms of mindfulness meditation, cognitive therapy, and mindfulness-based cognitive therapy for chronic low back pain. Clin J Pain 2020;36(10):740–9.
83. Ehde DM, Alschuler KN, Day MA, et al. Mindfulness-based cognitive therapy and cognitive behavioral therapy for chronic pain in multiple sclerosis: a randomized controlled trial protocol. Trials 2019;20(1):1–12.
84. Wandner LD, Prasad R, Ramezani A, et al. Core competencies for the emerging specialty of pain psychology. Am Psychol 2019;74(4):432.
85. Darnall BD, Scheman J, Davin S, et al. Pain psychology: a global needs assessment and national call to action. Pain Med 2016;17(2):250–63.
86. McKernan LC, Crofford LJ, Kim A, et al. Electronic delivery of pain education for chronic overlapping pain conditions: a prospective cohort study. Pain Med 2021;22(10):2252–62.
87. Tavallaei V. Rezapour-Mirsaleh Y. Rezaiemaram P. et al. Mindfulness for female outpatients with chronic primary headaches: an internet-based bibliotherapy, Eur J Transl Myol, 2018;28(2):175-184.
88. Veillette J, Martel M-E, Dionne F. A randomized controlled trial evaluating the effectiveness of an acceptance and commitment therapy–based bibliotherapy intervention among adults living with chronic pain. Canadian Journal of Pain 2019;3(1):209–25.

Ketamine for Complex Regional Pain Syndrome

A Narrative Review Highlighting Dosing Practices and Treatment Response

Theresa R. Lii, MD, MS[a], Vinita Singh, MD, MS[b,*]

KEYWORDS

- Causalgia • Chronic pain • Complex regional pain syndrome • CRPS • Infusion
- Ketamine • Reflex sympathetic dystrophy • RSD

KEY POINTS

- Intravenous ketamine at subanesthetic doses can produce long-lasting, but not permanent, pain relief in patients with complex regional pain syndrome.
- Clinical evidence across a variety of chronic pain conditions suggests that larger total doses of ketamine are correlated with longer periods of pain relief. However, very-high-dose infusions are often limited by financial cost and adverse effects.
- Subanesthetic doses (0.10–0.9 mg/kg/h) of intravenous ketamine given continuously over 5 days is the most commonly studied infusion regimen for complex regional pain syndrome and is most commonly reflected in clinical practice.
- Not all patients experience long-term (>1–3 months) pain relief from ketamine infusions; there appear to be responders and nonresponders to intravenous ketamine therapy.
- Further research is needed to identify the optimal dose and infusion protocol for intravenous ketamine, the utility of nonintravenous routes, as well as predictors of long-term response.

INTRODUCTION

Complex regional pain syndrome (CRPS) is a frequently debilitating pain condition affecting one or more limbs, which can develop with or without known trauma to the peripheral nervous system. CRPS has been described under other names, such as Sudeck's atrophy, algodystrophy, causalgia, and reflex sympathetic dystrophy.[1] Individuals with CRPS develop a constellation of signs and symptoms characterized

[a] Department of Anesthesiology, Perioperative and Pain Medicine, Stanford University, 450 Broadway Street, MC6343, Redwood City, CA 94063, USA; [b] Department of Anesthesiology, Emory University, 550 Peachtree Street, Emory University Hospital Midtown, Atlanta, GA 30308, USA
* Corresponding author.
E-mail address: vinita.singh@emory.edu

Anesthesiology Clin 41 (2023) 357–369
https://doi.org/10.1016/j.anclin.2023.03.005
anesthesiology.theclinics.com
1932-2275/23/

by autonomic and neuroinflammatory changes, such as redness and swelling, which can vary over time.[2]

The International Association of Pain (IASP) maintains the most up-to-date diagnostic criteria ("Budapest criteria") for CRPS.[3] The IASP also distinguishes between 3 subtypes: CRPS I ("type I"), which occurs without a known peripheral nerve lesion; CRPS II ("type II"), which is attributable to a discrete peripheral nerve lesion; and CRPS with remission of some features, which refers to patients who previously met full diagnostic criteria but no longer meet them.[4] For the purposes of this review, the authors address all 3 subtypes under the general term "CRPS."

The incidence of CRPS in a general population ranges from 5.5 to 20.6 per 100,000 person-years,[5,6] comparable to the incidence of trigeminal neuralgia.[7] Although CRPS accounts for only 1.2% of all pain diagnoses made in the United States,[8] the associated financial burden and amount of disability can be substantial. The mean lifetime medical costs of having CRPS is estimated to be $171,153 to $229,624 depending on therapy received.[9] In a cross-sectional study of patients with CRPS, 81% had stopped work owing to pain.[10] Disease duration can be quite long; a quarter of patients presenting to a pain clinic with CRPS might report at least 10 years of symptoms.[10]

Only 2 treatments have been approved for CRPS by the Food and Drug Administration: spinal cord stimulation (SCS) and dorsal root ganglion (DRG) stimulation.[11,12] One randomized controlled trial (RCT) for SCS in patients with CRPS found that it is effective for pain reduction; however, its advantage over physical therapy alone is lost 5 years after implantation.[13,14] A comparative effectiveness trial between SCS and DRG stimulation found that the proportion of patients with CRPS who reported pain relief at 12 months was higher in the DRG arm compared with the SCS arm.[15] However, much like SCS, the benefits of DRG stimulation are not experienced by all patients, or the effects tend to wane after a few years. In a longitudinal study of patients who received DRG stimulators for chronic intractable pain, 19% experienced no pain relief during the trial, and 10% had explants within the first 24 months owing to inadequate pain relief or the device could not provide enough current to maintain relief; 17% of the original cohort had later explants owing to inadequate pain relief or lead migration within 7 years of implantation.[16] Additional treatments for CRPS are needed, particularly for patients who have failed neuromodulation therapies.

EVIDENCE FOR KETAMINE IN COMPLEX REGIONAL PAIN SYNDROME

In this narrative review, the authors have included a summary table of retrospective and prospective studies involving the use of intravenous (IV) ketamine in patients with CRPS (**Table 1**), with a focus on dosages and response rates. They have excluded case reports and studies with mixed populations that include patients with non-CRPS pain conditions. Although intravenous ketamine has been described as a potential treatment for CRPS since the mid-1990s,[17] only 2 randomized placebo-controlled trials have tested ketamine in patients with CRPS. Schwartzman and colleagues[18] in the United States demonstrated that a 10-day series of outpatient subanesthetic infusions can result in superior analgesia for up to 12 weeks, compared with placebo infusions. Sigtermans and colleagues,[19] located in the Netherlands, showed that a 5-day continuous subanesthetic infusion delivered in an inpatient setting also showed analgesic superiority compared with placebo for up to 11 weeks.

Overall, the evidence for ketamine infusions in CRPS remains modest. A 2013 Cochrane review concluded that ketamine infusions had low-quality evidence backing its use, similar to the level of evidence for bisphosphonates, calcitonin, graded motor

Table 1
Characteristics of intravenous ketamine studies in patients with complex regional pain syndrome (primary analyses only)

Study and Year	Study Design	Sample Size	Setting	Drug	Infusion Rate	Treatment Duration, d	Duration of Pain Relief	Percent Responders	Definition of Responder	Medications to Control Side Effects
Correll et al,[75] 2004	Retrospective chart review	33	Inpatient	Racemic ketamine	10–50 mg/h	4.7	9.44 mo (mean duration of being pain free)	54	"Pain free" for ≥3 mo	Not reported
Goebel et al,[76] 2015	Open-label single-arm study	5	Inpatient	Racemic ketamine	0.15–0.9 mg/kg/h	5	6.7 wk (mean duration of "meaningful" pain relief)	20	"Meaningful" relief at 3 mo	Not reported
Goldberg et al,[77] 2010	Open-label single-arm study	16	Inpatient	Racemic ketamine	10–40 mg/h	5	—	60	"Meaningful pain relief" at 3 mo	Midazolam 2–4 mg intravenous (IV) q4h for restlessness, dysphoria, or hallucination, transdermal clonidine 0.1 mg/day
Kiefer et al,[51] 2008	Open-label single-arm study	20	Inpatient (intensive care)	Racemic ketamine	3–7 mg/kg/h	5	—	65	"Full remission" at 3 mo	Midazolam 0.15–0.4 mg/kg/h IV, clonidine 0.2–0.85 μg/kg/h IV
Mangnus et al,[56] 2021	Retrospective chart review	48	Inpatient	S(+)-ketamine	3–14 mg/h	7	—	48	Reduction of ≥2 points on the 0–10 Numeric Rating Scale pain scale at first follow-up (median 4 wk)	None (ketamine dose was reduced until side effects abated)

(*continued on next page*)

Table 1
(continued)

Study and Year	Study Design	Sample Size	Setting	Drug	Infusion Rate	Treatment Duration, d	Duration of Pain Relief	Percent Responders	Definition of Responder	Medications to Control Side Effects
Schwartzman et al,[18] 2009	Randomized placebo-controlled trial	26	Out patient	Racemic ketamine	0.175–0.35 mg/kg/h	10	Up to 12 mo (significant decrease compared with placebo)	—	—	Midazolam 2 mg IV before and after infusion, clonidine 0.1 mg PO before infusion
Sigtermans et al,[19] 2009	Randomized placebo-controlled trial	60	Inpatient	S(+)-ketamine	0.072–0.432 mg/kg/h	4.2	11 wk (significant decrease compared with placebo)	—	—	None (ketamine dose was reduced until side effects abated)

imagery, mirror therapy, and CRPS-focused physical and occupational therapy.[20] For context, many oral medications commonly used in CRPS—such as opioids, antidepressants, and antiepileptics—are not supported by randomized studies in CRPS. A more recent review authored by the American Society of Regional Anesthesia and Pain Medicine (ASRA), American Academy of Pain Medicine (AAPM), and the American Society of Anesthesiologists (ASA) argued that the use of intravenous ketamine in CRPS had grade B evidence, corresponding to low to moderate certainty.[21] A recent meta-analysis found that the available clinical evidence supports ketamine as a treatment for CRPS, although the investigators identified high heterogeneity between studies and high risk of publication bias.[22]

BRIEF OVERVIEW OF KETAMINE'S ANALGESIC MECHANISMS

Considering that the context-sensitive half-time of ketamine plateaus at around 1 hour,[23] it is remarkable that the analgesic effects of a prolonged ketamine infusion can last several weeks to months. The physiologic mechanism of ketamine's analgesic effect in CRPS is not well understood, although several mechanisms have been proposed.

First, ketamine is primarily known as an antagonist of the *N*-methyl-D-aspartate (NMDA) receptor, an excitatory glutamatergic ion channel expressed by neurons. NMDA receptors are necessary for long-term potentiation, a process by which neurons strengthen and increase signal transmission between each other with repetitive stimulation.[24] Long-term potentiation is thought to be a major mechanism underlying hyperalgesia, allodynia, and central sensitization,[25,26] which are seen frequently in CRPS; ketamine's antagonism of NMDA receptors is thought to reverse these phenomena.[27,28] The analgesic mechanism of action of ketamine may be much more complex, however, given that ketamine also interacts with several other receptors, including opioid, gamma-aminobutyric acid, dopamine, muscarinic, nicotinic, and L-type calcium channels.[29]

Neuroimmune modulation has also been proposed as a mechanism underlying ketamine's efficacy in CRPS. Inflammatory symptoms are a distinguishing feature of CRPS, especially in the acute stage. Patients with CRPS show changes in several immunologic markers within their cerebrospinal fluid,[30] indicating neuroinflammatory changes in the central nervous system as well. NDMA receptors are found on microglia and astrocytes, which are the immune cells of the central nervous system, and are thought to mediate the analgesic effects of ketamine on neuropathic pain.[31,32] Ketamine also exerts a variety of effects on peripheral markers of inflammation.[33] Ketamine can rapidly suppress proinflammatory cytokines in a variety of clinical populations, from patients undergoing major surgery[34,35] to patients with treatment-resistant depression with or without chronic pain.[36,37] Ketamine's complex effects on the neuroimmune system may in part explain ketamine's analgesic effects in CRPS.

The antidepressant effect of ketamine is well-documented in the psychiatric literature,[38] suggesting that ketamine may also impact the affective aspects of CRPS. Chronic pain and depression are known to be highly comorbid,[39,40] and there appears to be a bidirectional relationship between depression and pain severity.[41] In patients with CRPS, disability and pain severity were more strongly associated with anxiety and depression, in comparison to patients with low back pain.[42] Functional neuroimaging studies have found that ketamine exerts its effects in cortical areas that are similar between patients with major depressive disorder and CRPS. In depressed patients without chronic pain, ketamine increases the activity of the anterior cingulate gyrus and medial prefrontal cortex.[43] One functional magnetic resonance imaging study comparing a patient with CRPS with healthy subjects found evidence of post-ketamine normalization of resting state network activity in the anterior cingulate gyrus and prefrontal cortex.[44] The antidepressant effects of ketamine are thought to be mediated by a variety of mechanisms, including a glutamatergic surge associated with increased brain-derived neurotrophic factor, anti-inflammatory changes, and opioid receptor agonism.[45] Interestingly, the Sigtermans trial did not find changes in anxiety or depression in patients who received ketamine, whereas the Schwartzman trial did reveal significant decreases in the affective component of pain after ketamine infusion.[18,19] These differences may have arose from their different methods of measuring the emotional impact of pain.

KETAMINE DOSAGE AND DURATION OF PAIN RELIEF

To date, no randomized dose-ranging studies have been conducted for ketamine infusion therapy in patients with CRPS, or in any chronic pain condition. Several investigators have noted that, when comparing studies across all chronic pain conditions, the total dose of ketamine appears correlated with the duration of pain relief—with larger total doses resulting in longer-lasting analgesia.[21,46–48] In patients with fibromyalgia and chronic neuropathic pain, brief subanesthetic infusions (0.5 mg/kg over 30 minutes or 2 hours, respectively) do not produce analgesia lasting beyond 1 week.[49,50] Conversely, high-dose "ketamine comas" have been described in a series of 20 patients with CRPS who received a 5-day anesthetic ketamine infusion (up to 7 mg/kg/h), which required intubation and mechanical ventilation. Some patients experienced extraordinary results from this high-dose protocol, with about 50% of patients remaining completely pain-free for 5 to 11 years. Drawbacks of this approach include the high cost of intensive care and a high rate (20%) of iatrogenic complications, such as urinary and pulmonary infections.[51]

Not surprisingly, intermediate doses of intravenous ketamine have yielded intermediate lengths of pain relief. The RCTs conducted by Sigtermans and Schwartzman, separately, used similar subanesthetic infusion rates of ketamine, which were gradually raised over a few days. The Sigtermans trial started their infusions at 0.071 mg/kg/h and titrated the infusion rate 3 times daily up to 0.42 mg/kg/h, for an average of 4.2 continuous infusion days.[19] The Schwartzman trial initiated their ketamine infusions at 0.175 mg/kg/h on day 1, increased to 0.26 mg/kg/h on day 2, and reached their maximum dose of 0.35 mg/kg/h on day 3, and continued administering this dose 4 hours per day, for a total of 10 days.[18] Both studies demonstrated that a subanesthetic, multiday infusion regimen can yield 11 to 12 weeks of pain relief.

These intermediate doses of ketamine appear to be reflected in clinical practice as well. In a consensus survey of French pain physicians who are considered experts in ketamine therapy, the preferred dose of intravenous ketamine was 0.5 to 0.9 mg/kg per day, for 4 days of treatment.[52] Similarly, in a nationwide survey of pain clinics in the Netherlands, the median starting dose of intravenous ketamine in the outpatient setting was 5 mg/h; the median maximum dose was 27.5 mg/h, and the median infusion duration was 6 hours per day. The median starting dose in the inpatient setting was 5 mg/h; the median maximum dose was 25 mg/h, and the median days of infusion was 4 days.[53]

It is interesting to note that the Schwartzman trial infused ketamine for a total of 40 hours, whereas the Sigtermans trial infused ketamine for approximately 100 hours. Despite the Schwartzman trial having less than half the infusion hours with comparable infusion rates, the duration of pain relief obtained was similar to that of the Sigtermans trial. This might be attributed to the Schwartzman trial administering clonidine before and after each infusion; the investigators acknowledged that clonidine has been shown to potentiate the analgesic effects of ketamine.[54] An alternative explanation is that repeating multiple ketamine infusions in close succession, with daily breaks, might produce longer-lasting analgesia, compared with one continuous multiday infusion. More research into the optimal infusion regimen for intravenous ketamine is needed.

Based on the available data, an optimal balance of efficacy, cost, and safety likely lies between a single-day subanesthetic infusion (noneffective beyond 1 week) and a multiday anesthetic coma (high cost and high complication rate). Recent consensus guidelines from ASRA, AAPM, and ASA recommend starting with an outpatient infusion protocol that delivers a minimum dose of 80 mg infused over 2 hours or longer, and reassessing the patient before extending treatment.[21] Further dose-ranging studies will be necessary to establish an ideal dosing protocol.

RESPONSE RATE AND PREDICTORS OF KETAMINE RESPONSE

Researchers and clinicians have observed that the analgesic response to intravenous ketamine is highly variable.[55] In studies that report the percentage of treatment responders to ketamine, approximately one-half of patients with CRPS achieve some definition of long-term response to ketamine infusions. In a retrospective study of inpatients with CRPS who received a continuous subanesthetic ketamine infusion (3–14 mg/h, or 0.04–0.2 mg/kg/h for a 70-kg person) for up to 7 days, responders were defined as having at least a 2-point reduction in pain score on the 0 to 10 Numeric Rating Scale; in this study, 48% were still considered "responders" at 30 days postinfusion.[56] In the high-dose, open-label anesthetic infusion (3–7 mg/kg/h) study by Kiefer and colleagues,[51] 50% of participants experienced 5 to 11 years of complete pain relief.

Despite knowing such response variability exists, there are currently no well-established, replicated predictors of treatment response. In the 2 placebo-controlled RCTs for ketamine in CRPS, the investigators noted that the duration of disease did not correlate with analgesic response, which suggests that ketamine may remain a viable treatment even for patients with highly chronic, protracted disease.[18,19]

Various experimental biomarkers of ketamine response have been reported. Bosma and colleagues[57] explored whether quantitative sensory testing and functional neuroimaging could predict analgesic response to ketamine in patients with neuropathic pain; they found that treatment responders exhibited, at baseline, greater temporal summation of pain and increased dynamic functional connectivity between areas of the brain involved in the descending nociceptive pathway. The investigators proposed that dynamic functional connectivity mediates the relationship between temporal summation of pain and analgesic response to ketamine. From a practical standpoint, however, it may be more feasible to explore temporal summation of pain as a method of predicting treatment response to ketamine infusions in clinical populations.

Genomic markers have also been explored as potential predictors of ketamine response. In patients with CRPS, nonresponders to ketamine were found to have lower baseline levels of a specific microRNA (miR-548d-5p), which the investigators propose might increase glucuronosyltransferase activity, increasing levels of inactive conjugates, and thus potentially reducing the therapeutic efficacy of ketamine.[58]

Additional insights may be gleaned from studies of ketamine in major depressive disorder. In these studies, the most replicated predictors for the antidepressant response to ketamine include a family history of alcohol dependence and higher body mass index.[59] Increased heart rate and heart rate variation during ketamine infusion have also shown discriminative ability for predicting antidepressant response[60]—perhaps as a surrogate marker of increased physiologic sensitivity to ketamine's effects on the autonomic nervous system.

NONINJECTABLE FORMULATIONS OF KETAMINE

Oral and intranasal are the 2 most common nonparenteral routes of ketamine used.[16,56,57] The bioavailability is limited to less than 20% via the oral route owing to extensive hepatic metabolism.[58] Norketamine is the ketamine's metabolite formed via hepatic demethylation. It is 33% as potent as ketamine, has a longer half-life than ketamine (4 hours vs 2–3 hours), and is thought to contribute to oral ketamine's analgesic potential.[59,60,61] Some studies have reported successful long-term use of oral ketamine (>3 months) with a dosage ranging from 0.5 to 3 mg/kg in 3 to 4 divided dosages per day.[62,63] However, long-term use of ketamine needs to be under close supervision, with the eventual goal of discontinuation given the abuse potential and adverse effects associated with chronic use seen in ketamine abusers (cognitive impairment, ureteric metaplasia, and hepatic toxicity).[64,65]

The intranasal route has a higher bioavailability (up to 50%), as it avoids hepatic first-pass metabolism with absorption via the highly permeable and vascular nasal mucosa.[66,67] Most of the studies for the use of intranasal ketamine (usually 10–50 mg per spray, up to 1 mg/kg) for pain have been for intractable cancer pain, breakthrough pain, acute pain in the emergency room setting, or procedural sedation, especially in the pediatric population.[67–74] Recently published, multisociety consensus guidelines on the use of ketamine for chronic pain recommend that oral formulation can be used in lieu of serial infusion in those who respond positively to intravenous ketamine (grade B recommendation, low level of certainty). The guidelines also found moderate evidence (grade B recommendation, moderate level of certainty) for the use of intranasal ketamine preparation for breakthrough pain.

SUMMARY

CRPS is a frequently debilitating chronic pain condition with few evidence-based treatment options, and many patients with CRPS have intractable symptoms prompting the need for novel therapies. Intravenous ketamine has been investigated as a potential treatment for CRPS for over 20 years, with low to moderate levels of evidence. Current recommendations for initial ketamine dosing are to infuse at least 80 mg over a period of 2 hours or longer.[21] In addition, the current literature suggests that approximately one-half of patients with CRPS will experience long-term pain relief from a single ketamine infusion—although reliable predictors of treatment response are still unknown. Additional studies are needed to (1) identify doses and infusion protocols that strike an optimal balance between efficacy, cost, and safety; and (2) identify predictors of long-term analgesic response, in order to maximize the chance of treatment success in carefully selected patients.

CLINICS CARE POINTS

- Duration of complex regional pain syndrome has not been shown to affect analgesic response rates to ketamine infusion. Even patients with highly chronic complex regional pain syndrome refractory to other therapies should be considered for ketamine infusion. Conversely, ketamine may also be considered in patients with relatively acute presentations of complex regional pain syndrome.

- Meaningful pain relief lasting 1 to 3 months can be expected in 20% to 65% of patients with complex regional pain syndrome after a single ketamine infusion, if adequately dosed.
- The most studied ketamine infusion regimen is a subanesthetic dose (0.10–0.9 mg/kg/h) administered in a monitored inpatient setting over 5 consecutive days. Start at a lower dose and gradually uptitrate until analgesia is attained, or when adverse effects limit dose increases.
- Up to 10 days of outpatient infusions may be required to obtain a similar analgesic duration as 5 days of inpatient infusions; however, the ideal number of infusion days is unknown.
- With the first infusion, aim to give a total dose of at least 80 mg over a period of 2 hours or longer, as recommended by the American Society of Regional Anesthesia and Pain Medicine, the American Academy of Pain Medicine, and the American Society of Anesthesiologists. Assess patient response before repeating or lengthening treatment duration.
- Premedication or coadministration of intravenous midazolam (2–4 mg) and oral clonidine (0.1 mg) may be considered to limit the dissociative and sympathomimetic side effects of ketamine.

DISCLOSURES

The first author was supported by the National Institute on Drug Abuse of the National Institutes of Health, United States, under Award Number T32DA035165. The content is solely the responsibility of the authors and does not necessarily represent the official views of the National Institutes of Health, United States.

CONFLICTS OF INTEREST

The first author has no conflicts of interest to report. V. Singh: Stockholder, Releviate LLC.

REFERENCES

1. Iolascon G, de Sire A, Moretti A, et al. Complex regional pain syndrome (CRPS) type I: historical perspective and critical issues. Clin Cases Miner Bone Metab 2015;12(Suppl 1):4–10.
2. de Boer RDH, Marinus J, van Hilten JJ, et al. Distribution of signs and symptoms of Complex Regional Pain Syndrome type I in patients meeting the diagnostic criteria of the International Association for the Study of Pain. Eur J Pain 2011; 15(8):830.e1–8.
3. The International Association of Pain (IASP). ICD-11 Development Version Text relating to CRPS. Pain 2021. Available at: http://links.lww.com/PAIN/B358. Accessed August 30, 2022.
4. Goebel A, Birklein F, Brunner F, et al. The Valencia consensus-based adaptation of the IASP complex regional pain syndrome diagnostic criteria. Pain 2021; 162(9):2346–8.
5. Sandroni P, Benrud-Larson LM, McClelland RL, et al. Complex regional pain syndrome type I: incidence and prevalence in Olmsted County, a population-based study. Pain 2003;103(1):199–207.
6. de Mos M, de Bruijn AGJ, Huygen FJPM, et al. The incidence of complex regional pain syndrome: A population-based study. Pain 2007;129(1):12–20.
7. Manzoni GC, Torelli P. Epidemiology of typical and atypical craniofacial neuralgias. Neurol Sci 2005;26(Suppl 2):s65–7.

8. Murphy KR, Han JL, Yang S, et al. Prevalence of Specific Types of Pain Diagnoses in a Sample of United States Adults. Pain Physician 2017;20(2):E257–68.
9. Kemler MA, Furnée CA. Economic evaluation of spinal cord stimulation for chronic reflex sympathetic dystrophy. Neurology 2002;59(8):1203–9.
10. Schwartzman RJ, Erwin KL, Alexander GM. The Natural History of Complex Regional Pain Syndrome. Clin J Pain 2009;25(4):273–80.
11. Deer TR, Pope JE. Dorsal root ganglion stimulation approval by the Food and Drug Administration: advice on evolving the process. Expert Rev Neurother 2016;16(10):1123–5.
12. Walsh KM, Machado AG, Krishnaney AA. Spinal cord stimulation: a review of the safety literature and proposal for perioperative evaluation and management. Spine J 2015;15(8):1864–9.
13. Kemler MA, de Vet HCW, Barendse GAM, et al. Effect of spinal cord stimulation for chronic complex regional pain syndrome Type I: five-year final follow-up of patients in a randomized controlled trial. J Neurosurg 2008;108(2):292–8.
14. Kemler MA, Barendse GA, van Kleef M, et al. Spinal cord stimulation in patients with chronic reflex sympathetic dystrophy. N Engl J Med 2000;343(9):618–24.
15. Deer TR, Levy RM, Kramer J, et al. Dorsal root ganglion stimulation yielded higher treatment success rate for complex regional pain syndrome and causalgia at 3 and 12 months: a randomized comparative trial. Pain 2017;158(4):669–81.
16. Eldabe S, Copley S, Gulve A, et al. A prospective long-term follow-up of dorsal root ganglion stimulation for the management of chronic intractable pain. Pain 2022;163(4):702–10.
17. Backonja M, Arndt G, Gombar KA, et al. Response of chronic neuropathic pain syndromes to ketamine: a preliminary study. Pain 1994;56(1):51–7.
18. Schwartzman RJ, Alexander GM, Grothusen JR, et al. Outpatient intravenous ketamine for the treatment of complex regional pain syndrome: A double-blind placebo controlled study. Pain 2009;147(1):107–15.
19. Sigtermans MJ, van Hilten JJ, Bauer MCR, et al. Ketamine produces effective and long-term pain relief in patients with Complex Regional Pain Syndrome Type 1. Pain 2009;145(3):304.
20. O'Connell NE, Wand BM, McAuley JH, et al. Interventions for treating pain and disability in adults with complex regional pain syndrome- an overview of systematic reviews. Cochrane Database Syst Rev 2013;4.
21. Cohen SP, Bhatia A, Buvanendran A, et al. Consensus Guidelines on the Use of Intravenous Ketamine Infusions for Chronic Pain From the American Society of Regional Anesthesia and Pain Medicine, the American Academy of Pain Medicine, and the American Society of Anesthesiologists. Reg Anesth Pain Med 2018;1.
22. Zhao J, Wang Y, Wang D. The Effect of Ketamine Infusion in the Treatment of Complex Regional Pain Syndrome: a Systemic Review and Meta-analysis. Curr Pain Headache Rep 2018;22(2):12.
23. Kamp J, Olofsen E, Henthorn TK, et al. Ketamine Pharmacokinetics: A Systematic Review of the Literature, Meta-analysis, and Population Analysis. Anesthesiology 2020;133(6):1192–213.
24. Collingridge GL, Bliss TVP. NMDA receptors - their role in long-term potentiation. Trends Neurosci 1987;10(7):288–93.
25. Willis WD. Long-term potentiation in spinothalamic neurons. Brain Res Rev 2002;40(1):202–14.

26. Ruscheweyh R, Wilder-Smith O, Drdla R, et al. Long-Term Potentiation in Spinal Nociceptive Pathways as a Novel Target for Pain Therapy. Mol Pain 2011;7: 1744–8069.
27. Persson J, Axelsson G, Hallin RG, et al. Beneficial effects of ketamine in a chronic pain state with allodynia, possibly due to central sensitization. Pain 1995;60(2): 217–22.
28. Stubhaug A, Breivik H, Eide PK, et al. Mapping of punctuate hyperalgesia around a surgical incision demonstrates that ketamine is a powerful suppressor of central sensitization to pain following surgery. Acta Anaesthesiol Scand 1997;41(9): 1124–32.
29. Sleigh J, Harvey M, Voss L, et al. Ketamine – More mechanisms of action than just NMDA blockade. Trends in Anaesthesia and Critical Care 2014;4(2):76–81.
30. Alexander GM, Perreault MJ, Reichenberger ER, et al. Changes in immune and glial markers in the CSF of patients with Complex Regional Pain Syndrome. Brain Behav Immun 2007;21(5):668–76.
31. Hayashi Y, Kawaji K, Sun L, et al. Microglial Ca2+-Activated K+ Channels Are Possible Molecular Targets for the Analgesic Effects of S-Ketamine on Neuropathic Pain. J Neurosci 2011;31(48):17370–82.
32. Mei XP, Zhang H, Wang W, et al. Inhibition of spinal astrocytic c-Jun N-terminal kinase (JNK) activation correlates with the analgesic effects of ketamine in neuropathic pain. J Neuroinflammation 2011;8(1):6.
33. De Kock M, Loix S, Lavand'homme P. Ketamine and Peripheral Inflammation. CNS Neurosci Ther 2013;19(6):403–10.
34. Roytblat L, Talmor D, Rachinsky M, et al. Ketamine attenuates the interleukin-6 response after cardiopulmonary bypass. Anesth Analg 1998;87(2):266–71.
35. Yang Z, Chen ZQ, Jiang XQ. [Effects of subanesthetic dose of ketamine on perioperative serum cytokines in orthotopic liver transplantation]. Nan Fang Yi Ke Da Xue Xue Bao 2006;26(6):802–4.
36. Zhou Y, Wang C, Lan X, et al. Plasma inflammatory cytokines and treatment-resistant depression with comorbid pain: improvement by ketamine. J Neuroinflammation 2021;18:200.
37. Chen MH, Li CT, Lin WC, et al. Rapid inflammation modulation and antidepressant efficacy of a low-dose ketamine infusion in treatment-resistant depression: A randomized, double-blind control study. Psychiatr Res 2018;269:207–11.
38. Marcantoni WS, Akoumba BS, Wassef M, et al. A systematic review and meta-analysis of the efficacy of intravenous ketamine infusion for treatment resistant depression: January 2009 – January 2019. J Affect Disord 2020;277:831–41.
39. Bair MJ, Robinson RL, Katon W, et al. Depression and Pain Comorbidity: A Literature Review. Arch Intern Med 2003;163(20):2433–45.
40. Rayner L, Hotopf M, Petkova H, et al. Depression in patients with chronic pain attending a specialised pain treatment centre: prevalence and impact on health care costs. Pain 2016;157(7):1472–9.
41. Kroenke K, Wu J, Bair MJ, et al. Reciprocal Relationship Between Pain and Depression: A 12-Month Longitudinal Analysis in Primary Care. J Pain 2011; 12(9):964–73.
42. Bean DJ, Johnson MH, Kydd RR. Relationships Between Psychological Factors, Pain, and Disability in Complex Regional Pain Syndrome and Low Back Pain. Clin J Pain 2014;30(8):647–53.
43. McMillan R, Sumner R, Forsyth A, et al. Simultaneous EEG/fMRI recorded during ketamine infusion in patients with major depressive disorder. Prog Neuro Psychopharmacol Biol Psychiatr 2020;99:109838.

44. Becerra L, Schwartzman RJ, Kiefer RT, et al. CNS Measures of Pain Responses Pre- and Post-Anesthetic Ketamine in a Patient with Complex Regional Pain Syndrome. Pain Med 2015;16(12):2368–85.
45. Matveychuk D, Thomas RK, Swainson J, et al. Ketamine as an antidepressant: overview of its mechanisms of action and potential predictive biomarkers. Therapeutic Advances in Psychopharmacology 2020;10. 2045125320916657.
46. Maher DP, Chen L, Mao J. Intravenous Ketamine Infusions for Neuropathic Pain Management: A Promising Therapy in Need of Optimization. Anesth Analg 2017;124(2):661–74.
47. Noppers I, Niesters M, Aarts L, et al. Ketamine for the treatment of chronic non-cancer pain. Expert Opin Pharmacother 2010;11(14):2417–29.
48. Orhurhu V, Orhurhu MS, Bhatia A, et al. Ketamine Infusions for Chronic Pain: A Systematic Review and Meta-analysis of Randomized Controlled Trials. Anesth Analg 2019;129(1):241–54.
49. Noppers I, Niesters M, Swartjes M, et al. Absence of long-term analgesic effect from a short-term S-ketamine infusion on fibromyalgia pain: A randomized, prospective, double blind, active placebo-controlled trial. Eur J Pain 2011;15(9): 942–9.
50. Pickering G, Pereira B, Morel V, et al. Ketamine and Magnesium for Refractory Neuropathic Pain. Anesthesiology 2020;133(1):154–64.
51. Kiefer RT, Rohr P, Ploppa A, et al. Efficacy of Ketamine in Anesthetic Dosage for the Treatment of Refractory Complex Regional Pain Syndrome: An Open-Label Phase II Study. Pain Med 2008;9(8):1173–201.
52. Voute M, Riant T, Amodéo JM, et al. Ketamine in chronic pain: A Delphi survey. Eur J Pain 2022;26(4):873–87.
53. Mangnus TJP, Bharwani KD, Stronks DL, et al. Ketamine therapy for chronic pain in The Netherlands: a nationwide survey. Scandinavian Journal of Pain 2022; 22(1):97–105.
54. Jevtovic-Todorovic V, Wozniak DF, Powell S, et al. Clonidine potentiates the neuropathic pain-relieving action of MK-801 while preventing its neurotoxic and hyperactivity side effects. Brain Res 1998;781(1–2):202–11.
55. Kirkpatrick AF, Saghafi A, Yang K, et al. Optimizing the Treatment of CRPS With Ketamine. Clin J Pain 2020;36(7):516–23.
56. Blonk MI, Koder BG, van den Bemt PMLA, Huygen FJPM. Use of oral ketamine in chronic pain management: A review. Eur J Pain 2010;14(5):466–72.
57. Kronenberg RH. Ketamine as an Analgesic. J Pain Palliat Care Pharmacother 2002;16(3):27–35.
58. Clements JA, Nimmo WS, Grant IS. Bioavailability, pharmacokinetics, and analgesic activity of ketamine in humans. J Pharm Sci 1982;71(5):539–42.
59. White PF, Way WL, Trevor AJ. Ketamine–its pharmacology and therapeutic uses. Anesthesiology 1982;56(2):119–36.
60. Ebert B, Mikkelsen S, Thorkildsen C, Borgbjerg FM. Norketamine, the main metabolite of ketamine, is a non-competitive NMDA receptor antagonist in the rat cortex and spinal cord. Eur J Pharmacol 1997;333(1):99–104.
61. Holtman JR, Crooks PA, Johnson-Hardy JK, et al. Effects of norketamine enantiomers in rodent models of persistent pain. Pharmacol Biochem Behav 2008;90(4): 676–85.
62. Furuhashi-Yonaha A, Iida H, Asano T, et al. Short- and long-term efficacy of oral ketamine in eight chronic-pain patients. Can J Anaesth 2002;49(8):886–7.

63. Marchetti F, Coutaux A, Bellanger A, et al. Efficacy and safety of oral ketamine for the relief of intractable chronic pain: A retrospective 5-year study of 51 patients. Eur J Pain 2015;19(7):984–93.
64. Ke X, Ding Y, Xu K, et al. The profile of cognitive impairments in chronic ketamine users. Psychiatry Res 2018;266:124–31.
65. Bokor G, Anderson PD. Ketamine: An Update on Its Abuse. J Pharm Pract 2014; 27(6):582–6.
66. Yanagihara Y, Ohtani M, Kariya S, et al. Plasma concentration profiles of ketamine and norketamine after administration of various ketamine preparations to healthy Japanese volunteers. Biopharm Drug Dispos 2003;24(1):37–43.
67. Singh V, Gillespie TW, Harvey RD. Intranasal Ketamine and Its Potential Role in Cancer-Related Pain. Pharmacotherapy 2018;38(3):390–401.
68. Poonai N, Canton K, Ali S, et al. Intranasal ketamine for procedural sedation and analgesia in children: A systematic review. PLoS One 2017;12(3):e0173253.
69. Rocchio RJ, Ward KE. Intranasal Ketamine for Acute Pain. Clin J Pain 2021;37(4): 295–300.
70. Frey TM, Florin TA, Caruso M, et al. Effect of Intranasal Ketamine vs Fentanyl on Pain Reduction for Extremity Injuries in Children: The PRIME Randomized Clinical Trial. JAMA Pediatr 2019;173(2):140–6.
71. Pouraghaei M, Moharamzadeh P, Paknezhad SP, et al. Intranasal ketamine versus intravenous morphine for pain management in patients with renal colic: a double-blind, randomized, controlled trial. World J Urol 2021;39(4):1263–7.
72. Tongbua S, Sri-On J, Thong-On K, Paksophis T. Non-inferiority of intranasal ketamine compared to intravenous morphine for musculoskeletal pain relief among older adults in an emergency department: a randomised controlled trial. Age Ageing 2022;51(3):afac073.
73. Carr DB, Goudas LC, Denman WT, et al. Safety and efficacy of intranasal ketamine for the treatment of breakthrough pain in patients with chronic pain: a randomized, double-blind, placebo-controlled, crossover study. Pain 2004;108(1–2): 17–27.
74. Singh V, Gillespie TW, Lane O, et al. A dose-escalation clinical trial of intranasal ketamine for uncontrolled cancer-related pain. Pharmacotherapy 2022;42(4): 298–310.
75. Correll GE, Maleki J, Gracely EJ, et al. Subanesthetic Ketamine Infusion Therapy: A Retrospective Analysis of a Novel Therapeutic Approach to Complex Regional Pain Syndrome. Pain Medicine 2004;5(3):263–75.
76. Goebel A, Jayaseelan S, Sachane K, et al. Racemic ketamine 4.5-day infusion treatment of long-standing complex regional pain syndrome—a prospective service evaluation in five patients. Br J Anaesth 2015;115(1):146–7.
77. Goldberg ME, Torjman MC, Schwartzman RJ, et al. Pharmacodynamic Profiles of Ketamine (R)- and (S)- with 5-Day Inpatient Infusion for the Treatment of Complex Regional Pain Syndrome. Pain Physician 2010;13(4):379–87.

Blinded Pain Cocktails

A Reliable and Safe Opioid Weaning Method

Albert Hyukjae Kwon, MD[a,*], Luana Colloca, MD, PhD, MS[b], Sean C. Mackey, MD, PhD[c]

KEYWORDS

- Blinded pain cocktail • Opioid weaning • Methadone • Dose-extending placebo

KEY POINTS

- Managing chronic pain with chronic opioid therapy is a complex clinical problem owing to the inherent biopsychosocial model of pain.
- A blinded pain cocktail is an effective and safe method of weaning opioids in patients who struggle to wean opioids in the typical outpatient setting.
- Optimization of comorbid psychiatric conditions is associated with higher success of prolonged opioid abstinence.

INTRODUCTION

From 2001 to 2013, the worldwide use of opioid analgesic medications doubled, and among 214 countries, the United States had the highest opioid use.[1] A concurrent opioid crisis in the United States resulted in half a million deaths from illicit and prescribed opioid overdose between 1999 and 2019.[2] In 2015, 63.1% of 52,404 drug overdose deaths involved an opioid, reflecting a 15.6% increase compared with the year before.[3] This sharp increase in opioid-related deaths was driven by illicitly manufactured fentanyl and heroin; the rate of opioid prescriptions was already decreasing between 2012 and 2016.[4–6] Such troubling trends in the United States led to the Centers for Disease Control and Prevention (CDC) publishing a guideline for prescribing opioids for primary care in 2016 and a pocket guide on tapering opioids for chronic pain in 2017.[7–9] The federal government declared a public health emergency in 2017, and multiple states enacted a wide range of policies to limit opioid prescribing.[10–12]

In such a climate of varying guidance and state laws limiting opioid prescribing, opioid prescribing trends have abruptly shifted in the United States with nearly half of opioid prescribers indicating their rationale for tapering or discontinuing opioids

[a] Stanford University School of Medicine, 430 Broadway Street, Pavilion C, 3rd Floor, Redwood City, CA 94063, USA; [b] Pain and Translational Symptom Science, Placebo Beyond Opinions Center, School of Nursing, University of Maryland, Baltimore, 655 West Lombard Street, Room 729A, Baltimore, MD 21201, USA; [c] Stanford University School of Medicine, 1070 Arastradero Road, Suite 200, Palo Alto, CA 94304, USA
* Corresponding author.
E-mail address: alkwon@stanford.edu

Anesthesiology Clin 41 (2023) 371–381
https://doi.org/10.1016/j.anclin.2023.03.006 anesthesiology.theclinics.com
1932-2275/23/

in patient care was the 2016 CDC guidelines.[13] Although rate of opioid prescriptions was declining since 2012 at the rate of 5.2% annually, the rate of decline accelerated to 12.4% annually between 2016 and 2018 after the CDC opioid prescribing guideline was published.[6] Also, the rate of high-dose opioid prescriptions (>90 morphine milligram equivalents per day) decreased 66.1% from 2006 to 2018.[6] However, with approximately 19.0% of adults in the United States reporting persistent pain, inadequately treated chronic pain is a serious medical, ethical, and economic problem.[14] Opioid dose tapering among patients prescribed long-term opioids has been associated with overdose or mental health crises.[15] Therefore, primary care physicians who write most of the chronic opioid prescriptions struggle to wean patients who have been on high-opioid dosages.

Interdisciplinary opioid tapering programs[16] and patient-centered opioid tapering in the outpatient setting[17] are effective ways to wean high-dose opioids used for chronic pain. However, limited access to interdisciplinary opioid tapering programs and lack of training and confidence in the management of opioid-related care continue to pose a challenge to many clinicians, and pain medicine subspecialists are consulted.[18] As chronic pain is highly concomitant with mental health disorders, managing a patient on opioid therapy for chronic pain can potentially be a complex challenge.

The blinded pain cocktail method, a pharmacologic intervention described in the 1980s and 1990s, can be highly valuable when conventional outpatient tapering methods fail.[19–21] Today, the Stanford Comprehensive Interdisciplinary Pain Program, an inpatient medication-behavioral pain treatment program, frequently uses blinded pain cocktails to both taper opioids and define an optimal opioid dose to manage pain.

This review article aims to (1) outline psychosocial factors that may complicate opioid weaning, (2) describe clinical goals and how to use blinded pain cocktails in opioid tapering, and (3) summarize the mechanism of dose-extending placebos and ethical justification of its use in clinical practice. Although the authors also use blinded pain cocktails in their outpatient Stanford Pain Management Center for the same purposes outlined here, the scope of this article focuses on inpatient uses.

Psychosocial Factors that may Complicate Opioid Weaning: Interaction Between Opioid Signaling and Various Psychiatric Conditions

Adults who report a greater degree of anxiety, depression, and fatigue are far more likely to report persistent pain than those who report they never have anxiety, depression, or fatigue.[14] Common mental health disorders have been linked to a greater odds ratio of initiating opioid therapy and its continuation.[22] There are 5 known types of opioid receptors: mu receptor, kappa receptor, delta receptor, nociceptin receptor, and zeta receptor. Endogenous opioids that bind these receptors include enkephalins, endorphins, dynorphins, endomorphins, and nociceptin/orphanin FQ. PET[23,24] and postmortem human studies[25] have shown high opioid receptors in limbic and paralimbic regions that regulate emotions. Therefore, understanding the interaction between opioid signaling and various psychiatric conditions is relevant, and attention to these psychiatric disorders is essential in managing patients on chronic opioid therapy.

Anxiety Disorders

Opioids have an anxiety-suppressing effect in both animals and humans. The brain areas implicated in anxiety regulation, the amygdala, hypothalamus, and the midbrain, express opioid receptors.[26] In δ-opioid receptor knock-out mice, anxiogenic phenotypes were observed,[27] suggesting anxiety is modulated through the δ-opioid receptor. Endogenous opioids are released in stressful and anxiety-provoking situations to dampen anxiety behaviors. γ-Aminobutyric acid agonists are common antianxiolytics used in clinical practice. Naloxone has been shown to block the antianxiety effects of benzodiazepines.[28,29] Selective serotonin reuptake inhibitors (SSRIs) and serotonin noradrenaline reuptake inhibitors (SNRIs) are commonly used for the treatment of anxiety disorders. Serotonin facilitates endorphin release in the arcuate nucleus and nucleus accumbens and leads to antinociceptive effects of SSRIs and SNRIs.[30]

Anticipation of a future concern or potential threat leading to avoidance behaviors and fear responses is a common symptom in anxiety and pain disorders. Vocational performance and personal relationships can be negatively affected. When the worry is out of proportion to the situation and it hinders the patient's ability to function, the patient may meet criteria for an anxiety disorder (**Box 1**). Baseline anxiety and withdrawal symptoms from opioids precipitating aversive affective symptoms can contribute to maintenance of opioid use, escalation to compulsive opioid use, and relapse after a period of abstinence.[31] Therefore, uncontrolled anxiety disorders often complicate opioid tapering.

Depressive Disorders

Chronic pain, depression, and opioids are intertwined. In mice and rats, kappa-opioid receptors mediate affective component of pain, whereas mu-opioid receptors mediate pleasure sensations and blunt aversive behaviors.[32,33] Endogenous opioid response on mu-opioid receptors has been shown to be dysregulated in patients with major depressive disorder.[34] In clinical practice, higher doses and longer-term opioid therapy increase the likelihood of comorbid depression.[35,36] Also, patients with greater severity of depression are more likely to rely on chronic opioid therapy and higher opioid doses for chronic pain treatment.[36] The bidirectional risk of depression and chronic opioid therapy underscores the importance of surveilling patients on chronic opioid therapy for depressive symptoms.

This complex interaction between depression and opioids likely contributes to mental health crises and opioid overdose precipitated with tapering chronic opioid therapy in chronic pain patients.[15] Prolonged abstinence from opioids after weaning has been shown to be associated with control of comorbid depression.[37,38] Persistent feelings of sadness and worthlessness and lack of motivation or desire to engage in formerly pleasurable activities are characteristic of depressive disorders. The *Diagnostic and Statistical Manual of Mental Disorders* (Fifth Edition) defines 8 depressive disorders (**Box 2**). Therefore, treatment of comorbid depression is highly relevant to successful and safe opioid weaning and maintaining opioid abstinence.

Opioid Tolerance, Dependence, and Addiction

Chronic opioid treatments can lead to neurologic changes manifesting in opioid dependence, tolerance, and/or addiction. Understanding the neurobiology of these conditions is valuable to clinicians especially when trying to wean the dose.

Box 1
Anxiety disorders in *Diagnostic and Statistical Manual of Mental Disorders* (Fifth Edition)

Generalized anxiety disorder

Panic disorder

Specific phobia

Agoraphobia

Social anxiety disorder

Separation anxiety disorder

Box 2
Depressive disorders in *Diagnostic and Statistical Manual of Mental Disorders* (Fifth Edition)

Disruptive mood dysregulation disorder

Major depressive disorder

Persistent depressive disorder (dysthymia)

Premenstrual dysphoric disorder

Substance/medication-induced depressive disorder

Depressive disorder due to another medical condition

Other specific depressive disorder

Other unspecified depressive disorder

Opioid tolerance is a physiologic response to the continued use of opioids leading to the diminishing effectiveness of opioids. The patient developing opioid tolerance will report needing to increase opioid doses to achieve the same analgesic effect. Opioid receptors are inhibitory G protein–coupled receptors. Acute effects of opioids lead to decreased cyclic adenosine monophosphate (cAMP) signal transduction through an inhibitory regulative G-protein, adenylyl cyclase, protein kinase A, and cAMP phosphodiesterase. With chronic opioid therapy and chronic activation of opioid receptors, compensatory regulation of downstream signaling mediators offset the inhibitory effect of opioids. Through this offset compensatory mechanism, there is now a decreased response to an opioid dose that was previously effective.

Opioid dependence is a physical and/or psychological reliance on opioids leading to vulnerability to withdrawal when therapy is weaned or stopped. Locus coeruleus, a nucleus in the pons of the brainstem, regulates physiologic responses to stress and uses norepinephrine as its primary neurotransmitter. Mu-opioid receptors inhibit neuronal activity in the locus coeruleus and inhibit norepinephrine release. Through the same cellular mechanism of opioid tolerance, acute inhibitory effects of opioids on locus coeruleus also diminish with persistent opioid use. If chronic opioid therapy is decreased or discontinued, the inhibitory effect from opioid lessens, whereas downstream signaling mediators has been enhanced. This combination leads to excess norepinephrine release resulting in clinical symptoms of withdrawal: increased pain, tachycardia, anxiety, muscle cramps, sweating, shivering, and so forth.

Opioid addiction is characterized by cravings to use opioids and inability to control despite ongoing physical, social, and psychological harm. Mechanistically, opioids act on the brain's ventral tegmental area and release dopamine into the nucleus accumbens in the forebrain to activate the brain's reward system. This opioid-induced activation of the reward pathway produces the sensation of pleasure and promotes continued opioid use.

When a patient uses opioids in a manner incongruent with their prescriber's direction or aberrant behavior is detected, the patient should be assessed for opioid use disorder and referred to an addiction specialist if appropriate.

THE STANFORD BLINDED PAIN COCKTAIL PROTOCOL

When patients with chronic pain wish to wean opioids or the prescribing physician decides opioid taper to a lower dose is indicated to limit side effects of opioid therapy, a steady and gradual wean is attempted first while monitoring the patient's pain outcomes and functional status in the outpatient setting. When patients struggle to wean their opioids in the outpatient setting despite adding nonopioid multimodal analgesics, the blinded pain cocktail protocol in the Stanford Comprehensive Interdisciplinary Pain Program is offered as a medication-behavioral inpatient treatment option.[39] The primary goal of the blinded pain cocktail is to find a lower opioid dose that does not negatively impact the patient's functional outcome while leveraging dose-extending placebo effects, or in other words, to optimize opioid dosing. Dose-extending placebo effects are "placebos and/or subclinical dose of painkillers that are blended with treatments per reinforcement learning principles" (see later discussion).[40] During a 7- to 10-day hospital admission, pain psychology and physical therapy services are provided along with dose-extending placebos to address the patient's psychological vulnerabilities and pain behaviors.

The first step is to set proper expectations and to receive patient consent for blinding them to the pain cocktail contents and doses. Proper expectations are realistic expectations of outcomes that are achievable while their individual values, hopes, and desires are considered.

In terms of the informed consent process, patients are told they will receive a cocktail of opioid and nonopioid pain medications in the form of an oral liquid that will be mixed in a flavored syrup. The cocktail will have a total volume of liquid medications and syrup base that is kept constant at 25 mL, whereas the dose of medications can be adjusted daily. Some patients may be aware of the medication contents of the pain cocktail, but the dose of each medication is not shared with patients in all cases. Patients must consent to being blinded to the pain cocktail doses before admission. Alignment in treatment goals and approach is also key among the interdisciplinary pain team, hospital pharmacists, and bedside nurses to help patients cope with any increases in pain and obtain meaningful functional gain.

A critical step is the shift to methadone administration. Upon admission, if the patient does not have contraindications to methadone, the patient's home opioid is converted to methadone with the total daily dose equivalent to 50% to 80% of the patient's total opioid daily dose. Methadone is administered in 2 to 3 divided doses, and the home opioid is discontinued. In addition, a "blinding" agent is added to the cocktail to mask the central nervous system effects of subsequent titration. Typically, the authors use baclofen as a blinding agent. However, other medications (eg, antihistamines) can be used as well.

The initial methadone dose is maintained for the first 2 days, while monitoring for analgesic effect and daily baseline function. The methadone dose may be adjusted higher on the second day if analgesic effect is inadequate. The patient must perceive equal or better pain relief with the pain cocktail compared with home opioids before starting the weaning process. Therefore, an additional day may be required to establish a methadone dose with adequate analgesia. Other nonopioid home medications that patients take before admission can also be included in the pain cocktail if a liquid formulation of the medication is available.

Starting on the third or fourth hospital day, methadone is weaned by a 10% to 20% increment every day. The pain cocktail is adjusted daily with options to add nonopioid analgesics (**Table 1**) to the pain cocktail to manage the patient's pain and withdrawal symptoms. The total volume of the cocktail is kept constant so that weaning of active ingredients is not apparent to the patient and so it provides a perception of continued medication administration. Clonidine and/or ondansetron are commonly added to address mild or moderate opioid withdrawal symptoms. One or 2 extra pain cocktails containing low-dose short-acting opioid may be administered as needed to address

Table 1
Nonopioid adjunct medications that can be added in pain cocktail

Nonsteroidal anti-inflammatory drugs	Ibuprofen, Naproxen, Meloxicam
Barbiturate	Phenobarbital
Alpha-2 agonist	Clonidine
Gabapentinoids	Gabapentin, Pregabalin
Muscle relaxants	Baclofen, Cyclobenzaprine, Diazepam
Antidepressants	Sertraline, Venlafaxine, Mirtazapine, Trazodone
Anticonvulsants	Carbamazepine, Lamotrigine, Primidone
Antihistamine	Hydroxyzine, Diphenhydramine
Antipsychotics	Quetiapine, Ziprasidone

severe opioid withdrawal symptoms. Consistent requirement of additional short-acting opioids may indicate that the patient needs a slower methadone taper.

Although each patient's needs and clinical scenario determine how long the tapering period lasts, most patients can wean off methadone or wean down to a much lower dose within 7 to 10 days. Patients who remain on a lower methadone dose may continue a slower weekly wean as an outpatient to ultimately achieve opioid abstinence. Alternatively, a subset of patients may remain on a small dose of methadone or another opioid agonist to maintain an adequate level of daily function. At the end of the blinded pain cocktail protocol, patients may be unblinded to the content and doses of the pain cocktail, or some, interestingly, decide to remain blinded and continue taking the pain cocktail as an outpatient therapy indefinitely. Oftentimes at the end of the blinded pain cocktail protocol, patients are taking an opioid-free pain cocktail.

USE OF DOSE-EXTENDING OPEN-LABEL PLACEBOS IN THE PAIN COCKTAIL PROTOCOL

Human studies on placebo-mediated analgesia suggest the placebo mechanism lies with opioid receptor signaling pathways.[41,42] More specifically, dose-extending placebos can treat physiologic and psychological dependence on opioids and other potentially habit-forming analgesics.[40] Murine studies have shown that conditioning with morphine and contextual cues can lead to enhanced pain tolerance even with saline (placebo) given with the same contextual cues.[43,44] Dose-extending placebo activates endogenous pain modulatory systems mediated through the mu-opioid receptor,[45,46] and placebo-induced pain tolerance enhancement can be reversed by naloxone, a mu-opioid antagonist.[47]

Open-label placebo refers to placebo medications presented to patients without deception and in a positive context with their full knowledge that no active pharmacologic compound exists in the medication they receive. This was used in treating irritable bowel syndrome (IBS) in 2010. Patients were told that the open-label placebo pills are "placebo pills made of an inert substance, like sugar pills, that have been shown in clinical studies to produce significant improvement in IBS symptoms through mind-body self-healing processes."[48] The use of open-label placebo in IBS showed significantly higher mean global improvement scores in IBS compared with treatment as usual. Open-label placebo was also used successfully in treatment of chronic low back pain. Adding an open-label placebo to treatment as usual showed a statistically greater reduction in low back pain score and pain-related disability.[49]

Research on dose-extending open-label placebo indicates that placebos can be used without deceiving the patient and with patient's informed consent are ethical and effective in symptom management. Recent studies have shown that a dose-extending placebo can decrease the total dose of active medications required for a clinical response. A reduction of medication has been documented for opioids in the context of spinal cord injury,[50] stimulants for attention-deficit/hyperactivity disorder,[51] corticosteroids for psoriasis,[52] zolpidem for insomnia,[53] desloratadine for allergic rhinitis,[54] and immune suppressive drugs for renal transplant.[55]

During the pain cocktail protocol, it is not uncommon to have patients who report adequate analgesic effects to pain cocktails without any active ingredient (flavored syrup only) or subtherapeutic doses of an opioid or nonopioid analgesic. Some patients remain on placebo pain cocktails for a couple of days before revealing the pain cocktail ingredients at the end of the hospitalization.

EFFECTIVENESS OF BLINDED PAIN COCKTAIL IN OPIOID REDUCTION

The success rate of weaning off opioids using this method is reported to be high and safe. Of 124 patients, 107 patients admitted to an inpatient multidisciplinary pain service were weaned off opioids over about a weeklong taper with methadone.[20] Also, only 4 of 124 patients had objective problems of withdrawal or excessive dosing of active ingredients, demonstrating how safe this protocol is. Multidisciplinary pain rehabilitation programs using a pain cocktail blinded to dose of analgesics showed more than a doubling of increased activity levels, and analgesic doses decreased by 80% on average in 36 patients.[56] Although these were retrospective studies conducted more than 20 years ago, the large number of patients and the authors' experience at Stanford demonstrate that pain cocktails using methadone as the opioid agonist is an effective tool in achieving an opioid reduction or abstinence while maintaining or even improving daily function.

One may ask whether blinding patients is advantageous, as one may feel uncomfortable with the notion of using placebos. When comparing the pain cocktail method with patient-controlled reduction methods of opioid reduction among 108 chronic pain patients over 4 weeks, 89% of patients treated with the pain cocktail method were abstinent of opioids compared with 68% of patient-controlled reduction method.[21] However, there were no differences in the rates of continued opioid abstinence between the pain cocktail method and patient-controlled reduction method at 1- and 6-month follow-ups. Nevertheless, patients can be ethically informed that the pain cocktails will aim to wean patients off opioids with safe lower doses. Patients will be informed that the opioids will decrease overall but will not be aware of the exact time of the reduction. Patients can be educated about the power of pharmacologic conditioning, which allows them to harness beneficial outcomes while the risks associated with the opioids are minimized.[57] Ethically permissible approaches to weaning opioids have been indicated using preauthorization requests that are part of the informed consent.[57] The authorized approach can be complemented with educational videos created to inform patients. It is important to remember that a patient-authorized blinded pain cocktail protocol is advantageous in weaning patients off opioids or to a safer, lower dose. Maintaining long-term opioid abstinence is associated with how well their comorbid psychosocial factors are managed.[37]

SUMMARY

With the opioid epidemic and federal and state regulations put in place in response to the opioid epidemic, there is greater avoidance of opioid therapy for the treatment of chronic pain. For many patients who have been on chronic opioid therapy, opioid doses are being weaned or stopped abruptly at the cost of significant physical and psychological suffering. Because of the biopsychosocial model of chronic pain, weaning opioids is often a complicated clinical problem, and the typical physician-patient directed opioid weaning strategy is often not successful, possibly owing to the patient's comorbid psychosocial conditions. Preauthorized blinded pain cocktail protocol can be an effective and safe alternative method to weaning opioids rapidly in an inpatient interdisciplinary pain program or even on an outpatient basis over 1 to 2 months.

CLINICS CARE POINTS

- A preauthorized consent process to blind the pain cocktail should be adopted.
- Patients should be educated, and realistic expectations should be set.
- If weaning of opioids is implemented in an inpatient setting, the first 2 to 3 days should be used to transition home opioids to methadone dosed at 50% to 80% of the home opioid daily dose.
- Subsequently, methadone should be weaned daily by 10% to 20% increments while adding nonopioid analgesics and other medications to counteract withdrawal symptoms.
- Psychotherapy and rehabilitative care should be provided to support the patient throughout the hospitalization.
- Adequate management of comorbid psychiatric conditions is associated with achieving prolonged opioid abstinence.

DISCLOSURE

All three authors (A.H. Kwon, L. Colloca, S. Mackey) do not have any conflicts of interests nor grant support to disclose in regards to this work.

REFERENCES

1. Berterame S, Erthal J, Thomas J, et al. Use of and barriers to access to opioid analgesics: a worldwide, regional, and national study. Lancet 2016;387(10028):1644–56.
2. Centers for Disease Control. Wide-ranging online data for epidemiologic research (WONDER). https://wonder.cdc.gov. Accessed August 7, 2022.
3. Rudd RA, Seth P, David F, et al. Increases in Drug and Opioid-Involved Overdose Deaths - United States, 2010-2015. MMWR Morb Mortal Wkly Rep 2016;65(50–51):1445–52.
4. Gladden RM, Martinez P, Seth P. Fentanyl Law Enforcement Submissions and Increases in Synthetic Opioid-Involved Overdose Deaths - 27 States, 2013-2014. MMWR Morb Mortal Wkly Rep 2016;65(33):837–43.
5. Peterson AB, Gladden RM, Delcher C, et al. Increases in Fentanyl-Related Overdose Deaths - Florida and Ohio, 2013-2015. MMWR Morb Mortal Wkly Rep 2016;65(33):844–9.
6. Centers for Disease Control and Prevention UDOHAHS. Annual surveillance report of drug-related risks and outcomes. United States surveillance special report; 2019. https://www.cdc.gov/drugoverdose/pdf/pubs/2019-cdc-drug-surveillance-report.pdf. Accessed July 31, 2022.

7. Frieden TR, Houry D. Reducing the Risks of Relief–The CDC Opioid-Prescribing Guideline. N Engl J Med 2016;374(16):1501–4.
8. Dowell D, Haegerich TM, Chou R. CDC Guideline for Prescribing Opioids for Chronic Pain - United States, 2016. MMWR Recomm Rep (Morb Mortal Wkly Rep) 2016;65(1):1–49 [published correction appears in MMWR Recomm Rep. 2016;65(11):295].
9. Pocket CDC. Guide: Tapering Opioids for Chronic Pain. 2017. https://www.cdc.gov/drugoverdose/pdf/clinical_ pocket_guide_tapering-a.pdf. Accessed August 13, 2022.
10. Danielson EC, Harle CA, Silverman R, et al. Assessing Variation in State Opioid Tapering Laws: Comparing State Laws with the CDC Guideline. Pain Med 2021;22(12):2941–9.
11. Heins SE, Frey KP, Alexander GC, et al. Reducing High-Dose Opioid Prescribing: State-Level Morphine Equivalent Daily Dose Policies, 2007-2017. Pain Med 2020; 21(2):308–16.
12. Davis CS, Lieberman AJ, Hernandez-Delgado H, et al. Laws limiting the prescribing or dispensing of opioids for acute pain in the United States: A national systematic legal review. Drug Alcohol Depend 2019;194:166–72.
13. Persico AL, Bettinger JJ, Wegrzyn EL, et al. Opioid Taper Practices Among Clinicians. J Pain Res 2021;14:3353–8.
14. Kennedy J, Roll JM, Schraudner T, et al. Prevalence of persistent pain in the U.S. adult population: new data from the 2010 national health interview survey. J Pain 2014;15(10):979–84.
15. Agnoli A, Xing G, Tancredi DJ, et al. Association of Dose Tapering With Overdose or Mental Health Crisis Among Patients Prescribed Long-term Opioids. JAMA 2021;326(5):411–9 [published correction appears in JAMA. 2022 Feb 15;327(7):688] [published correction appears in JAMA. 2022 Feb 15;327(7):687].
16. Sullivan MD, Turner JA, DiLodovico C, et al. Prescription Opioid Taper Support for Outpatients With Chronic Pain: A Randomized Controlled Trial. J Pain 2017;18(3): 308–18.
17. Darnall BD, Ziadni MS, Stieg RL, et al. Patient-Centered Prescription Opioid Tapering in Community Outpatients With Chronic Pain [published correction appears in JAMA Intern Med. 2022 Jun 1;182(6):690]. JAMA Intern Med 2018; 178(5):707–8.
18. Kirane H, Drits E, Ahn S, et al. Addressing the opioid crisis: An assessment of clinicians' training experience, practices, and attitudes within a large healthcare organization. J Opioid Manag 2019;15(3):193–204.
19. Murphy JL, Clark ME, Banou E. Opioid cessation and multidimensional outcomes after interdisciplinary chronic pain treatment. Clin J Pain 2013;29(2):109–17.
20. Buckley PF, Sizemore WA, Charlton EJ. Medication management in patients with chronic non-malignant pain. A review of the use of a drug withdrawal protocol. Pain 1986;26(2):153–65.
21. Ralphs JA, de C Williams AC, Richardson PH, et al. Opiate reduction in chronic pain patients: a comparison of patient-controlled reduction and staff controlled cocktail methods. Pain 1994;56(3):279–88.
22. Sullivan MD, Edlund MJ, Zhang L, et al. Association between mental health disorders, problem drug use, and regular prescription opioid use. Arch Intern Med 2006;166(19):2087–93.
23. Frost JJ, Douglass KH, Mayberg HS, et al. Multicompartmental analysis of [11C]-carfentanil binding to opiate receptors in humans measured by positron emission tomography. J Cereb Blood Flow Metab 1989;9(3):398–409.

24. Melichar JK, Nutt DJ, Malizia AL. Naloxone displacement at opioid receptor sites measured in vivo in the human brain. Eur J Pharmacol 2003;459(2–3):217–9.
25. Pilapil C, Welner S, Magnan J, et al. Autoradiographic distribution of multiple classes of opioid receptor binding sites in human forebrain. Brain Res Bull 1987;19(5):611–5.
26. Peckys D, Landwehrmeyer GB. Expression of mu, kappa, and delta opioid receptor messenger RNA in the human CNS: a 33P in situ hybridization study. Neuroscience 1999;88(4):1093–135.
27. Filliol D, Ghozland S, Chluba J, et al. Mice deficient for delta- and mu-opioid receptors exhibit opposing alterations of emotional responses. Nat Genet 2000; 25(2):195–200.
28. Soubrié P, Jobert A, Thiebot MH. Differential effects on naloxone against the diazepam-induced release of behavior in rats in three aversive situations. Psychopharmacology (Berl) 1980;69(1):101–5.
29. Duka T, Millan MJ, Ulsamer B, et al. Naloxone attenuates the anxiolytic action of diazepam in man. Life Sci 1982;31(16–17):1833–6.
30. Singh VP, Patil CS, Jain NK, et al. Paradoxical effects of opioid antagonist naloxone on SSRI-induced analgesia and tolerance in mice. Pharmacology 2003;69(3):115–22.
31. Aston-Jones G, Harris GC. Brain substrates for increased drug seeking during protracted withdrawal. Neuropharmacology 2004;47(Suppl 1):167–79.
32. Peciña S, Berridge KC. Hedonic hot spot in nucleus accumbens shell: where do mu-opioids cause increased hedonic impact of sweetness? J Neurosci 2005; 25(50):11777–86.
33. Massaly N, Copits BA, Wilson-Poe AR, et al. Pain-Induced Negative Affect Is Mediated via Recruitment of The Nucleus Accumbens Kappa Opioid System. Neuron 2019;102(3):564–73.e6.
34. Kennedy SE, Koeppe RA, Young EA, et al. Dysregulation of endogenous opioid emotion regulation circuitry in major depression in women. Arch Gen Psychiatry 2006;63(11):1199–208.
35. Scherrer JF, Svrakic DM, Freedland KE, et al. Prescription opioid analgesics increase the risk of depression. J Gen Intern Med 2014;29(3):491–9.
36. Scherrer JF, Salas J, Lustman PJ, et al. Change in opioid dose and change in depression in a longitudinal primary care patient cohort. Pain 2015;156(2): 348–55.
37. Huffman KL, Sweis GW, Gase A, et al. Opioid use 12 months following interdisciplinary pain rehabilitation with weaning. Pain Med 2013;14(12):1908–17.
38. Juurlink DN, Dhalla IA. Dependence and addiction during chronic opioid therapy. J Med Toxicol 2012;8(4):393–9.
39. Prasad R, Coleman S. The Stanford Opioid Management Model. Pract Pain Manag 2014;14(5).
40. Colloca L, Enck P, DeGrazia D. Relieving pain using dose-extending placebos: a scoping review. Pain 2016;157(8):1590–8.
41. Amanzio M, Benedetti F. Neuropharmacological dissection of placebo analgesia: expectation-activated opioid systems versus conditioning-activated specific subsystems. J Neurosci 1999;19(1):484–94.
42. Wager TD, Scott DJ, Zubieta JK. Placebo effects on human mu-opioid activity during pain. Proc Natl Acad Sci U S A 2007;104(26):11056–61.
43. Guo JY, Wang JY, Luo F. Dissection of placebo analgesia in mice: the conditions for activation of opioid and non-opioid systems. J Psychopharmacol 2010;24(10): 1561–7.

44. Nolan TA, Price DD, Caudle RM, et al. Placebo-induced analgesia in an operant pain model in rats. Pain 2012;153(10):2009–16.
45. Colagiuri B, Schenk LA, Kessler MD, et al. The placebo effect: From concepts to genes. Neuroscience 2015;307:171–90.
46. Zhang RR, Zhang WC, Wang JY, et al. The opioid placebo analgesia is mediated exclusively through μ-opioid receptor in rat. Int J Neuropsychopharmacol 2013;16(4):849–56.
47. Benedetti F, Pollo A, Colloca L. Opioid-mediated placebo responses boost pain endurance and physical performance: is it doping in sport competitions? J Neurosci 2007;27(44):11934–9.
48. Kaptchuk TJ, Friedlander E, Kelley JM, et al. Placebos without deception: a randomized controlled trial in irritable bowel syndrome. PLoS One 2010;5(12):e15591.
49. Carvalho C, Caetano JM, Cunha L, et al. Open-label placebo treatment in chronic low back pain: a randomized controlled trial. Pain 2016;157(12):2766–72 [published correction appears in Pain. 2017 Feb;158(2):365].
50. Morales-Quezada L, Mesia-Toledo I, Estudillo-Guerra A, et al. Conditioning open-label placebo: a pilot pharmacobehavioral approach for opioid dose reduction and pain control. Pain Rep 2020;5(4):e828.
51. Sandler AD, Bodfish JW. Open-label use of placebos in the treatment of ADHD: a pilot study. Child Care Health Dev 2008;34(1):104–10.
52. Ader R, Mercurio MG, Walton J, et al. Conditioned pharmacotherapeutic effects: a preliminary study. Psychosom Med 2010;72(2):192–7.
53. Perlis M, Grandner M, Zee J, et al. Durability of treatment response to zolpidem with three different maintenance regimens: a preliminary study. Sleep Med 2015;16(9):1160–8.
54. Goebel MU, Meykadeh N, Kou W, et al. Behavioral conditioning of antihistamine effects in patients with allergic rhinitis. Psychother Psychosom 2008;77(4):227–34.
55. Kirchhof J, Petrakova L, Brinkhoff A, et al. Learned immunosuppressive placebo responses in renal transplant patients. Proc Natl Acad Sci U S A 2018;115(16):4223–7.
56. Kraft GH. Treatment strategies of operant conditioning in rehabilitation. The prevention and management of disability due to chronic pain following industrial injuries. J Occup Med 1975;17(10):658–62.
57. Colloca L, Kisaalita NR, Bizien M, et al. Veteran engagement in opioid tapering research: a mission to optimize pain management. Pain Rep 2021;6(2):e932.

Transitional Pain Medicine; New Era, New Opportunities, and New Journey

Abdullah Sulieman Terkawi, MD, MS(Epi)*, Einar Ottestad, MD[1], Omar Khalid Altirkawi, MD[2], Vafi Salmasi, MD, MS(Epi)[3]

KEYWORDS

• Transitional pain • Chronic • Persistent • Postsurgical pain

KEY POINTS

- Chronic postsurgical pain (CPSP) is pain that develops or increases in intensity after a surgical procedure and lasts more than 3 months.
- Transitional pain medicine is the medical field that focuses on understanding the mechanisms of CPSP and finding out risk factors and preventive treatments.
- Lessening the incidence, and maybe the severity, of CPSP can be potentially achieved by implementing multidisciplinary perioperative service (ie, transitional pain service).

The International Association for Study of Pain defines chronic postsurgical pain (CPSP) as the following: "chronic pain that develops or increases in intensity after a surgical procedure."[1] CPSP is also known as persistent postsurgical pain (PPSP). CPSP refers to persistent pain that continues more than 3 months after surgery and excludes other causes of pain (eg, infection, malignancy, preexisting pain, and so forth).[2] We want to extrapolate from the aforementioned definitions to introduce a new terminology: "transitional pain medicine," which is the medical field that focuses on understanding the mechanisms of CPSP and elucidating the risk factors and preventive and treatment measures.

INCIDENCE OF CHRONIC POSTSURGICAL PAIN

We searched PubMed using the following search strategies: (("Pain, Postoperative"[-Mesh]) AND "Chronic Pain"[Mesh]) AND "Incidence"[Mesh]. We did not restrict our

Department of Anesthesiology, Perioperative and Pain Medicine, Stanford University School of Medicine, Palo Alto, CA, USA
[1] Present address: 127 Elliott Drive, Menlo Park, CA 94025.
[2] Present address: 280 West California Avenue, Apartment 107, Sunnyvale, CA 94086.
[3] Present address: 1070 Arastradero Road Suite 200, Palo Alto, CA 94304.
* Corresponding author. 1070 Arastradero Road Suite 200, Palo Alto, CA 94304.
E-mail address: aterkawi@stanford.edu

Anesthesiology Clin 41 (2023) 383–394
https://doi.org/10.1016/j.anclin.2023.03.007
anesthesiology.theclinics.com
1932-2275/23/

search to time or language. We also searched the references that were used on the selected studies. We identified 93 relevant references. We also searched the references that were used on the selected studies. **Fig. 1** summarizes the incidence of CPSP after different surgeries. The highest incidence (>20%) of CPSP is reported after thoracic, breast, inguinal hernia, lumbar spine, and hip/knee arthroplasty surgery.[3,4] It is important to highlight that overall, this is a poorly studied area, and further research is recommended.

MECHANISMS AND CHARACTERISTICS

The transition from acute to chronic pain is complex; inflammatory and immune response to nerve and tissue damage can result in both peripheral (at the level of injury; peripheral nervous system) and central (spinal cord and brain) sensitization.[2–4,35,36]

CPSP can occur secondary to perioperative nerve or muscle injury. These injuries are not always due to direct trauma (eg, nerve cut or electrocautery), but they can occur secondary to ischemic injury from prolonged retraction, use of a tourniquet, or tight belt as well as entrapment from developing scar tissue. The mechanism and the degree of injury may determine the severity and duration of the pain. After the initial injury, peripheral and central sensitization may develop, which can cause CPSP (**Table 1**).[2–4,35–37] As such, we appreciate the importance of applying "preventive analgesia" to avoid such sensitizations and subsequently CPSP.

Another important theory for transitioning from acute to chronic pain is "conditional pain modulation." Normally, we live in a balanced state between the pronociceptive and antinociceptive systems. Surgical injury activates the pronociceptive systems, which our body soon counteracts with the antinociceptive system. The imbalance between these 2 systems (ie, stronger pronociceptive) can lead to persistent postsurgical pain. This imbalance can happen secondary to defects in the recruitment of antinociceptive systems (eg, the pain is so severe and so prolonged that the endogenous system is exhausted) or latent pain sensitization. The latter typically happens in patients with chronic pain and opioid users who develop an imbalance between the 2 systems (eg, hyperalgesia). Therefore, surgical pain can quickly exhaust the antinociceptive systems.[4] Understanding the aforementioned theory will help explain why "preventive analgesia" is a critical factor in preventing CPSP. In order to optimize preventive analgesia, the following needs to be satisfied: the depth of analgesia must be adequate to block all nociceptive input during surgery; the analgesic technique must cover the entire surgical field; and the duration of analgesia must cover the entire perioperative period.

Clinical presentation of central and peripheral sensitization is similar to other neuropathic pain conditions. It includes hyperalgesia, allodynia, dysesthesia, and other conditions.[37] Incidence of chronic neuropathic pain varies widely based on procedure-specific aspects of surgery (eg, injury to intercostal nerves during thoracotomy or brachial plexus during mastectomy). Neuropathic CPSP results in higher rate of disability and higher pain intensity with reduced quality of life.[1,2,38]

RISK FACTORS

Early identification of patients with risk factors enables us to implement preventive measures and thus decrease the incidence of CPSP. These risk factors are related to the surgical procedure or patient characteristics and condition.

We searched PubMed using the following search strategies: ((("Pain, Postoperative"[Mesh]) AND "Chronic Pain"[Mesh])) AND "Risk Factors"[Mesh]. We also searched the references that were used on the selected studies. We did not restrict our search

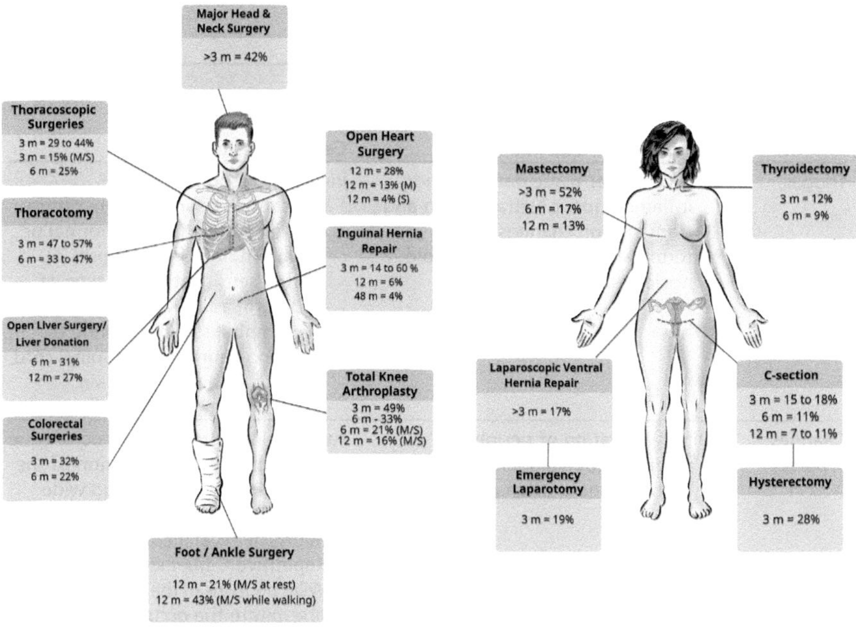

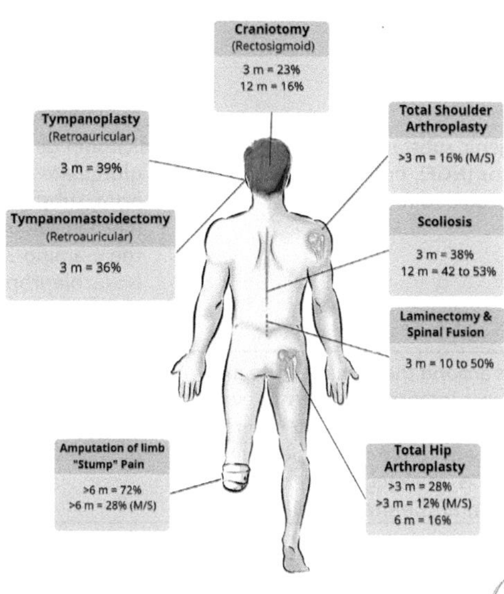

Fig. 1. Summary of the incidence of CPSP after different surgeries, based on our search findings. References: Thoracoscopic surgery[5,6]; Thoracotomy[5,7]; Colorectal surgery[8]; C-section[9,10]; Thyroidectomy[11]; Tympanoplasty (retroauricular incision)[12]; Tympanomastoidectomy (retroauricular incision)[12]; Inguinal hernia repair[13,14]; Breast surgery[15,16]; Open liver surgery—liver donation[17]; Foot/Ankle surgery[18]; Laparoscopic ventral hernia repair[19]; Scoliosis surgery[20,21]; Laminectomy and spinal fusion[22]; Major head and neck surgery[23]; Total knee arthroplasty (TKA)[24–26]; Total hip arthroplasty (THA)[27,28]; Total shoulder arthroplasty (TSA)[29]; Emergency Laparotomy[30]; Hysterectomy[31]; Open heart surgery[32]; Craniotomy (retrosigmoid approach)[33]; Amputation of limb "stump" pain.[34] Unless indicated the incidence for any severity of pain. m, months; M, moderate; S, severe.

Table 1
Peripheral and central sensitization

	Peripheral Sensitization	Central Sensitization
Trigger	It occurs after tissue damage and inflammation; posttranslation and transcription changes in the terminal ends of high-threshold nociceptors	Increased responsiveness of nociceptive neurons in the central nervous system to their normal or subthreshold afferent input. Central sensitization is a type of long-term adaptive neuroplasticity that amplifies pain signaling by affecting neurons in the spinal cord, resulting in a form of "pain memory."
Changes places	Direct activation of peripheral receptors (polymodal C fibers and high-threshold mechanoreceptors)	At the spinal cord and CNS; occurs due to windup and sensitization of the second-order neurons and wide dynamic ranges (WDR) through neurochemical mediators. Repetitive C-fiber stimulation of WDR neurons in the dorsal horn can precipitate the occurrence of windup and central sensitization. Long lasting effects (and maintenance of central sensitization) can be due to alterations in microglia, astrocytes, gap junctions, membrane excitability, and gene transcription.
Chemical mediators	Algogenic substances: nerve growth factor (NGF), bradykinin, prostaglandin, substance P	Calcitonin gene–related peptide, glutamate release from the dorsal horn, substance P, and NMDA mechanisms increased expression of the α-amino-3-hydroxy-5-methyl-4-isoxazolepropionic acid (AMPA) receptor and brain-derived neurotrophic factor (BDNF) release.
Lead to	Events around the damaged site allow a lower intensity stimulus to evoke an action potential in the fibers. This leads to *primary hyperalgesia*, which is an exaggerated response to pain at the site of injury	Allodynia and *secondary hyperalgesia*, which is an increased pain response evoked by stimuli outside the area of injury
Example	Hyperalgesia at the site of the injury	Complex regional pain syndrome (CRPS)

to time or language. We found 175 relevant references. We also searched the references that were used on the selected studies. **Fig. 2** summarizes risk factors for developing CPSP. Many of these factors can be potentially better controlled to prevent CPSP or reduce its severity.

Surgery-Related Risk Factors

CPSP incidence varies widely by type of surgery: anatomic location, extent of surgical trauma, and type of tissue injured. Surgical complications also increase the risk of CSPS including reoperation, infection, and so forth.[1–4]

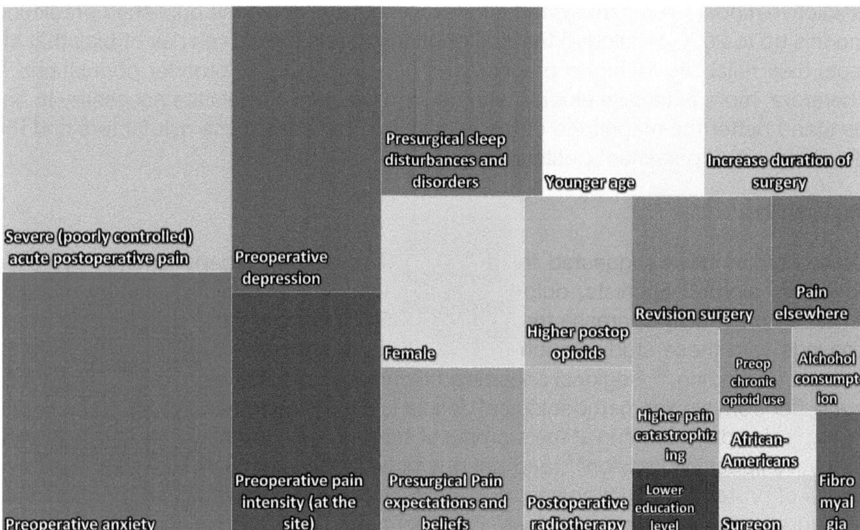

Fig. 2. Summary of the most important risk factors for chronic postsurgical pain. The square size correlate with the number of times we found this specific risk factor in our systematic search. This may be a good indicator of how much this factor is important, but unless they are all compared in one large study this cannot be taken as a proof.[6,8,9,15,17,18,20,21,23–25,30,31,39–45]

Higher intensity of acute pain after surgery seems to be one of the most important risk factors for CPSP and prolonged opioid use. Duration of severe pain and trajectory of pain are also important in predicting incidence of CPSP.[46–50] Higher intensity of neuropathic-like or visceral pain (more than incisional pain) is also predictive of higher risk of CSPS.[47,51–53]

Patient-Related Risk Factors

Preexisting chronic pain, more specifically at the surgical site, predicts higher incidence of CPSP. Preoperative opioid use is also associated with higher risk of CPSP and prolonged postoperative opioid use.[3,47,54] Other chronic pain conditions (eg, fibromyalgia, migraine, low back pain, and other conditions) also increase the risk of CPSP.[3,47]

Psychological comorbidities are associated with increased prevalence of CPSP and prolonged postoperative opioid use. Anxiety is highlighted as the main psychosocial risk factor, whereas catastrophizing, reduced ability to cope with pain, depression, hypervigilance, and other psychosocial distress also increase the risk of CPSP.[3,4,36,47,55]

Other patient-related risk factors include younger (adult) age, female sex, high body mass index, lower level of education, and socioeconomic status.[3,4,47,56] Some studies suggested polymorphism at certain genes (eg, catechol-O-methyltransferase, melanocortin-1 receptor, and so forth) can increase the risk of CPSP but the predictive value is poor.[3,4,47]

PREDICTION

The risk factors mentioned earlier may be used to predict which patient will develop CPSP and therefore selectively apply transitional pain services. Many risk factors can be treated or controlled before surgery. Multiple attempts were done to build predictive models. A recent systematic review that evaluated the published prediction models up to 2020 concluded that the existing models are at high risk of bias that affects their reliability to inform practice and generalizability to broader populations.[57] Therefore, more extensive studies with better prediction models are necessary to understand better the magnitude of the relationship between these risk factors and the development of persistent postsurgical pain.

PREVENTION

Some studies have suggested that the use of ketamine, gabapentinoids, systemic lidocaine, alpha-2 agonists, duloxetine, and nonsteroidal antiinflammatory medications can potentially decrease the chance of CPSP; however, there are certain shortcomings with these studies such as small sample size, lack of appropriate control groups, or blinding.[58] Regional anesthesia techniques provide more promising results but suffer from similar methodological deficiencies.[58,59] Perioperative oral pregabalin, 75 mg, twice daily, starting at the morning of surgery and continuing for 1 week[60]; perioperative lidocaine infusion[61]; and perioperative ketamine infusion,[62] all showed evidence of protective effect against postmastectomy pain. However, the optimal dose and duration is yet to be determined. Behavioral therapy has been shown to decrease postoperative opioid use, but its effect on developing CPSP is yet to be studied.[63,64] Preoperative opioid use increases the incidence of persistent postoperative pain[55,65]; decreasing opioids preoperatively can improve outcomes 6 to 12 months after surgery.[48] Reducing perioperative use of opioids by application of multimodal and regional techniques could potentially reduce the risk of CPSP.[37] Keeping in mind the "preventive analgesia" concept we discussed earlier is a key success with any analgesic modality someone must choose. This concept is further supported by the fact that most of the positive studies used longer duration treatment than negative studies.

Postoperative Opioid Use

When patients complain about persistent postoperative pain after discharge, providers often represcribe opioids to address this in the acute postoperative setting. Represcribing opioids is usually done without a long-term plan or sometimes even appropriate risk stratification and follow-up.[66–70] One study showed that patients who received a second prescription of opioids within the first postoperative week had almost 50% increased chance of still taking an opioid medication 1 year after surgery.[67]

Considering these risks and the potential for poor outcomes of chronic opioid use, it is important to appropriately manage persistent pain in this patient population instead of relying solely on opioids. In addition to following-up with surgeons and primary care physicians, a pain specialist needs to be involved in addressing pain better and developing a plan to appropriately wean off opioid medications.[66,71–73]

ROLE OF TRANSITIONAL PAIN SERVICE

A transitional pain service is a multidisciplinary team of specialists established to optimize pain control, monitor, appropriately wean off opioids, prevent unnecessary readmissions, and reduce the incidence of disabilities resulting from CPSP. The role of a transitional pain service starts preoperatively by identifying patients at high risk of CPSP. These patients can be optimized by decreasing opioid medications, delivering appropriate education, applying behavioral therapy to decrease anxiety around the event of surgery, and setting appropriate expectations. Transitional pain service

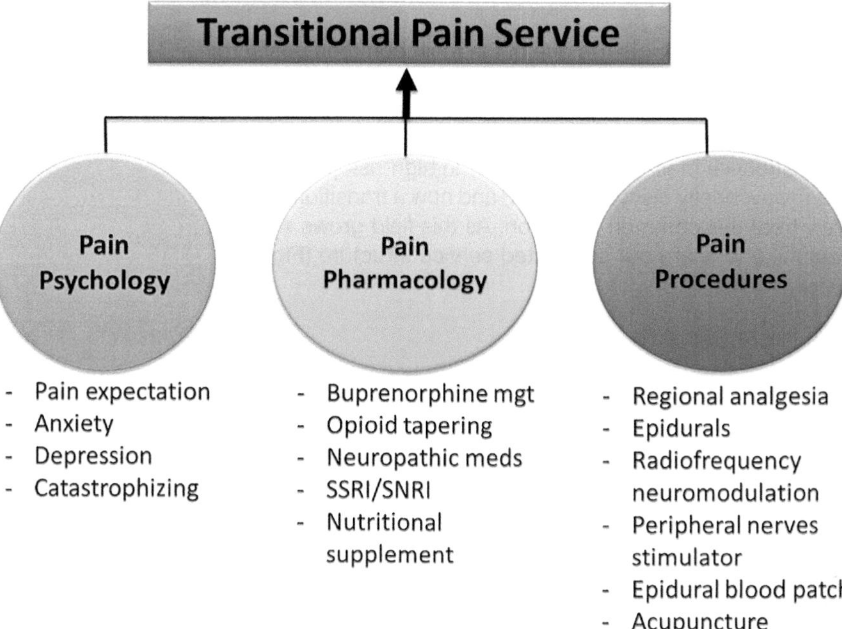

Fig. 3. Suggested multidisciplinary transitional pain service. Each discipline can potentially deliver the services listed later. This model is built with intention to cover all the risk factors and use intervention that has been proved to reduce the incidence and severity of chronic postsurgical pain. SNRI, serotonin and norepinephrine reuptake inhibitors; SSRI, selective serotonin reuptake inhibitors.

continues to work with these patients to optimize perioperative pain control by use of appropriate multimodal and regional techniques and managing opioid medications. The postoperative pain management strategy should always include a plan to wean opioids after achieving appropriate pain control. Improving coping and functioning is a key aspect of this phase. Based on these goals, an efficient transitional pain service includes pain specialists, pain psychologists, and physical/occupational therapists.

Box 1
To help building this field, we recommend adopting those goals for any study

Fundamental outcome measures (goals) for the transitional pain service (TPS):

Primary:

- Incidence of persistant postsurgical pain (PPSP) at 3 months[a]
- Incidence of persistant postsurgical opioid use (PPSO) at 3 months[a]

Secondary

- Length of hospital stay
- Emergency room visits/admissions for uncontrolled pain
- Functional outcomes[b]

This will help standardizing the data for future comparisons.[a]Three months will satisfy the definition of chronic postsurgical pain; however, for secondary outcomes someone may add 6 and 12 months.[b]Functional outcomes is important, and we recommend using validated tools to measure them (eg, the NIH PROMIS questionnaires).

FUTURE DIRECTIONS

Postsurgical pain (CPSP) is one of the most common postsurgical complications with mean incidence of 20% to 30% (ranging from 5% to 85% in different types of surgery).[1,46] Incorrect treatment with opioids without proper follow-up is common.[74] Chronic pain is a costly disease costing the economy more than $600 billion yearly, and ineffective management of CPSP in high-risk patients exacerbates the problem. This review briefly discusses CPSP and how a transitional pain service can more effectively treat this common condition. As this field grows and becomes established, we would like to share our suggested service structure (**Fig. 3**) and intended outcomes measure (**Box 1**).

CLINICS CARE POINTS

- Chronic postsurgical pain (CPSP) is more common than previously expected and ranges between 10% and 50% depending on the type of surgery.
- CPSP can occur secondary to perioperative nerve or muscle injury. These injuries are not always due to direct trauma (eg, nerve cut or electrocautery), but they can occur secondary to ischemic injury from prolonged retraction, use of tourniquet, or tight belt as well as entrapment from developing scar tissue.
- Depending on the underlying cause, these pain syndromes tend to improve with time.
- Unfortunately, one great challenge is that these patients commonly end up opioid dependent.
- Multiple risk factors have been discovered, with the most common, and modifiable, being uncontrolled acute postoperative pain; preoperative anxiety and depression; and preoperative site pain, chronic pain, and opioid use.

DISCLOSURE

A.S. Terkawi: none. E. Ottestad: Consultant for BioVentus, Nalu, SPR Therapeutics, Coloplast, Invicta (equity), Abbott, and Medtronic. Grants and research support from Bioness. O.K. Altirkawi: none. V. Salmasi: Consultant for AppliedVR. Funding from NINDS, United States as K23 (1K23NS120039–01A1).

REFERENCES

1. Schug SA, Lavand'homme P, Barke A, et al. The iasp classification of chronic pain for icd-11: Chronic postsurgical or posttraumatic pain. Pain 2019;160:45–52.
2. Rosenberger DC, Pogatzki-Zahn EM. Chronic postsurgical pain - update on incidence, risk factors and preventive treatment options. BJA Educ 2022;22:190–6.
3. Glare P, Aubrey KR, Myles PS. Transition from acute to chronic pain after surgery. Lancet 2019;393:1537–46.
4. Richebé P, Capdevila X, Rivat C. Persistent postsurgical pain: Pathophysiology and preventative pharmacologic considerations. Anesthesiology 2018;129:590–607.
5. Bayman EO, Parekh KR, Keech J, et al. A prospective study of chronic pain after thoracic surgery. Anesthesiology 2017;126:938–51.
6. Zhang Y, Zhou R, Hou B, et al. Incidence and risk factors for chronic postsurgical pain following video-assisted thoracoscopic surgery: A retrospective study. BMC Surg 2022;22:76.

7. Bayman EO, Brennan TJ. Incidence and severity of chronic pain at 3 and 6 months after thoracotomy: Meta-analysis. J Pain 2014;15:887–97.
8. Jin J, Chen Q, Min S, et al. Prevalence and predictors of chronic postsurgical pain after colorectal surgery: A prospective study. Colorectal Dis 2021;23: 1878–89.
9. Jin J, Peng L, Chen Q, et al. Prevalence and risk factors for chronic pain following cesarean section: A prospective study. BMC Anesthesiol 2016;16:99.
10. Weibel S, Neubert K, Jelting Y, et al. Incidence and severity of chronic pain after caesarean section: A systematic review with meta-analysis. Eur J Anaesthesiol 2016;33:853–65.
11. Wattier JM, Caïazzo R, Andrieu G, et al. Chronic post-thyroidectomy pain: Incidence, typology, and risk factors. Anaesth Crit Care Pain Med 2016;35:197–201.
12. Güven M, Kara A, Yilmaz MS, et al. Comparison of incidence and severity of chronic postsurgical pain following ear surgery. J Craniofac Surg 2018;29: e552–5.
13. Bande D, Moltó L, Pereira JA, et al. Chronic pain after groin hernia repair: Pain characteristics and impact on quality of life. BMC Surg 2020;20:147.
14. Takata H, Matsutani T, Hagiwara N, et al. Assessment of the incidence of chronic pain and discomfort after primary inguinal hernia repair. J Surg Res 2016;206: 391–7.
15. Berger JM, Longhitano Y, Zanza C, et al. Factors affecting the incidence of chronic pain following breast cancer surgery: Preoperative history, anesthetic management, and surgical technique. J Surg Oncol 2020;122:1307–14.
16. Schreiber KL, Zinboonyahgoon N, Flowers KM, et al. Prediction of persistent pain severity and impact 12 months after breast surgery using comprehensive preoperative assessment of biopsychosocial pain modulators. Ann Surg Oncol 2021; 28:5015–38.
17. Holtzman S, Clarke HA, McCluskey SA, et al. Acute and chronic postsurgical pain after living liver donation: Incidence and predictors. Liver Transpl 2014;20: 1336–46.
18. Remérand F, Godfroid HB, Brilhault J, et al. Chronic pain 1 year after foot surgery: Epidemiology and associated factors. Orthop Traumatol Surg Res 2014;100: 767–73.
19. Liang MK, Clapp M, Li LT, et al. Patient satisfaction, chronic pain, and functional status following laparoscopic ventral hernia repair. World J Surg 2013;37:530–7.
20. Chidambaran V, Ding L, Moore DL, et al. Predicting the pain continuum after adolescent idiopathic scoliosis surgery: A prospective cohort study. Eur J Pain 2017;21:1252–65.
21. Julien-Marsollier F, David R, Hilly J, et al. Predictors of chronic neuropathic pain after scoliosis surgery in children. Scand J Pain 2017;17:339–44.
22. Derbent A, Yilmaz B, Uyar M. [chronic pain following spine surgery]. Agri 2012; 24:1–8.
23. Terkawi AS, Tsang S, Alshehri AS, et al. The burden of chronic pain after major head and neck tumor therapy. Saudi J Anaesth 2017;11:S71–9.
24. Gungor S, Fields K, Aiyer R, et al. Incidence and risk factors for development of persistent postsurgical pain following total knee arthroplasty: A retrospective cohort study. Medicine (Baltim) 2019;98:e16450.
25. Rice DA, Kluger MT, McNair PJ, et al. Persistent postoperative pain after total knee arthroplasty: A prospective cohort study of potential risk factors. Br J Anaesth 2018;121:804–12.

26. Sugiyama Y, Iida H, Amaya F, et al. Prevalence of chronic postsurgical pain after thoracotomy and total knee arthroplasty: A retrospective multicenter study in japan (japanese study group of subacute postoperative pain). J Anesth 2018; 32:434–8.
27. Nikolajsen L, Brandsborg B, Lucht U, et al. Chronic pain following total hip arthroplasty: A nationwide questionnaire study. Acta Anaesthesiol Scand 2006;50: 495–500.
28. Pagé MG, Katz J, Curtis K, et al. Acute pain trajectories and the persistence of postsurgical pain: A longitudinal study after total hip arthroplasty. J Anesth 2016;30:568–77.
29. Best MJ, Harris AB, Bansal A, et al. Predictors of long-term opioid use after elective primary total shoulder arthroplasty. Orthopedics 2021;44:58–63.
30. Tolstrup MB, Thorup T, Gögenur I. Chronic pain, quality of life and functional impairment after emergency laparotomy. World J Surg 2019;43:161–8.
31. Han C, Ge Z, Jiang W, et al. Incidence and risk factors of chronic pain following hysterectomy among southern jiangsu chinese women. BMC Anesthesiol 2017; 17:103.
32. Meyerson J, Thelin S, Gordh T, et al. The incidence of chronic post-sternotomy pain after cardiac surgery–a prospective study. Acta Anaesthesiol Scand 2001; 45:940–4.
33. Harner SG, Beatty CW, Ebersold MJ. Headache after acoustic neuroma excision. Am J Otol 1993;14:552–5.
34. Ehde DM, Czerniecki JM, Smith DG, et al. Chronic phantom sensations, phantom pain, residual limb pain, and other regional pain after lower limb amputation. Arch Phys Med Rehabil 2000;81:1039–44.
35. Pogatzki-Zahn E, Segelcke D, Zahn P. Mechanisms of acute and chronic pain after surgery: Update from findings in experimental animal models. Curr Opin Anaesthesiol 2018;31:575–85.
36. Chapman CR, Vierck CJ. The transition of acute postoperative pain to chronic pain: An integrative overview of research on mechanisms. J Pain 2017;18: 359.e1–38.
37. Pogatzki-Zahn EM, Segelcke D, Schug SA. Postoperative pain-from mechanisms to treatment. Pain Rep 2017;2:e588.
38. Haroutiunian S, Nikolajsen L, Finnerup NB, et al. The neuropathic component in persistent postsurgical pain: A systematic literature review. Pain 2013;154: 95–102.
39. Wang Y, Liu Z, Chen S, et al. Pre-surgery beliefs about pain and surgery as predictors of acute and chronic postsurgical pain: A prospective cohort study. Int J Surg 2018;52:50–5.
40. Habib AS, Kertai MD, Cooter M, et al. Risk factors for severe acute pain and persistent pain after surgery for breast cancer: A prospective observational study. Reg Anesth Pain Med 2019;44:192–9.
41. Hruschak V, Cochran G. Psychosocial predictors in the transition from acute to chronic pain: A systematic review. Psychol Health Med 2018;23:1151–67.
42. Skrejborg P, Petersen KK, Kold S, et al. Presurgical comorbidities as risk factors for chronic postsurgical pain following total knee replacement. Clin J Pain 2019; 35:577–82.
43. Varallo G, Giusti EM, Manna C, et al. Sleep disturbances and sleep disorders as risk factors for chronic postsurgical pain: A systematic review and meta-analysis. Sleep Med Rev 2022;63:101630.

44. Willingham MD, Vila MR, Ben Abdallah A, et al. Factors contributing to lingering pain after surgery: The role of patient expectations. Anesthesiology 2021;134: 915–24.
45. Yoon S, Hong WP, Joo H, et al. Long-term incidence of chronic postsurgical pain after thoracic surgery for lung cancer: A 10-year single-center retrospective study. Reg Anesth Pain Med 2020;45:331–6.
46. Fletcher D, Stamer UM, Pogatzki-Zahn E, et al. Chronic postsurgical pain in europe: An observational study. Eur J Anaesthesiol 2015;32:725–34.
47. Lavand'homme P. Transition from acute to chronic pain after surgery. Pain 2017; 158(Suppl 1):S50–4.
48. Steyaert A, Lavand'homme P. Prevention and treatment of chronic postsurgical pain: A narrative review. Drugs 2018;78:339–54.
49. Lavand'homme PM, Grosu I, France MN, et al. Pain trajectories identify patients at risk of persistent pain after knee arthroplasty: An observational study. Clin Orthop Relat Res 2014;472:1409–15.
50. Hah JM, Cramer E, Hilmoe H, et al. Factors associated with acute pain estimation, postoperative pain resolution, opioid cessation, and recovery: Secondary analysis of a randomized clinical trial. JAMA Netw Open 2019;2:e190168.
51. Martinez V, Ammar SB, Judet T, et al. Risk factors predictive of chronic postsurgical neuropathic pain: The value of the iliac crest bone harvest model. Pain 2012;153:1478–83.
52. Beloeil H, Sion B, Rousseau C, et al. Early postoperative neuropathic pain assessed by the dn4 score predicts an increased risk of persistent postsurgical neuropathic pain. Eur J Anaesthesiol 2017;34:652–7.
53. Blichfeldt-Eckhardt MR, Ording H, Andersen C, et al. Early visceral pain predicts chronic pain after laparoscopic cholecystectomy. Pain 2014;155:2400–7.
54. Hah JM, Sharifzadeh Y, Wang BM, et al. Factors associated with opioid use in a cohort of patients presenting for surgery. Pain Res Treat 2015;2015:829696.
55. Pagé MG, Kudrina I, Zomahoun HTV, et al. A systematic review of the relative frequency and risk factors for prolonged opioid prescription following surgery and trauma among adults. Ann Surg 2020;271:845–54.
56. Schnabel A, Yahiaoui-Doktor M, Meissner W, et al. Predicting poor postoperative acute pain outcome in adults: An international, multicentre database analysis of risk factors in 50,005 patients. Pain Rep 2020;5:e831.
57. Papadomanolakis-Pakis N, Uhrbrand P, Haroutounian S, et al. Prognostic prediction models for chronic postsurgical pain in adults: A systematic review. Pain 2021;162:2644–57.
58. Carley ME, Chaparro LE, Choiniere M, et al. Pharmacotherapy for the prevention of chronic pain after surgery in adults: An updated systematic review and meta-analysis. Anesthesiology 2021;135:304–25.
59. Weinstein EJ, Levene JL, Cohen MS, et al. Local anaesthetics and regional anaesthesia versus conventional analgesia for preventing persistent postoperative pain in adults and children. Cochrane Database Syst Rev 2018;4:CD007105.
60. Reyad RM, Omran AF, Abbas DN, et al. The possible preventive role of pregabalin in postmastectomy pain syndrome: A double-blinded randomized controlled trial. J Pain Symptom Manage 2019;57:1–9.
61. Terkawi AS, Sharma S, Durieux ME, et al. Perioperative lidocaine infusion reduces the incidence of post-mastectomy chronic pain: A double-blind, placebo-controlled randomized trial. Pain Physician 2015;18:E139–46.

62. Kang C, Cho AR, Kim KH, et al. Effects of intraoperative low-dose ketamine on persistent postsurgical pain after breast cancer surgery: A prospective, randomized, controlled, double-blind study. Pain Physician 2020;23:37–47.
63. Darnall BD, Ziadni MS, Krishnamurthy P, et al. My surgical success": Effect of a digital behavioral pain medicine intervention on time to opioid cessation after breast cancer surgery-a pilot randomized controlled clinical trial. Pain Med 2019;20:2228–37.
64.. Ziadni MS, You DS, Keane R, et al. My surgical success": Feasibility and impact of a single-session digital behavioral pain medicine intervention on pain intensity, pain catastrophizing, and time to opioid cessation after orthopedic trauma surgery-a randomized trial. Anesth Analg 2022;135(2):394–405.
65. Brown CR, Chen Z, Khurshan F, et al. Development of persistent opioid use after cardiac surgery. JAMA Cardiol 2020;5:889–96.
66. Mikhaeil J, Ayoo K, Clarke H, et al. Review of the transitional pain service as a method of postoperative opioid weaning and a service aimed at minimizing the risk of chronic postsurgical pain. Anaesthesiol Intensive Ther 2020;52:148–53.
67. Alam A, Gomes T, Zheng H, et al. Long-term analgesic use after low-risk surgery: A retrospective cohort study. Arch Intern Med 2012;172:425–30.
68. Gomes T, Redelmeier DA, Juurlink DN, et al. Opioid dose and risk of road trauma in canada: A population-based study. JAMA Intern Med 2013;173:196–201.
69. Dhalla IA, Mamdani MM, Sivilotti ML, et al. Prescribing of opioid analgesics and related mortality before and after the introduction of long-acting oxycodone. CMAJ (Can Med Assoc J) 2009;181:891–6.
70. Lugoboni F, Mirijello A, Zamboni L, et al. High prevalence of constipation and reduced quality of life in opioid-dependent patients treated with opioid substitution treatments. Expert Opin Pharmacother 2016;17:2135–41.
71. Katz J, Weinrib AZ, Clarke H, et al. Chronic postsurgical pain: From risk factor identification to multidisciplinary management at the toronto general hospital transitional pain service a systematic review of the relative frequency and risk factors for prolonged opioid prescription following surgery and trauma among adults. Can J Pain 2019;3:49–58.
72. Gomes T, Mamdani MM, Dhalla IA, et al. The burden of premature opioid-related mortality. Addiction 2014;109:1482–8.
73. Jones MR, Viswanath O, Peck J, et al. A brief history of the opioid epidemic and strategies for pain medicine. Pain Ther 2018;7:13–21.
74. Bicket MC, Long JJ, Pronovost PJ, et al. Prescription opioid analgesics commonly unused after surgery: A systematic review. JAMA Surg 2017;152:1066–71.

Review of Ultrasound-Guided Procedures in the Management of Chronic Pain

Anuj K. Aggarwal, MD[a,1], Einar Ottestad, MD[a,2], Kayla E. Pfaff, BA[a,2], Alice Huai-Yu Li, MD[a,3], Lei Xu, MD[a,3], Ryan Derby, MD[a,2], Daniel Hecht, MD[a,2], Jennifer Hah, MD, MS[a,4], Scott Pritzlaff, MD[b,5], Nitin Prabhakar, MD[c,2], Elliot Krane, MD, FAAP[a,6], Genevieve D'Souza, MD, FASA[a,6], Yasmine Hoydonckx, MD, MSc[d,7,*]

KEYWORDS

- Ultrasound guidance • Peripheral nerve • Nerve block
- Pulsed radiofrequency ablation • Fascial plane • Chronic pain

KEY POINTS

- The use of ultrasound in chronic pain treatment has gained popularity and applicability in the past decade.
- This review synthetizes the available evidence for ultrasound-guided nerve and plane blocks for chronic pain management.

Continued

INTRODUCTION

There has been an explosion in the number of publications that relate to the use of ultrasound (US) for guiding interventional procedures to relieve acute and chronic pain.

---

[a] Department of Anesthesiology, Perioperative and Pain Medicine, Stanford University, Stanford, CA, USA; [b] Department of Anesthesiology and Pain Medicine, University of California, Davis, Sacramento, CA, USA; [c] Division of Physical Medicine and Rehabilitation, Department of Orthopedic Surgery, Stanford University, Stanford, CA, USA; [d] Department of Anesthesia and Pain Management, University of Toronto, Toronto, ON, Canada
[1] Present address: 450 Broadway Street Pavilion A, Redwood City, CA 94063, USA.
[2] Present address: 430 Broadway Street, Pavilion C, 3rd Floor, MC6343, Redwood City, CA 94063, USA.
[3] Present address: 300 Pasteur Drive, Room H3536, Stanford, CA, 94305, USA.
[4] Present address: 1070 Arastradero Road, Suite 200, Palo Alto, CA 940304, USA.
[5] Present address: 4860 Y Street, Suite 3020 Sacramento, California 95817, USA.
[6] Present address: 453 Quarry Road Stanford, CA 94305-5663, USA.
[7] Present address: 399 Bathurst Street, McL 2-405, Toronto, ON M5T 2S8, Canada.
* Corresponding author. Department of Anesthesia and Pain Management, University of Toronto, 399 Bathurst Street, McL 2-405, Toronto, ON M5T 2S8, Canada
E-mail address: Yasmine.hoydonckx@uhn.ca

Anesthesiology Clin 41 (2023) 395–470
https://doi.org/10.1016/j.anclin.2023.02.003
1932-2275/23/

Continued

- A positive effect for the majority of the included blocks was found, with strongest evidence for greater occipital nerve and genicular nerve blocks.
- Due to enhanced safety and precision, ultrasound-guided chronic pain blocks are helpful in diagnostics and have proven to be capable of treating previously intractable pain syndroms.
- The paucity of high quality evidence makes it hard to draw firm treatment recommendations presently.
- There is a need for prospective comparative effectiveness studies to further establish the efficacy and better safety profile of USG nerve and plane blocks for the indication of chronic pain.

Guidance with US is now used to perform procedures focused on peripheral nerves, the spine, and the musculoskeletal system. The published literature on these procedures has examined the domains of accuracy, efficacy, and safety conferred by the use of US. However, there is a need for a comprehensive systematic effort to synthesize the available evidence for US-guided nerve blocks for chronic pain management.

This narrative review focuses on the evidence for US-guided procedures on the following peripheral nerves and fascial planes to relieve chronic pain: greater occipital nerve (GON), trigeminal nerve and sphenopalatine ganglion, stellate ganglion, suprascapular nerve (SSN), median nerve, radial nerve, ulnar nerve, transversus abdominis plane, quadratus lumborum, rectus sheath, anterior cutaneous abdominal nerves, pectoralis and serratus plane (PEC), erector spinae plane, ilioinguinal nerve (ILN) and iliohypogastric nerve (IHN), genitofemoral nerve (GFN), lateral femoral cutaneous nerve (LFCN), foot and ankle nerves, and genicular nerves (GNs). Blocks that focus on treatment of musculoskeletal or spine pain were not included.

MATERIAL AND METHODS

Data Sources and Search

We conducted comprehensive, serial searches of the literature from inception to April 17, 2021, with the assistance of a medical information specialist. The following databases were searched: EMBASE, 1947 onward; MEDLINE, 1946 onward; MEDLINE In-Process and Other Non-Indexed Citations (all using the OvidSP Platform); and Cochrane Database of Systematic Reviews. PROSPERO and Cochrane Central Register of Controlled Trials were included to identify reviews or trials that may have been published but missed during the initial search on MEDLINE and EMBASE. Papers in all languages were included when it was possible to translate them into English language. Specific search terms used include names of the anatomic structures of interest that were combined with "ultrasound" and "pain" using Boolean operators (AND, OR). The scope of studies included randomized controlled trials (RCTs), systematic reviews, observational or cohort studies, case-control studies, case series/reports, and conference abstracts.

Inclusion Criteria and Study Selection

We prespecified eligibility criteria using the population, intervention, comparator, and outcomes model as follows:

Population: Studies included in the clinical analysis focused on humans.

Intervention: The intervention of interest was US-guided interventional procedures for chronic nerve pain.

Comparator: Comparators included placebo treatment or conventional medical management.

Outcome: Our primary outcome was change in intensity of pain assessed on a numerical rating scale (NRS) or visual analog scale (VAS) after the intervention. Secondary outcomes of interest included functional outcomes, quality of life, and patient satisfaction or global impression of change. Sustainability of analgesic benefit and adverse effects were also noted.

Titles, abstracts, and when required, full text of the papers identified from the initial search were examined for relevance as per the inclusion criteria for this review. Only studies that met the above-mentioned criteria were included for data extraction. We completed the search by reviewing the bibliographies of every selected article to look for possible additional articles that were not identified by the initial search.

Data Extraction

The reference data, populations, and outcomes were extracted from the articles into prespecified tables using a standardized data extraction form. The data collection form was pilot-tested before its use. We extracted information on studies' source (study ID and reviewer ID), number of patients, type of study, patient characteristics, details of intervention, comparator group where reported, previous treatments, follow-up time points, outcomes, and adverse effects of the intervention.

Data Synthesis

Our synthesis of clinical studies was anticipated to focus on results from RCTs followed by prospective trials or case series or reports. A meta-analysis was not planned due to the limited number, clinical heterogeneity, methodological diversity, and paucity of clinical trials. We synthesized the results of each anatomic structure of interest under the following headings: anatomy and technique, evidence and indications for use of US, complications and adverse effect, and a summary of the findings. A grade was assigned for the evidence for performing US-guided intervention for each procedure to relieve pain. This grading system categorized evidence on a scale

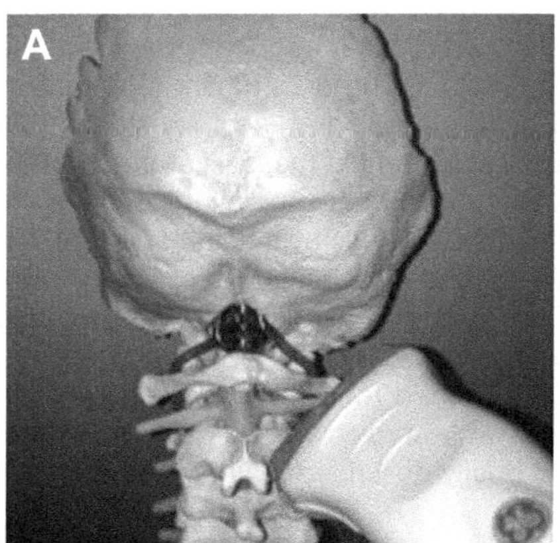

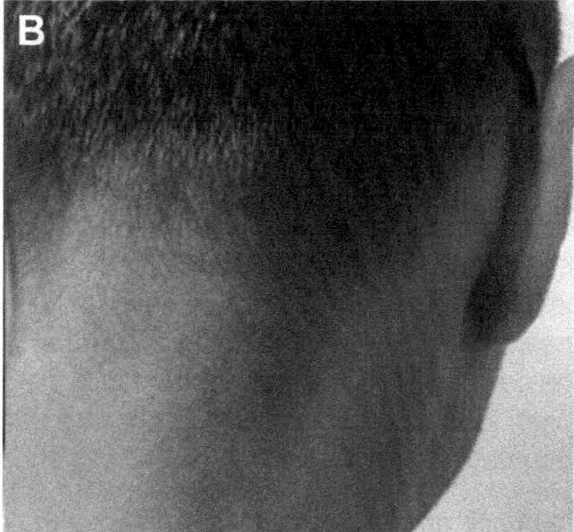

Fig. 1. GON block. (*A*) Proximal approach. Positioning of the ultrasound probe at the level of the C2 spinous process and slightly rotated in a cranial direction to bring the transducer parallel to the obliquus capitis inferior and optimize visualization of the occipital nerve. (*B*) Surface anatomy.

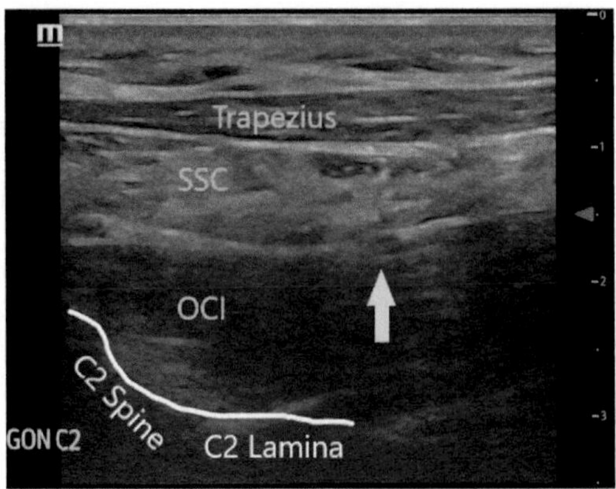

Fig. 2. GON block proximal approach. Visualization of the GON (*arrow*) at the C1-C2 level, lying in a plane between semispinalis capitis muscle (SSC), and the trapezius muscle can be seen overlying the semispinalis capitis. The block needle can be introduced lateral to medial, medial to lateral, or out of plane and 2 to 3 mL LA with/without steroid is injected in the plane between the obliquus capitis inferior (OCI) muscle and the semispinalis capitis muscle.

from A to D, or as I (insufficient), according to the US Preventative Services Task Force grading of evidence guidelines.[1] This system was chosen because of its flexibility, which permits high-grade recommendations in the absence of high-quality level 1 studies, which are challenging to conduct for interventional procedures.[2]

RESULTS

Greater Occipital Nerve

Anatomy and technique

The GON provides sensation to the skin in the posterior skull, temporal areas, and vertex. The GON also provides motor innervation to the semispinalis capitis muscle (SSC). The GON arises from the medial branch of the dorsal ramus of the second cervical (C2) nerve that runs deep to the SSC and becomes superficial above the superior nuchal line.[3] The nerve is highly variable in its course, but it frequently traverses the SSC and the trapezius muscle aponeurosis (TMA). Using a landmark (LM)-guided (LMG) technique, the GON can be blocked by the injection of local anesthetic (LA) and/or steroids just medial to the palpated occipital artery at the level of the superior nuchal line (distal approach). Given the variable course of the nerve in relation to the artery, the results of LMG injections can be inconsistent. However, ultrasound-guided (USG) technique has made the GON block (GONB) more specific and clinical studies have shown more favorable results of the GONB using USG technique.[3–5] By targeting the nerve more proximal in its course, at the level of C2, one can inject medication at the common areas of entrapment including the SSC and TMA. The proximal approach might confer more sustained relief in patients with chronic migraines.[6] The GONB technique is discussed in several papers and briefly described in **Figs. 1** and **2**.[6]

Evidence and indications for ultrasound

Multiple systematic reviews and meta-analyses have demonstrated LMG GONB to be effective in the treatment of (chronic) primary headaches, like chronic migraine[7–11] or cluster headache,[12,13] by significantly reducing pain score, number of headache days, and medication consumption.

Table 1
Overview of literature of ultrasound-guided blocks of the head and upper limb

First Author, Year, Number of Patients, Type of Study	Pain Syndrome	Ultrasound-Guided Intervention (Nerve Block/Neurolysis/RFA), Comparator, Injectate, Number of Blocks (Single/Series), Outcomes Measured, FU Time Points	Outcomes
GON			
Shim et al,[4] 2011 (n = 45) RCT	Occipital headache	• Nerve block • US vs LM • LA + DXM • Single • VAS • 4 wk	Mean (SD) VAS score at baseline and at 4 wk: • US group: 6.4 (0.2) to 2.3 (0.2) • LM group: 6.5 (0.2) to 3.8 (0.3) $P = .0003$ No difference in side effects between groups
VanderHoek et al,[14] 2013 (n = 2) CR	Occipital neuralgia	• Nerve block/pulsed RFA • N/A • Methylprednisolone (MP) + BUP 0.25%/N/A • Single • NRS • 4–6 wk	• Patient 1: NRS 3–7/10. Duration of relief several months • Patient 2: pain relief for 4–6 mo
Pingree et al,[15] 2017 (n = 14) P	Primary headaches	• Proximal GONB at C2 • N/A • LA + BET + BUP • Single • NRS • 30 min and 2–4 wk	Mean decrease of NRS • At 30 min: 3.78 ($P < .001$) • At 2 wk: 2.64 ($P = .006$) • At 4 wk: 2.21 No adverse events
Akyol et al,[17] 2015 (n = 21) CS	Postdural puncture headache	• Nerve block • N/A • BUP 0.25% 4 mL • Series • VAS • 24 h	• Significant pain reduction up to 24 h postprocedure.

(*continued on next page*)

Table 1
(continued)

First Author, Year, Number of Patients, Type of Study	Pain Syndrome	Ultrasound-Guided Intervention (Nerve Block/Neurolysis/RFA), Comparator, Injectate, Number of Blocks (Single/Series), Outcomes Measured, FU Time Points	Outcomes
Sahai-Srivastava and Subhani,[16] 2010 (n = 89) R	Occipital neuralgia	• Nerve block • N/A • LA (5 vs 1%) • Single • Adverse effects • 2 y	• 9% Of patients had adverse effects following GONB • Trend to have more side effects with lidocaine 5% ($P = .07$) compared with 1% ($P = .33$)
Flamer et al,[6] 2019 (n = 40) RCT	Chronic migraines	• Nerve block • Proximal vs distal • BUP + EPI + MP • Single • NRS • 3 mo	• At 1 wk: NRS significantly reduced in both cohorts • At 1 wk: sleep significantly improved in both groups • At 1 mo: number of headache days significantly reduced at in both groups • At 3 mo: NRS significantly reduced in proximal group
Stellate			
Aleanakian et al,[37] 2020 (n = 105) R	CRPS Neuropathic pain	• USG SGB • N/A • LA ± clonidine • VAS/temperature/complications • 7 d	• Significant immediate reduction of pain by 2.1 points on NRS (SD: 2.6, $P < .001$) • No correlation of pain relief with change in temperature or Horner
Yoo et al,[39] 2012 (n = 20) RCT	Poststroke pain	• USG SGB • LMG SGB • LA • Single • VAS • 2–4 wk	• Both blocks significantly decreased VAS at weeks 2 and 4 • USG block showed more significant pain improvement than blind ($P < .05$) VAS difference at week 2 (US vs LM): 2.61 (1.09) vs 1.88 (0.62) VAS difference at week 4 (US vs LM): 3.67 (1.03) vs 3.13 (0.62)

Wei et al,[38] 2014 (n = 16) R	CRPS	• Nerve block • N/A • BUP 0.5% • Series (range 4–19 per patient) • NRS • Unclear timing: "after last SGB block"	Significant reduction in pain compared with baseline • Spontaneous pain: Mean (SD) baseline 3.3 (2.8) to 1.5 (2.3) $P < .001$ • Evoked pain: Mean (SD) baseline 6.7 (2.2) to 3.8 (2.3) $P < .001$ Relative pain reduction not associated with duration of CRPS pain symptoms Transient side effects in 13% of patients (hoarseness, dysphagia, increased pain)
Ghai et al,[40] 2016 (n = 20) P	Chronic pain head/neck/arm	• Nerve block • N/A • BUP 0.25% + TC 40 mg • Single • NRS/temperature/ROM/vasomotor changes/quality of block • 30 min	• NRS significant decrease at 30 min up to 3 mo • Temperature rise significant increase up to 2 wk • Edema significant decrease up to 3 mo • ROM improved in 10 patients • No complication, hoarseness in 20% of patients • Quality of block excellent (15%) and good (85%)
Suprascapular nerve			
Aydın et al,[42] 2019 (n = 42) CS	Hemipleg c shoulder	• Nerve block + home exercise program • No SSNB + home exercise program • Betamethasone dipropionate plus betamethasone sodium phosphate (6.43 mg/mL + 2.63 mg/mL; 1 mL), 10% lidocaine (2 mL), and physiologic serum (2 mL) • Single • VAS • 1 wk, 1 mo, 3 mo	• Intervention group: VAS significantly decreased at 1 mo compared with control group

(*continued on next page*)

Table 1
(continued)

First Author, Year, Number of Patients, Type of Study	Pain Syndrome	Ultrasound-Guided Intervention (Nerve Block/Neurolysis/RFA), Comparator, Injectate, Number of Blocks (Single/Series), Outcomes Measured, FU Time Points	Outcomes
Wu et al,[43] 2014 (n = 42) RCT	Adhesive capsulitis	• (p)RFA • PT only • 180 s (2 Hz, 30-m pulse width, 42°C) • Single • VAS • 1, 4, 8, 12 wk	• Intervention group: shorter time to onset of significant pain relief ($P < .001$) • Intervention group: significant reduction of VAS score at week 1 (40% vs 4.7%) ($P < .001$).
Abdelshafi et al,[44] 2011 (n = 50) CS	Chronic shoulder pain	• Continuous USG SSNB + rehab • Intra-articular steroid injection + rehab VS rehab only • 3 mL marcaine; the injection continued every 12 h for 2 wk; 2 doses of Depo medrol 40 mg was injected at interval of 2 wk • Continuous • SPADI • 1, 4, and 12 wk	• Group 1 had more improvement in pain scores, disability scores, and range of movement data compared with groups 2 and 3
Median			
Chen et al,[56] 2015 (n = 36) RCT	CTS	• pRFA + night splint • Night splint • Steroid • Single • VAS • 1, 4, 8, 12 wk	• Significant shorter onset time in intervention group (mean of 2 d vs 14 d) • Significant lower VAS in intervention vs comparator up to 12 wk: 1.1 ± 0.8 vs 3.0 ± 1.2 ($P < .001$)
Radial			
Zhang et al,[59] 2017 (n = 12) CS	Painful stump neuroma	• RFA • N/A • N/A • Series • NRS • 6 mo	• Decrease in median NRS score for intermittent sharp pain assessment from 10.0 ± 0.5 to 2.0 ± 0.9 and for continuous burning pain assessment from 7.0 ± 1.0 to 2.0 ± 1.0

Oh et al,[60] 2016 (n = 2) CS	Intractable lateral epicondylitis	• RFA • N/A • N/A • Single • VAS • 12 wk	• Case 1: after 1 wk, the VAS pain score was 3–5/10 and was not exacerbated by light activities of daily living 1 wk later • Case 2: a 70% reduction in pain was evident after 1 wk
Guo et al,[58] 2019 (n = 9) CS	Residual limb neuroma in individuals with limb amputation	• RFA • N/A • N/A • Single • NRS • 1 d, 2 d, 2 wk, 3 mo	• Six patients reported significant reduction in pain scores (defined as at least 50% reduction) and an improvement in comfort/ease of wearing their prosthetic limb, with no adverse effects • All 9 patients NRS baseline 9.56 ± 1.01; 3 mo 3.56 ± 4.1; *P* = .0156
Ulnar			
Zhang et al, 2017 (n = 12) CS	Painful stump neuroma and postamputation pain	• RFA • N/A • N/A • Series • NRS • 6 mo	• Decrease in median NRS score for intermittent sharp pain assessment from 10.0 ± 0.5 to 2.0 ± 0.9 and for continuous burning pain assessment from 7.0 ± 1.0 to 2.0 ± 1.0.
Mizuno et al,[66] 2001 (n = 1) CR	Postherpetic neuralgia and CRPS	• Nerve block • N/A • NP • NP • NP • NP	• Reduction of pain and edema as well as improvement in mobility of each joint of her right upper extremity was observed

(*continued on next page*)

Table 1
(continued)

First Author, Year, Number of Patients, Type of Study	Pain Syndrome	Ultrasound-Guided Intervention (Nerve Block/Neurolysis/RFA), Comparator, Injectate, Number of Blocks (Single/Series), Outcomes Measured, FU Time Points	Outcomes
Yadav et al,[67] 2010 (n = 1) CR	Chemotherapy-induced peripheral neuropathy	• RFA • N/A • N/A • Single • NRS • Immediately following procedure	• 80% Relief in symptoms, and the onset of that relief was within hours of the procedure
Kwak et al,[68] 2019 (n = 2) CR	Cubital tunnel syndrome	• (p)RFA • N/A • N/A • Single • NRS • 2 wk, 1, 2, 3, 6 mo	• Patient 1: complete pain relief for at least 6 mo • Patient 2: complete pain relief until week 2, then 60% pain reduction from baseline for at least 6 mo
Trigeminal			
Nader et al,[22] 2013 (n = 1) CR	Trigeminal neuralgia (V2)	• Nerve block • N/A • BUP + MP • Series • NRS • 2 wk	• Sustained pain relief in V2 and 60% relief in V3 for 2 wk
Nader et al,[26] 2015 (n = 1) CR	Trigeminal neuralgia (V2)	• pRFA • N/A • BUP + MP • Series • NRS • 6 mo	• Immediate pain relief postprocedure, sustained for > 6 mo. No neurologic side effects reported

Gupta et al,[27] 2018 (n = 1) CR	Oral cancer	• Nerve block • N/A • BUP 0.25% + TC • Single • NRS • 2 wk	• NRS 3/10 after 30 min of procedure • No data of outcome at 2 wk • No complications
Nader et al,[25] 2013 (n = 15) CS	Trigeminal neuralgia (V2)	• Nerve block • N/A • BUP 0.25% + steroid • Series • NRS • 15 mo	• 80% Loss of sensation 15 min after injection • 14 Of 15 patients had good pain relief after one or several injections • Range of duration of relief: 1 wk – 13 mo (after repeated injections)

Abbreviations: BET, betamethasone; BUP, bupivacaine; CR, case report; CS, case series; CTS, carpal tunnel syndrome; FU, follow-up; MP, methylprednisolone; N/A, not applicable; P, prospective; (p)RFA, (pulsed) radiofrequency ablation; PT, physiotherapy; R, retrospective; rehab, rehabilitation; ROM, range of motion; SPADI, shoulder pain and disability index.

However, the number of studies on US-guided GONB for primary headaches is surprisingly limited to 6 papers (2 RCTs, 2 observational studies, 1 case series, 1 case report; total of 211 patients)[4,6,14–17] (**Table 1**).

We found one study that demonstrated increased efficacy of GONB using USG compared with LMG techniques presumably due to real-time needle visualization, visualization of surrounding structures, and LA spread around the target.[4]

A cadaver study of Greher and colleagues[5] investigated the accuracy of GONB and visibility of the GON at the proximal and distal nerve block site, demonstrating that the proximal approach has a higher success rate and should allow a more precise blockade of the GON. This fact was clinically tested by Flamer and colleagues[6] who compared the efficacy of proximal versus distal USG GONB in patients with chronic migraine. Both approaches significantly reduced headache pain and frequency at 1 week and 1 month; however, the proximal approach seemed to have a long-lasting effect until end of the third month.[6]

Despite frequent clinical use, we could only find 3 small studies (1 prospective, 1 retrospective study, 1 case report; 105 patients) on the utility and safety of USG GONB for occipital neuralgia and cervicogenic headache.[14–16] Pingree and colleagues[15] demonstrated sustained pain relief up to 4 weeks following a USG proximal GONB at the level of C2. A small case series of 21 patients with postdural puncture headache reported GONB to provide significant pain relief up to 24 hours.[17]

Complications and safety

USG GONB has demonstrated to be safe in the treatment of different headache syndromes.[15,16] Apart from the standard risks of bleeding, infection, damage to surrounding structures, transient site pain, and bradycardia are reported, as well as dizziness, slurred speech, headache, and vision changes. One study demonstrated that a higher rate of these side effects occurred with increased strength of LA used (1% vs 5%), although the difference was not significant.[16]

Summary

Although there are strong data that LMG GONB is effective for the treatment of primary headaches, the literature on the use of US for GONB is limited.

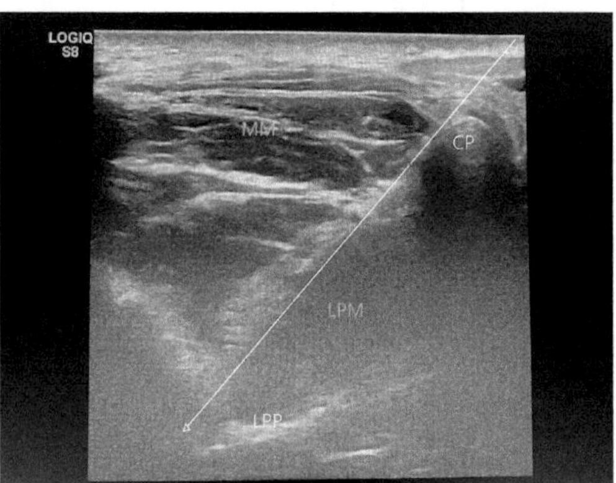

Fig. 3. Sphenopalatine ganglion block. Ultrasound probe is placed over mandibular notch inferior to the zygomatic arch. Mouth open, moving coronoid process out of the way. The needle is introduced in-plane parallel to the transducer probe, and advanced lateral to medial, posterior to anterior toward the pterygopalatine fossa (*white arrow*). The injectate is deposited deep to the lateral pterygoid muscle and plate. CP, condylar process; LPM, lateral pterygoid muscle; LPP, lateral pterygoid plate; MM, masseter muscle.

There is limited evidence that USG GONB has an increased efficacy in successfully targeting the GON with a lower rate of adverse effects, compared with the LMG approach.[4–6]

Based on the available evidence, the authors' recommendation for use of US in GONB for primary headaches is grade A, higher level of certainty. There is need for more RCTs to demonstrate the efficacy and superiority over LMG approach.

Trigeminal Nerve and Sphenopalatine Ganglion

Anatomy and technique

The trigeminal nerve (V) is a major conduit for sensory innervation to the face and head region, along with minor motor contributions to the jaw. The nerve consists of 3 major branches: the ophthalmic (V1), maxillary (V2), and mandibular (V3) nerves. From the trigeminal ganglion located within the Meckel cave, these 3 nerves arise and exit through different foramina within the skull. The V1 division, along with cranial nerves III, IV, and VI, exits the cavernous sinus anteriorly through the superior orbital fissure into the orbit. The V2 division travels within the lateral wall of the cavernous sinus and exits through the foramen rotundum. The V2 nerve then crosses the pterygopalatine fossa, enters the orbit through the inferior orbital fissure, runs forward on the floor of the orbit, and then emerges through the infraorbital foramen, terminating into inferior palpebral, lateral nasal, and superior labial branches. In the pterygopalatine fossa, the maxillary nerve is connected to the sphenopalatine ganglion, a large parasympathetic ganglion that is involved in the pathophysiology of primary headaches. The V3 division, the only branch with motor innervation, exits through the foramen ovale.[18,19]

Traditionally, the trigeminal nerve and sphenopalatine ganglion block have been performed under computed tomography (CT) or fluoroscopy guidance. Recently, literature emerged about use of US for maxillary nerve block with sphenopalatine ganglion block in the pterygopalatine fossa.[20–22] Three different USG approaches have been described by Nader and colleagues[22,23] (**Fig. 3**). This block is indicated for the treatment of trigeminal neuralgia and atypical face pain. The procedure is discussed in **Fig. 3**.[22,23]

Evidence and indications for ultrasound

In a cadaver dye study by Kampitak and colleagues[24] USG maxillary nerve block was attempted using the lateral pterygoid plate as LM to reach the pterygopalatine fossa. This study demonstrated a high degree of accuracy and feasibility.[24] We did not find any studies comparing US with other image guidance techniques.

Only 4 case reports (total of 17 patients) have been published in regard to the clinical use of USG for maxillary nerve/pterygopalatine ganglion block in patients with refractory trigeminal neuralgia[22,25–27] (see **Table 1**). Unilateral block was performed in all cases, with LA and steroids. Outcomes were evaluated immediately postprocedure up to 15 months. The range of duration of therapeutic effect after a USG trigeminal nerve block (TNB) was from 2 weeks (single injection) to 13 months (after repeated injections).[22,25,26] Pulsed radiofrequency ablation (pRFA), combined with injection of LA with steroid, was performed in 1 patient with sustained pain relief over 6 months.[26] We found 1 case report on a patient with facial pain from an oral carcinoma reported who underwent a USG pterygopalatine block.[27] This USG technique could be especially useful in cancer cases, given the improved visualization of the nerve structures despite possible distortion of anatomy.

Complications and safety

Compared with fluoroscopy, the USG technique can be challenging. Awareness of the proximity of the facial nerve, parotid gland, and superior maxillary artery is required.[23]

Summary

One cadaver study suggests that US can be used to effectively target the maxillary nerve and sphenopalatine ganglion. There is weak evidence that USG maxillary nerve/sphenopalatine ganglion block is effective in treating refractory trigeminal nerve pain.

Based on the available evidence, the authors' recommendation for performing US trigeminal nerve block for facial pain is grade I, insufficient. This intervention should be investigated in larger (randomized controlled) trials. This intervention could be offered bedside to patients in refractory pain who require quick pain relief.

Stellate Ganglion

Anatomy and technique

The first thoracic segments of the spinal cord contribute sympathetic fibers to the head, neck, upper limbs, and heart. These sympathetic fibers synapse in the superior, middle, and inferior cervical ganglions after ascending through the sympathetic chain in the paravertebral space. The stellate ganglion exists in approximately 80% of the general population and commonly consists of a fusion of the inferior cervical ganglion and the first thoracic ganglion, although variations exist. This ganglion is commonly located just anterior to the transverse process of the sixth (C6) and extends caudad to the neck of the first rib. Image reconstruction using 3D sonography shows that the cervical sympathetic trunk is located posterolaterally to the prevertebral fascia on the surface of the longus colli muscle. The carotid artery runs lateral and anterior to the stellate ganglion. Other relevant anatomy includes the vertebral artery, which runs deep to the stellate ganglion, and the thyroid gland, which sits anterior and medial to the stellate ganglion.[28,29] The inferior thyroid artery also courses in the area of the stellate ganglion, originating from the thyrocervical trunk and passing anteriorly to the vertebral artery and the longus colli muscle at C7 level. The course of this vessel is often tortuous and variable, and therefore identification by US is crucial. Another

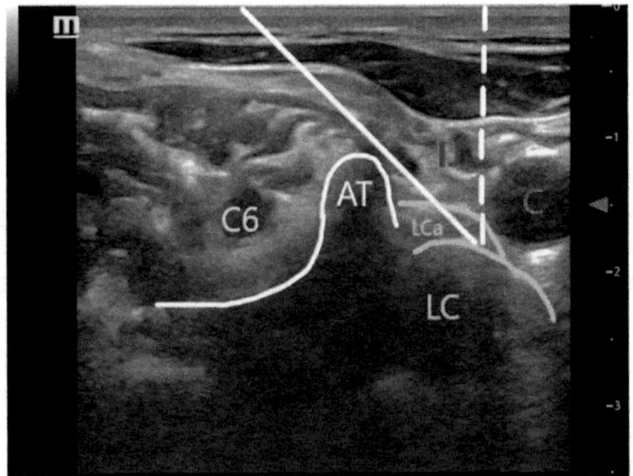

Fig. 4. Stellate ganglion block. Transverse view at C6. The patient is positioned supine with neck rotated to the contralateral side. The needle paths of anterior and lateral approaches are marked by long solid and dotted lines, respectively. Right side of the picture is medial. The block can be performed in an in-plane (lateral to medial) technique. The target is the prevertebral fascia between the longus capitis and longus colli muscles. The tip should reach the prevertebral fascia of the longus colli at the tip of the C6 anterior tubercle. AT, anterior tubercle; C, carotid artery; C6, C6 spinal nerve.IJ, internal jugular vein (compressed); LC, longus colli muscle; LCa, longus capitis muscle.

anatomic consideration for stellate ganglion block (SGB) is to understand that there are individuals in whom the branches from the second thoracic spinal nerve join the first thoracic spinal nerve. These fibers, called Kuntz nerves, join the brachial plexus and bypass the stellate ganglion entirely. If an SGB provides incomplete or poor relief, one must consider that the patient may have an anatomic variant described earlier.[30] The SGB can be performed in in-plane (lateral to medial) and out-of-plane techniques. Details are shown in **Fig. 4**.[31]

Evidence and indications for ultrasound

Traditionally, sympathetic-mediated pain of the head, neck, upper thorax, and upper extremities has been successfully managed using LMG and fluoroscopic-guided SGB.[32] These syndromes would include complex regional pain syndrome (CRPS) and postherpetic neuralgia.[33–36] More atypical indications for SGB are emerging, like alleviating symptoms of posttraumatic stress disorder.[37]

The authors found 4 papers on the use of US for SGB (1 RCT, 1 prospective, and 2 retrospective studies; 161 patients in total)[37–40] (see **Table 1**). In all studies, the injectates used were LAs only. One RCT compared USG SGB with LMG in patients with poststroke pain: both groups had significant improvement after SGB at weeks 2 and 4 postprocedure. However, the USG group showed a larger change in pain reduction compared with the LMG.[39] In a small prospective study by Ghai and colleagues[40] 20 patients received a single USG SGB with bupivacaine and steroid. The investigators noted sustained pain relief, improved temperature, vasomotor changes, and range of motion up to 3 months postprocedure, presumably due to addition of steroids.[40] A large retrospective study by Aleanakian and colleagues[37] investigated the effectiveness, safety, and predictive potential of USG SGB in sympathetically mediated pain. The investigators concluded that immediate pain reduction after a series of blocks was highly significant and that there was no correlation of efficacy with change of temperature, vital signs, or presence of Horner syndrome.[37] Last, in a small retrospective case series a significant reduction in spontaneous and evoked pain compared with baseline was found.[38]

Complications and safety

USG SGB increases safety by providing real-time visualization of needle trajectory, and increased accuracy allows the use of smaller volumes of LA.[29] Transient hoarseness (3.9%) occurs secondary to blockade of the recurrent laryngeal nerve. Specific complications for this block include pneumothorax, nerve injury, hematoma (0.6%) by puncture of surrounding vessels, esophageal or tracheal puncture, and thyroid injury. Epidural or intrathecal injection can also occur. Overall, the incidence of complications is lower than in non-USG techniques.[37,38]

Summary

Current evidence suggests that USG SGB enhances accuracy and safety, but more robust comparative studies are needed to demonstrate superiority. Based on the available evidence, the authors' recommendation for use of USG SGB is grade B, moderate level of certainty.

Suprascapular Nerve

Anatomy and technique

The SSN serves both sensory and motor functions. In addition to innervating the scapula, subacromial bursa, coracoclavicular ligament, and glenohumeral and acromioclavicular joints, it provides motor innervation for the supraspinatus and infraspinatus muscles.[41] Anatomically, the SSN originates from the C4-C6 nerve roots of the upper

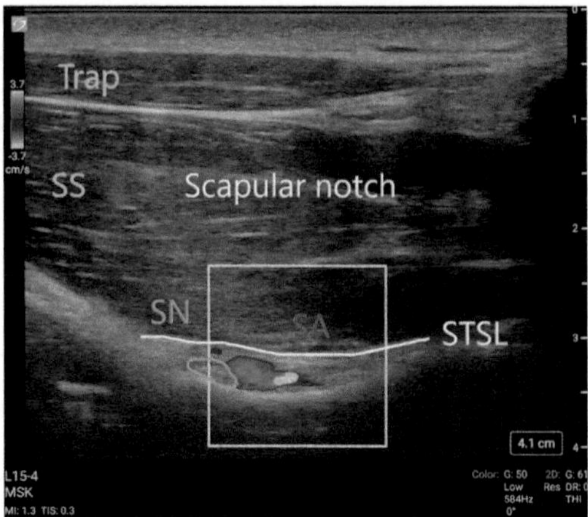

Fig. 5. Suprascapular nerve block. Transverse view over suprascapular notch in supraspinatus fossa. After palpating the scapular spine, the probe is placed on the patient to obtain a transverse view of the scapular spine; this allows for US visualization of the suprascapular notch. The suprascapular artery can be identified with color Doppler and typically runs medial to the SSN. The needle is directed toward the notch medial to lateral to avoid acromion, with an in-plane approach. Typically 2.5 to 5 mL of a long-lasting local anesthetic is injected to minimize spread back toward the brachial plexus. SA, suprascapular artery; SN, suprascapular nerve; SS, supraspinatus; STSL, superior transverse scapular ligament. Trap, trapezius.

trunk of the brachial plexus. The SSN subsequently runs under the omohyoid muscle in the posterior triangle of the neck, posteriorly toward the suprascapular notch, deep to the superior transverse scapular ligament, through the scapular foramen into the supraspinous fossa, laterally to the spinoglenoid notch, and exits into the infraspinous fossa.

Multiple sites for the SSN block have been described.[41–43] One technique involves blocking superiorly as the SSN runs into the suprascapular notch. The advantage of this location is the nerve fibers supplying both the supraspinatus and infraspinatus muscles are blocked. This approach is in contrast to the posterior site of the SSN, which involves blocking the SSN posteriorly as it passes into the spinoglenoid notch and only blocks the nerve fibers supplying the infraspinatus muscle.[41]

Although various techniques have been reported, a standard SSN technique is described in **Fig. 5**.

Evidence and indications for ultrasound

Given the wide range of causes of chronic shoulder pain, various studies have been conducted on USG SSN block for different pain conditions. However, most of the evidence stems from case series and reports with limited RCTs. A 2014 RCT assessed the efficacy of USG pRFA of the SSN for adhesive capsulitis. Twenty-one patients completed the study as the interventional group, which received a 1-time treatment of USG pRFA of the SSN followed by 12 weeks of physical therapy, and 21 patients completed the study as the control group, which only received 12 weeks of physical therapy. The investigators found the interventional group required a significantly shorter length of time to achieve pain relief and reported lower VAS pain scores compared with the control group.[43] There were no adverse events reported.

A 2019 study evaluating the efficacy of USG SSN block for painful hemiplegic shoulder randomized 42 patients to either receive a USG SSN block (n = 21) with a home exercise program or home exercise program only (n = 21). At 1 week, 1 month, and 3 months postdischarge, the investigators evaluated shoulder range of motion (ROM) and VAS for pain in addition to other metrics and found that the USG SSN group significantly increased shoulder ROM at 1 to 3 months, and decreased pain VAS at 1 month.[42]

A 2011 study compared 3 different modalities for the treatment of chronic shoulder pain by randomly dividing 50 patients (with a total of 63 shoulders) into 3 groups: group 1 (n = 23 shoulders) received continuous SSN block under USG in addition to a rehabilitation program, group 2 (n = 20 shoulders) received intra-articular injection of steroid in addition to a rehabilitation program, and group 3 (n = 20 shoulders) received only the rehabilitation program. Follow-up at 1, 4, and 12 weeks revealed that group 1 had the most improvement compared with groups 2 and 3 regarding pain scores, disability, and range of movement data.[44]

Complications and safety

USG SSN has a much lower incidence of nerve damage to the SSN, pneumothorax, and intravascular injection, compared with non-USG SSN.[41] Furthermore, various studies have noted the favorable safety profile of USG SSN including additional factors such as avoidance of exposing staff to unnecessary radiation compared with fluoroscopy-guided SSN block.[45] Additional studies evaluating the efficacy of USG SSN have not reported complications.[42–44]

Summary

According to the most recent evidence, the authors' recommendation for performing USG SSN in the treatment of shoulder pain, including causes such as hemiplegic shoulder and adhesive capsulitis, is grade C, moderate level of certainty. Despite few RCTs, most data are specific to various shoulder pain causes and primarily consist of case series and case reports. Although there seems to be a favorable adverse effect profile, more work is needed to elucidate the efficacy of USG SSN for shoulder pain and its various causes.

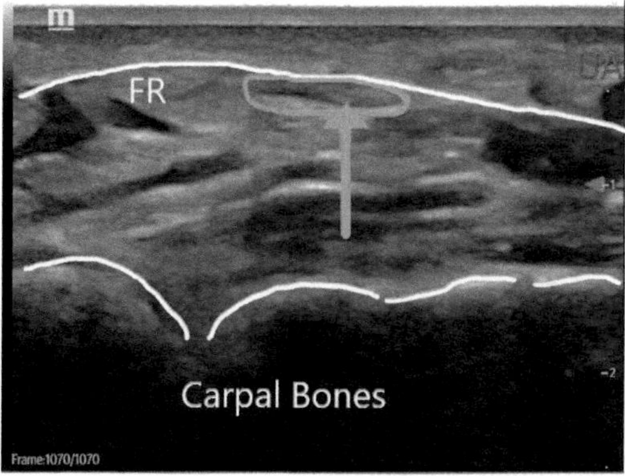

Fig. 6. Transverse view of median nerve at the level of carpal tunnel. The median nerve (*arrow*) lies under the flexor retinaculum (FR). The ulnar artery (UA) is shown on the medial side (right side of the sonogram). The US probe is placed transversely at the first carpal crease, and the needle is inserted perpendicular to the US plane.

Median Nerve

Anatomy and technique

The median nerve is a terminal branch of the brachial plexus, formed by the lateral (C5, C6 roots) and medial cords (C8, T1 roots). After arising in the axilla, the median nerve transverses the arm giving off the muscular and anterior interosseous nerve branches in the proximal forearm. The median nerve innervates the superficial and deep groups of muscles in the anterior compartment of the forearm (with the exception of flexor carpi ulnaris) and supplies the distal radioulnar joint and wrist joint. The median nerve also gives off sensory branches to the forearm. The median nerve enters the hand via the carpal tunnel. The nerve gives off recurrent (muscular) branch, which supplies the thenar muscles, and digital cutaneous branches, which supply the radial side of the palm, and the palmar surface of the index finger, long finger, and radial half of the ring finger. The nerve also supplies the dorsal surface of the index and long fingers and the radial half of the distal ring finger.[46]

The ideal site for median nerve blockade is at the level of the carpal tunnel, given its superficial nature and minimal risk for vascular injury.[47] The original LMG technique is associated with an increased risk of postoperative neurologic complications.[48] Recent studies have demonstrated that use of US is a safer and more efficient alternative.[49,50] Using a high-frequency linear US probe, placed transversely at the first carpal crease, the needle is inserted perpendicular, in an out-of-plane approach. A small amount of LA should be sufficient to ensure a circumferential spread around the nerve.[50] Dextrose 5% has also been proved to have an outstanding effect on peripheral entrapment neuropathy[51] (**Fig. 6**).

Evidence and indications for ultrasound

In a cadaveric study by To and colleagues,[52] the accuracy of carpal tunnel injections was compared with and without use of US. The USG carpal tunnel injections had significantly higher accuracy rates.[52] There are several prospective trials on the use of USG forearm blocks in the perioperative pain setting that clearly demonstrate faster onset time, more efficient pain control, and increased duration of sensory block.[46,50–54] However, there is paucity of literature on the use of USG for median nerve blocks in patients with chronic pain. The authors found that 1 case report on the use of USG median and ulnar nerve blocks in the forearm with onabotulinum toxin A injection for palmar hyperhidrosis was published.[55] The investigators concluded that using US helped them minimize the number in injections and therefore reduce risk of mechanical or neural damage.

In a single-blind RCT, the therapeutic efficacy of USG pRFA treatment of the median nerve combined with night splint was compared with night splint alone in patients with carpal tunnel syndrome[56] (see **Table 1**). The USG cohort demonstrated lower VAS scores and stronger finger pinch compared with the control group over the entire study.

Complications and safety

Extrapolating from the literature on the perioperative use of USG median nerve blocks, the authors note no published complications or adverse events. Given the proximity to the radial and ulnar arteries, there is a risk a vascular puncture and these vessels should be avoided. The ulnar nerve also travels superficially with the ulnar artery and should be visualized before injection.

Summary

Several prospective perioperative and cadaver studies have demonstrated greater efficacy, patient satisfaction, and better pain control with USG blocks. However, the use of USG median nerve block for chronic pain setting is limited to 1 RCT. Based on the current evidence, the evidence for use of US for median nerve block is grade I, insufficient.

Radial Nerve

Anatomy and technique

The radial nerve is a terminal branch of the posterior cord of the brachial plexus and carries fibers of spinal nerves C5-T1. The nerve runs alongside the axillary artery in the axilla, entering the posterior compartment of the arm. The proximal radial nerve provides muscular branches for the triceps muscle, brachialis, brachioradialis, and extensor carpi radialis longus. The nerve also provides sensory innervation to the posterior part of the arm and forearm through the posterior cutaneous nerve of the arm and the forearm. The radial nerve also supplies the elbow joint. It runs down in the spiral groove of the humerus, between the lateral and medial head of the triceps muscle, until it reaches the lateral epicondyle of the humerus, where it terminates into a superficial and deep branch and runs further down into the forearm.

The deep branch or posterior interosseous nerve (PIN), passes laterally to the neck of the radius and enters the dorsal compartment of the forearm, innervating the majority of the extensor muscles and providing articular branches to the wrist and carpal joints. The PIN typically pierces the supinator muscle along its proximal course, and this is a common site of entrapment. The nerve further divides into 4 terminal branches that can typically be compressed at 1 of 4 other sites as well. These 4 sites are the fibrous bands around the radial head, the recurrent radial vessels, the arcade of Frohse at the supinator, and/or the tendinous margin of the extensor carpi radialis brevis. The superficial radial nerve (SRN) provides cutaneous innervation to the lateral two-thirds of the dorsum of the hand and lateral two and one-half proximal phalanges. Compression of the SRN in the tunnel region beneath the tendon of the brachioradialis muscle is an uncommon cause of SRN neuropathy. This condition, known as *cheiralgia paresthetica*, is characterized by pain in the hand with no significant motor weakness.

The radial nerve can be blocked proximally at the spiral groove or more distally at the elbow. Distal to the crease of the elbow, the nerve divides into the superficial

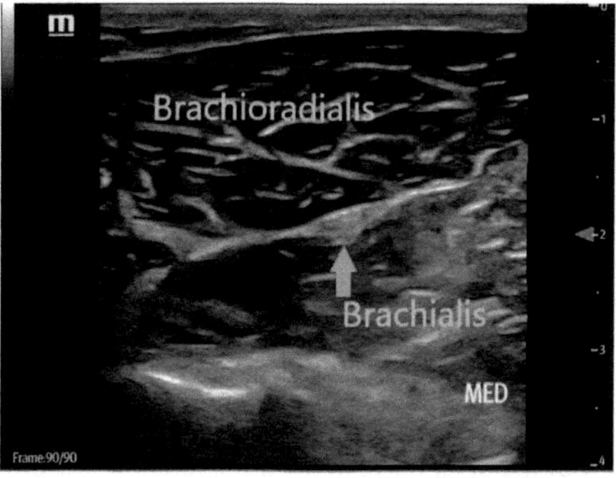

Fig. 7. Sonogram of radial nerve (*arrow*) at the elbow, 3 cm proximal to the elbow crease. The US probe is placed 3 to 4 cm above the crease of the elbow in a transverse orientation. The radial nerve can be seen between the brachioradialis (laterally) and the brachialis muscle (medially).

and deep branches, making blockade of the nerve at this site suboptimal unless block of one of these branches is required.[57] The technique is discussed in **Fig. 7**.

Evidence and indication for ultrasound

We found 3 case series on the use of US for pRFA of the radial nerve (total of 23 patients) (see **Table 1**). Guo and colleagues[58] reported on the efficacy of upper extremity continuous RFA for residual neuromas in individuals with limb amputations and postamputation pain. About 66% of patients who underwent the procedure reported more than 50% reduction in pain scores. Meanwhile, a similar study reported that 100% of patients achieved symptom relief from postamputation pain after a combination of alcohol injection followed by RFA, if necessary.[59] A case report involving 2 subjects with intractable lateral epicondylitis underwent pRFA of the radial nerve with significant reduction in pain reported over the following 12 weeks.[60]

Complications and safety

The risk of complication of USG radial nerve block is low. One case report describes compartment syndrome as a complication of a combined median, ulnar, and radial nerve block using liposomal bupivacaine. Other complications include infection, hematoma, vascular puncture, and nerve injury.[61]

Summary

The radial nerve is best visualized for USG intervention just proximal to the elbow in between the brachialis and brachioradialis muscles or at the spiral groove. USG radial nerve block and/or RFA have been used with success for postamputation pain, lateral epicondylitis, radial tunnel syndrome, and entrapment of the SRN or PIN. The risk of complications from radial nerve block is low. Based on the current evidence, the authors' recommendation for performing USG radial nerve blocks for chronic pain indication is I, insufficient.

Ulnar Nerve

Anatomy and technique

The ulnar nerve is the terminal branch of the medial cord of the brachial plexus and is derived from spinal nerves C8-T1. The nerve runs along the medial side of the humerus

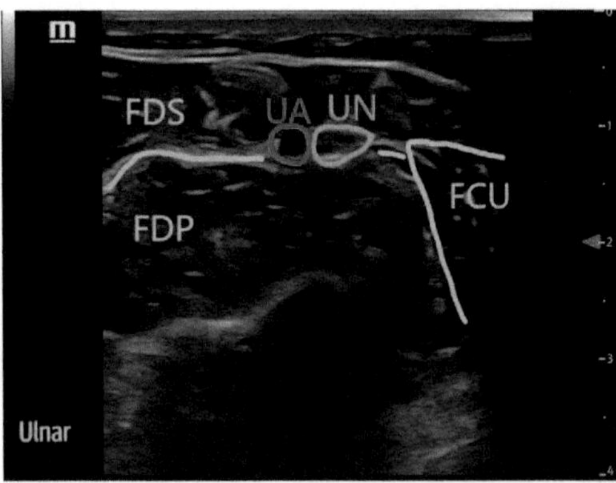

Fig. 8. Transverse view of the ulnar nerve in the distal forearm. The ulnar artery (UA) is seen medial to the ulnar nerve (UN). The ulnar nerve runs just deep to the flexor digitorum superficialis (FDS), superficial to the flexor digitorum profundus (FDP), and medial to the flexor carpi ulnaris (FCU) at this location. The block needle is introduced in-plane with the needle tip advanced just deep to the ulnar nerve.

and enters the cubital tunnel at the posteromedial elbow between the olecranon process of the ulna and the medial epicondyle. After traversing the cubital tunnel, it enters the flexor compartment of the forearm, passing between the ulnar and humeral heads of the flexor carpi ulnaris muscle, which it lies deep to as it runs through the proximal part of the forearm. The nerve can be visualized in close proximity to the ulnar artery, usually medial to the vessel. Near the wrist, the ulnar nerve passes superficially to the flexor retinaculum and enters the palm of the hand through Guyon canal.[62] Proximal to the wrist the ulnar nerve gives off the dorsal cutaneous branch to the dorsum of the hand. The nerve block is performed at the level of the proximal forearm (**Fig. 8**). The ulnar nerve should not be blocked at the level of the elbow, due to the surrounding of bony structures at this location, thereby increasing the likelihood of compression injury after injection into a fixed space.

Evidence and indications for ultrasound

Multiple studies have shown that LMG ulnar nerve block leads to high rates of vascular puncture or intraneural injection. One study showed that 50% of block passes resulted in ulnar artery puncture when the proceduralist used the traditional volar approach for ulnar nerve block by placing the block needle just lateral to the tendon of the flexor carpi ulnaris.[63] A similar cadaveric study also found high rates of arterial puncture and intraneural injection while using the LMG approach.[54]

Meanwhile, one study found that USG ulnar nerve block reduced the ED95 dose of 1% mepivacaine to block the ulnar nerve at the forearm to 0.7 mL, a far smaller volume than is typically used for blind or LM-based approaches.[64] This study gives evidence that US increases accuracy tremendously. Another study did not find a difference in required injection volume between US and nerve stimulation-guided block.[65]

Indications for USG ulnar nerve interventions for chronic pain are limited and typically are combined with median and radial nerve interventions (see **Table 1**). One study showed that USG alcohol injection and RFA of the upper-extremity nerves is an effective treatment of postamputation pain; 100% patients in the study achieved symptom relief from either alcohol injection alone or injection followed by RFA.[59] Meanwhile, a case report elucidates the efficacy of ulnar nerve block in combination with SGB and continuous epidural block for a patient with postherpetic neuralgia and CRPS of the upper extremity. The patient had a reduction of pain and edema and had increased mobility of the affected limb following these interventions.[66]

Another case report outlines the efficacy of ulnar and median nerve RFA in a patient with severe, debilitating chemotherapy-induced peripheral neuropathy. The patient had 80% relief in symptoms, and the onset of that relief was within hours of the procedure.[67] Another case report describes the use of pRFA of the ulnar nerve for cubital tunnel syndrome. One patient has complete pain relief for at least 6 months. In the second patient, the pain returned after 2 weeks; however, it remained significantly reduced (60% from baseline) up to the end of the study at 6 months.[68]

Complications and safety

The risk of complications of USG ulnar nerve block is low as demonstrated by the studies discussed.

Summary

Studies have demonstrated increased safety and accuracy of USG blocks compared with LMG. Although multiple case reports exist regarding the efficacy of peripheral nerve blocks to treat various chronic neuralgias, no controlled studies exist at this time. Of the existing case reports, most subjects had positive results and decreased

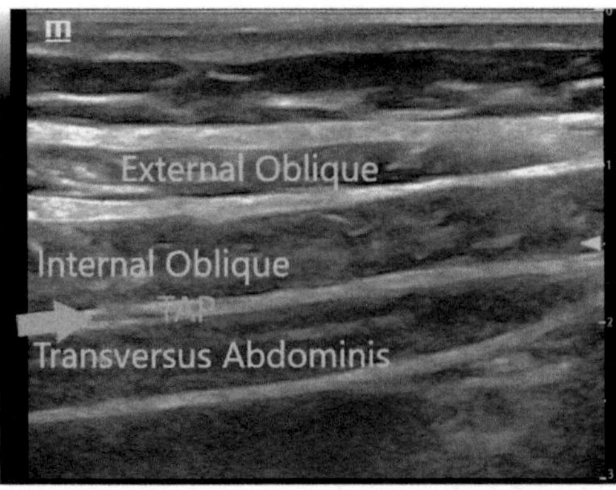

Fig. 9. Sonogram of the abdominal wall layers. The US probe is positioned 3 finger breaths superior and posterior to the ASIS. Using an in- or out-of-plane approach, the needle tip is positioned in the TAP, between internal oblique and transversus abdominis muscles, and its placement is confirmed with hydrodissection followed by injection of the LA. Arrow points to neurovascular structure in plane.

pain after the intervention with almost half reporting complete pain relief.[69] The evidence for use of USG ulnar nerve block for chronic pain is I, insufficient.

Transversus Abdominus Plane Block

Anatomy and technique

The thoracolumbar nerves that innervate the anterior abdominal wall (T6-L1) course through the transversus abdominus plane (TAP) between the internal oblique and transverse abdominus muscles to their eventual area of innervation.[70] These nerves communicate with one another creating a wide plexus at 3 predictable locations including anterolaterally, traveling with the deep circumflex iliac artery, and the deep inferior epigastric artery.

Initial USG approaches to blocking these nerves, referred to as the *midaxillary*, *anterior*, or *lateral* approaches, resulted in incomplete blockade of sensory innervation to the abdomen above the umbilicus. Attempts to account for this difference have since been made and have resulted in the "subcostal" approach first described by Hebbard and colleagues[71] in 2009 and the quadratus lumborum block (QLB) first described by Blanco in 2007.[72,73]

Several studies have attempted to define the spread of dye injected into the TAP as well as to characterize the resulting sensory distribution. These studies have confirmed the observation that LA injected using the traditional midaxillary and the subcostal approach does not reliably spread above the T10 level.[74,75] Støving and colleagues[76] investigated the cutaneous sensory block of 20 mL ropivacaine injected into the TAP in the midaxillary approach in healthy volunteers and concluded that the block is located predominantly lateral to a line through the anterior superior iliac spine (ASIS) and does not cross the midline. Mapping of the sensory loss showed great variability and patchiness on the anterior abdominal wall. At present, the LMG technique is no longer recommended because of large variation of anatomy, ambiguity of the procedure, and risk of peritoneal perforation.[77,78]

Compared with LMG, USG TAP blocks are safer and more accurate and considered the gold-standard technique.[79] The TAP block technique[31] is illustrated by **Fig. 9**.

Table 2
Overview of literature of ultrasound-guided abdominal plane blocks

First Author, Year, Number of Patients, Type of Study	Pain Syndrome	Ultrasound-Guided Intervention (Block/Neurolysis/RFA), Comparator, Injectate, Blocks (Single/Series), Outcomes Measured, FU Time Points	Outcomes
TAP			
Covotta et al,[80] 2020 (n = 96) RCT	Postsurgical pain after robotic partial nephrectomy	• Nerve block • GA • Ropivacaine 0.5% • Single • NRS and morphine consumption • 24 h, 3, 6, 12 mo	• At 24 h: median morphine consumption: 14.16 mg vs 10.6 mg, $P < .008$ (no TAP vs TAP) • At all FU times: significant NRS score difference at all follow-ups (favoring TAP) except at 12 mo
Moeschler et al,[81] 2021 (n = 60) RCT	Chronic abdominal wall pain	• Nerve block • TPI • BUP 0.25% 10 mL + TC 20 mg (TAP) vs BUP 0.25% 5 mL + TC 20 mg (TPI) • Single • NRS • 3 mo	• Mean baseline pain: 5.5 vs 4.7 (TAP vs TPI) • At 3 mo: NRS between-group difference was 1.7 (95% CI, 0.3–3.0) favoring TPI group
Niraj and Kanel,[82] 2020 (n = 54) P	Chronic abdominal pain secondary to chronic pancreatitis	• TAP block: LA + steroids • TAP PRF • BUP 0.25% + MP • Single • NRS • 6 mo	• NRS scores: TAP block: 8.3 ± 1.0 (baseline) vs 5.8 ± 2.3 (at 6 mo) $P < .001$ PRF: 8.6 ± 0.5 (baseline) vs 5.4 ± 2.6 (at 6 mo) $P = .07$
Baciarello et al,[83] 2018 (n = 5) CS	Chronic postoperative abdominal wall pain	• Nerve block • N/A • LA + steroids • Single • NRS • 7 days- 1 y	• 4 of 5 patients: ≥50% pain relief within hours of the procedure • 2 of 5: low NRS up to 6 and 12 mo

(*continued on next page*)

Table 2
(continued)

First Author, Year, Number of Patients, Type of Study	Pain Syndrome	Ultrasound-Guided Intervention (Block/Neurolysis/RFA), Comparator, Injectate, Blocks (Single/Series), Outcomes Measured, FU Time Points	Outcomes
Abd-Elsayed et al,[84] 2020 (n = 92) R	Chronic abdominal pain	• Nerve block • N/A • 0.25% BUP + TC • Single • NRS • 3 mo	• The procedure improved pain in 81.9% of TAP blocks performed. • Mean NRS 6.1 vs 2.5 (baseline vs 3 mo)
Sahoo and Nair,[89] 2015 (n = 2) CR	ACNES	• Nerve block • N/A • MP + ropivacaine • Single • VAS • 6–12 mo	• Case 1: baseline 7/10 VAS, complete pain relief at 12 mo • Case 2: Complete relief and without any further injection 6 mo later
Gebhardt and Wu,[85] 2013 (n = 1) CR	Abdominal sarcoma	• Neurolysis • N/A • Phenol • Single • NRS/analgesic intake • 45 d	• Mean baseline NRS: 5/10. • Mean NRS at day 1: 2/10; day 28, 1/10; day 45, 2/10.
Restrepo-Garces et al, [86] 2014 (n = 1) CR	Abdominal wall cancer pain	• Neurolysis • N/A • Phenol • Single • VAS/analgesic intake • 2 mo	• NRS reduction of 70% (dynamic) and 100% (static) up to 2 mo • 50% decrease opioid reduction up to 2 mo.

Sakamoto et al,[87] 2012 (n = 1) CR	Metastatic colon cancer	• Neurolysis • N/A • Ethanol and ropivacaine • Single • NRS • 4 d	• Baseline patient's pain score was 7/10 at rest, which increased to 10/10 on any movement. • Pain scores were 0–5/10 d 1, 7/10 d 2, 0/10 d 3 & 4.
Lee et al,[88] 2020 (n = 1) CR	Gastrostomy site pain in a patient with cancer	• Neurolysis • N/A • Phenol • Single • NRS • 4 mo	• NRS Baseline: 9/10 • NRS Immediate post-procedure: 0/10 • NRS at 1 wk: NRS 3/10. • NRS at 4 mo: NRS 2/10, no opioids.
Sahoo and Nair,[89] 2015 (n = 2) CR	ACNES	• TAP block • N/A • Ropivacaine 0.375% + methylprednisolone 20 mg • Single • Pain relief • 12 mo; 6 mo	• >80% pain relief
Gulur et al,[116] 2014 (n = 3) CR	ACNES	• TAP block • N/A • Lidocaine 1% and triamcinolone 40 mg • Single for 1 patient; series for the other 2 patients • Pain relief, functional status • 4 mo; 20 mo; 2 mo	• Pain relief, functional status
Imajo,[117] 2016 (n = 1) CR	ACNES	• TAP + rectus sheath block • N/A • Mepivacaine 0.5% • Single • NRS • None	• NRS improvement from 4 to 0

(continued on next page)

Table 2
(continued)

First Author, Year, Number of Patients, Type of Study	Pain Syndrome	Ultrasound-Guided Intervention (Block/Neurolysis/RFA), Comparator, Injectate, Blocks (Single/Series), Outcomes Measured, FU Time Points	Outcomes
QL			
Fernandez,[103] 2020 (n = 4) CS	Hip OA	• Nerve block • N/A • LA + DXM • Single • NRS • 6 mo	• NRS: significant decrease up to 6 mo
Carvalho et al,[104] 2017 (n = 1) CR	NP postabdominal hernia repair	• Nerve block • N/A • LA + MP • Single • NRS • 6 mo	• Immediate postprocedural pain relief. • At 6 mo: still significant reduction in allodynia without compromising the quality of life.
Rectus sheath block			
None			
PECS1, PECS2, serratus plane			
Fujii et al,[130] 2019 (n = 80) RCT	Postmastectomy pain	• PEC2 block • SPB • Ropi 0.5% 30 mLs • single • NRS, incidence chronic pain • 6 mo	• Immediate post-procedure NRS similar in both groups • At 6 mo: PEC2 significantly reduced the rate of patients in moderate/severe pain compared to serratus block (10% vs 33% *P* = .03, adjusted odds ratio (95% CI) 0.23 (0.07–0.80), *P* = .02. • At 6 mo: proportion of painfree patients 25% vs 48% (serratus vs PEC2) *P* = .06, adjusted OR (95% CI) 2.9 (1.1–7.5), *P* = .03 • At 6 mo: QoL was similar in both groups

Zocca et al,[131] 2016 (n = 8) CS	Postmastectomy pain	• SPB • N/A • 0.25% BUP + MP • Single • NRS • 12 wk	• Immediate pain relief in 8/8 patients from 25% to 100%. • Range of duration of pain relief: 2 d to 12 wk
Sir et al,[132] 2019 (n = 1) CR	Intercostal neuralgia	• SPB • N/A • LA + steroid • Series • VAS • 6 mo	• At 1 mo after 1st injection: VAS 2/10 • After 2nd injection: no pain until 6 mo
Takimoto et al,[133] 2016 (n = 1) CR	Postmastectomy pain	• SPB • N/A • LA • Series • NRS • 11 mo	• VAS 10 of 10 vs 6/10 vs 4 of 10 (baseline vs after first block vs second block) • Patient did not require further intervention in the remaining 11 mo follow-up period
Bawany et al,[134] 2020 (n = 1) CR	Postmastectomy pain	• PEC1 & PEC2 • N/A • 0.25% BUP + DMX • Single • NRS/ROM • 4 mo	• NRS baseline 8 of 10 • NRS at 24 h: 0 of 10 • ROM: 70% improvement up to 4 mo
Erector spinae block			
Piraccini et al,[150] 2020 (n = 1) CR	Postmastectomy pain syndrome	• ESPB • N/A • BUP + TC • Series • NRS • 3 mo	• Baseline NRS: 10 of 10 • At 7 d after first block: 8 of 10 • At 7 d after second block: 5 of 10 • At 3 mo: 2 of 10 • Stop of intake of analgesics up to 3 mo

(*continued on next page*)

Table 2
(continued)

First Author, Year, Number of Patients, Type of Study	Pain Syndrome	Ultrasound-Guided Intervention (Block/Neurolysis/RFA), Comparator, Injectate, Blocks (Single/Series), Outcomes Measured, FU Time Points	Outcomes
Hasoon et al,[148] 2020 (n = 1) CR	Postmastectomy pain syndrome	• ESPB • N/A • 0.25% BUP + MP • Single • NRS • 3 mo	• Immediately after procedure: NRS 0 of 10 • At 1 mo: NRS reduction 70% and opioid usage reduction 50% • At 3 mo: continued pain relief and significant improvement in her QOL
Rispoli et al,[149] 2019 (n = 5) CS	Thoracic spinal tumor-related pain	• ESPB • N/A • 0.25% BUP + DMP • Single • VAS • 1 mo	• At 1 mo: significant difference in pain scores: range 0–7 of 10
Abdominal cutaneous nerve block			
Chrona,[113] 2013 (n = 1) CR	ACNES	• Abdominal cutaneous nerve block • N/A • Lidocaine 1% initial block; subsequent blocks TC 20 mg + ropivicaine 0.2% • Series • NRS • 2 mo	• Immediately after first procedure: NRS 0 of 10 • Patient had 4 consecutive blocks (2 with TC) every ~7–10 d. • At 2 mo: NRS 2 to 10

Jacobs et al,[111] 2021 (n = 117) RCT	ACNES	• Abdominal cutaneous nerve block • Freehand technique • Lidocaine 1% • Series • NRS • Immediate, 6 wk, 3 mo	• No significantly different rate of successful responses between US and freehand group • No significantly different rate of successful responses (defined as proportion of injections yielding >50% reduction in pain) between the time immediately after the injection regimen compared with 3 mo postblock • Subcutaneous tissue thickness was not found to influence the rate of successful blocks
Kanakarajan et al,[115] 2011 (n = 9) CS	ACNES	• Abdominal cutaneous nerve block • N/A • Bupivacaine 0.5% + TC 40 mg • Single • NRS • 12 wk	• 6 responders with >50% pain relief

Abbreviations: ACNES, anterior cutaneous nerve entrapment syndrome; CI, confidence interval; CS, case series; CR, case report; DPM, depomedrol; DXM, dexamethasone; ESPB, erector spinae plane block; FU, follow-up; GA, general anesthetic; MP, methylprednisone; N/A, not applicable; NP, not provided; OA, osteoarthritis; PECS, pectoralis nerve; QL, quadratus lumborum; QOL, quality of life; RSB, rectus sheath block; TC, triamcinolone; TPI, trigger point injections.

Evidence and indications for ultrasound

We found 10 papers on the use of USG TAP block for chronic abdominal wall pain (CAWP) (2 RCT, 2 observational trial, 1 case series, 5 case reports) (**Table 2**).[80,89] There is significant heterogeneity in terms of technique, volume of injectate, and pain indication. One RCT investigated the effect of TAP block in prevention of CAWP after robotic partial nephrectomy compared with placebo. At 3 and 6 months postsurgery, the incidence of CAWP in the TAP group was lower than that in the comparator group.[80] Moeschler and colleagues[81] compared US TAP block versus US trigger point injections in 60 patients with CAWP. At 3 months follow-up, the TAP block group showed significantly lower pain scores.[81] In a prospective trial of 54 patients with chronic abdominal pain secondary to chronic pancreatitis, Niraj and Kamel[82] concluded that US-TAP block with steroids was effective in managing myofascial pain up to 6 months postprocedure. However, there was only limited and short-lasting effect of 2 to 3 weeks on the visceral pain component. The investigators concluded that TAP block is ineffective in providing pain relief of the ongoing pancreatic inflammation process, but can help with the myofascial pain component.[82]

A small case series of 5 patients with CAWP following surgery received TAP blocks with LA and steroid. Although 4 patients had 50% or more pain relief postprocedure, only 2 patients maintained pain relief up to 12 months follow-up.[83]

A retrospective series on 92 patients with chronic abdominal pain receiving TAP blocks with steroids showed significant improvement in abdominal pain scores up to 3 months.[84] Three case reports were published on the use of TAP neurolysis for cancer-related abdominal wall pain. All 3 patients showed sustained pain relief and less opioid requirement until time of death (up to 2 months).[85–87,89] One case reported on neurolytic TAP block combined with rectus sheath neurolysis for intractable gastrostomy pain in a patient with cancer, who had significant pain relief for over 4 months.[88] Finally, 1 case report documented on use of TAP block in 2 patients with anterior cutaneous nerve entrapment syndrome (ACNES) with 6 to 12 months of pain relief.[89]

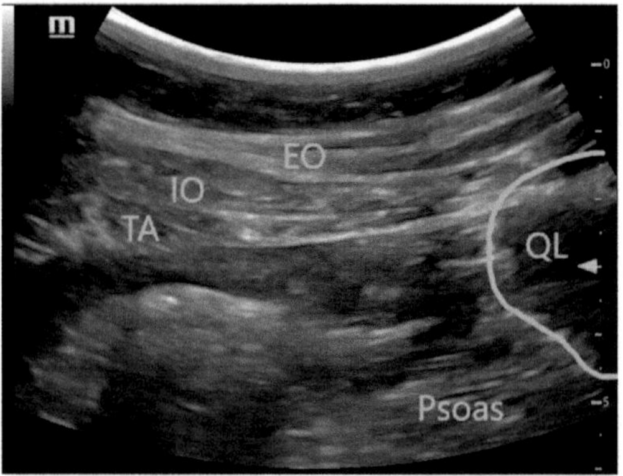

Fig. 10. Ultrasound image for quadratus lumborum block. The technique consists of an in-plane, anterior-to-posterior needle trajectory. For the lateral QLB, LA is deposited at the lateral border of the QL muscle, after penetrating the transversus abdominis aponeurosis.EO, external oblique muscle; IO, internal oblique muscle; QL, quadratus lumborum; TA, transversus abdominis muscle.

Complications and safety

Complications from USG TAP blocks are rare. Studies have demonstrated that the use of US reduces the incidence of inadvertent peritoneal placement of the needle.[90] Despite an improvement in the accuracy of block placement using US, there has been a case report of liver injury after TAP block with US.[91] Based on several reviews, use of US is concluded to be superior to LMG techniques for TAP block and reduces risk of intraperitoneal injection.[92,93]

Summary

USG TAP blocks and neurolysis are superior in terms of safety compared with LMG techniques and offer effective analgesia to patients suffering from chronic abdominal wall pain. Based on anatomic and dye studies, it is likely that the most benefit will be observed with the subcostal approach. Based on the available evidence, the authors' recommendation for performing USG TAP block for chronic abdominal pain is grade A, high level of certainty.

Quadratus Lumborum Block

Anatomy and technique

The QLB was first developed by Blanco and colleagues[94] in 2007 as a posterior approach to the TAP block, which intended to resemble the original LMG technique using the triangle of Petit. This approach was further developed by El-Boghdadly and colleagues[95] and others and has resulted in multiple proposed injection sites, sometimes referred to as the *lateral*, *posterior*, and *anterior* approaches to the QLB, which refer to their position in relation to the quadratus lumborum muscle. Dye studies suggest possible spread posteriorly into the paravertebral or epidural space when injected in the QL plane offering it advantages over the TAP block and possibly more extensive craniocaudal spread.[96] It has been suggested that a posterior QLB provides the greatest coverage spreading from T7-L1. The lateral/posterior QLB technique is discussed in **Fig. 10**.

Evidence and indications for ultrasound

Although several RCTs have been performed that help inform our understanding of the usefulness of the USG QLB in the perioperative pain setting,[94,97–102] the evidence for USG QLB for chronic pain is scarce. Second, there is no consensus as to the optimal approach to the QLB and the lack of agreement is reflected in the heterogeneity of the existing studies.

The authors only found 2 case reports (see **Table 2**). One patient with chronic hip osteoarthritis pain received a QLB with LA and dexamethasone and showed significant pain decrease for more than 6 months.[103] Another patient with chronic postabdominal hernia repair pain got a bilateral QLB with LA and methylprednisone and had significant reduction in allodynia up to 6 months.[104]

Complications and safety

No studies have looked specifically at complications related to USG QLB, and the complication rate has been inferred from studies on TAP blocks, which may not accurately approximate the risk. In addition, as described earlier, because the term "QLB" refers to multiple different injection sites it is difficult to make an educated estimate of its general risk. It should be noted, however, that the branches of the lumbar arteries, which emerge from the abdominal aorta, travel laterally and posterior to the QL muscle. One case report has been published describing 2 cases of hematoma resulting from QLB.[105] However, the rate of complications in QLB is generally considered to be low based on the lack of reported adverse events.

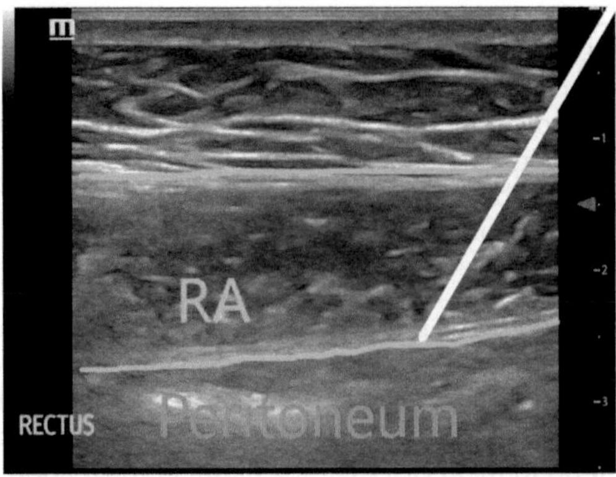

Fig. 11. Ultrasound anatomy of rectus abdominis sheath. With the patient in supine position, the probe is placed immediately lateral to the umbilicus in transverse position. The needle is inserted in an in-plane orientation, piercing through the anterior rectus sheath, and advanced through the body of muscle until the needle tip reaches the posterior rectus sheath (*white line*). The spread of LA should be visualized in the sheath and not inside the muscle. RA, rectus abdominis.

Summary

Although the bulk of evidence of USG QLB for perioperative pain setting, the indication for USG QLB for chronic pain is less established. There are no concerns in terms of safety. The authors rate the current evidence for USG QLB I. The USG QLB can be selectively offered to individual patients based on professional judgment.

Rectus Sheath Block

Anatomy and technique

Rectus sheath blocks (RSB) provide cutaneous analgesia to the midline anterior abdominal wall. The RSB was first described by Schleich in 1899 who targeted the ventral rami of the seventh to twelfth intercostal nerves by injecting LA in the potential space between the rectus abdominus muscles and the posterior aspect of the rectus sheath.[106] With the advent of US, the preferred approach to this block is to inject in the most lateral aspect of the rectus abdominus muscle to avoid injuring the deep inferior epigastric artery, which runs in the muscle belly and is often difficult to visualize even with US. Because this block is performed in the compartment of the rectus abdominus sheath it is expected to have its effects predominantly in the medial most aspects of the abdominal wall[106] (**Fig. 11**).

Evidence and indications for ultrasound

Based on a review by Abrahams and colleagues,[92] there are only few trials that have investigated the efficacy of RSB. However, the limited literature comparing outcomes in USG and LMG injections gives strong support for the use of US.[92] These trials, however, were on perioperative abdominal pain but showed significant decrease in postoperative pain and analgesic intake.[106–109] The authors did not find any literature in chronic pain setting.

Complications and safety

The limited number of studies on RSB did not identify any adverse events.

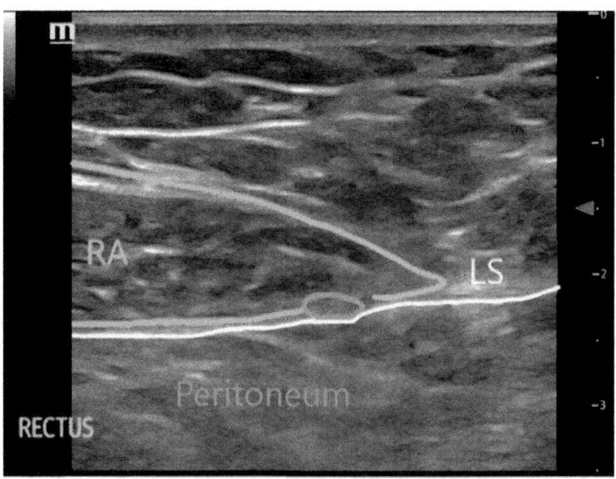

Fig. 12. Ultrasound image of ACNES block. The anterior cutaneous nerve travels in the transversus abdominis plane in the flank and then passes through the linea semilunaris (LS) under the rectus abdominis (RA) in the same fascial plane. The nerve is seen as a swelling in the fascia that enters the deep portion of the lateral rectus abdominis and then passes through the muscle to become superficial. Upon identification of the abdominal cutaneous nerve, a sterile spinal needle (typically 22G, 1.5-inch long) should be advanced in the longitudinal view toward the targeted nerve. A preliminary test of 0.5 mL should be injected to confirm solution spread around the nerve, followed by volume of up to 3 mL to obtain uniform vertical spread of solution within the musculature.

Summary

Although literature on the use of RSB for perioperative abdominal pain looks promising, there are no data on the use of RSB for chronic pain treatment. The available evidence for recommending RSB for chronic pain is I, insufficient.

Anterior Cutaneous Nerve Entrapment Syndrome Block

Anatomy and technique

ACNES refers to the severe, refractory chronic pain stemming from entrapment of the cutaneous branches of the lower thoracoabdominal intercostal nerves, typically T8-T12, at the lateral border of the rectus abdominis muscle.[110] Anatomically, innervation of the rectus abdominis muscle begins during the embryonic stage, when segmental myotomes polymerize to form the rectus abdominis muscle and are innervated by 8 separate neurovascular bundles originating from the T5-T12 thoracic vertebra.[111] Each somatic nerve includes 3 branches: a dorsal branch that innervates the back muscles and lateral and ventral branches that together innervate the abdominal wall muscles.[112] Superficial to this, the skin overlying the abdominal wall is supplied with sensory innervation from the lower 6 intercostal nerves (T7-T12). Importantly, these branches are termed the *anterior cutaneous intercostal nerve* branches and run through subcutaneous fascia to terminate at the skin. Furthermore, each nerve has specific anchoring points: at the spinal cord where the posterior and lateral branch take off, at the opening to the rectus muscle channel where the nerve turns sharply, at where the nerve passes through the anterior rectus sheath, and at the skin. When viewed from a cephalad to caudad direction, the lower thoracoabdominal intercostal nerves course between the internal oblique and transversus abdominus muscles, but upon reaching the rectus abdominis they make a sharp turn to enter 1 of 5 rectus channels, typically one per T8-T12. It has been postulated that the acute angle of this turn is responsible for the nerve entrapment that causes the symptoms of ACNES. Support for this anatomic theory stems from the observation that ACNES pain is often exacerbated by abdominal muscle contraction, because this would further entrap the lower thoracoabdominal intercostal nerves.[113]

Various US techniques have been used to treat ACNES; the most common is discussed in **Fig. 12**.

Evidence and indications for ultrasound

A 2021 multicenter nonblinded RCT compared ACNES between USG abdominal wall infiltration and a freehand technique in 117 patients. After 4 injections at 2-week intervals, patients were followed up at 6 weeks and 3 months postblock. The investigators did not find a significantly different rate of successful responses (defined as >50% reduction in pain per NRS) neither between the US and freehand group nor between the time immediately after the injection regimen and 3 months postblock. Subcutaneous tissue thickness was also not found to influence the rate of successful blocks.[111]

A 2013 case report found that in a 37-year-old woman who had undergone an elective myomectomy complicated by intractable pain (mean NRS of 8 of 10), she had complete pain relief after 30 minutes postinjection. Pain reoccurred after 1.5 days, and the block was repeated 4 more times every 7 to 10 days with pain relief progressively longer than the previous one so that after 2 months of therapy the patient had significant pain relief to a mean NRS of 2 of 10.[114]

A 2011 case series found that among 9 patients with ACNES who had been treated with USG abdominal cutaneous nerve injections with a median follow-up of 12 weeks, 6 responders reported at least 50% pain relief.[115]

Alternatively, there have also been limited case reports on the TAP block as a treatment option for ACNES (see section Transversus Abdominus Plane Block). One 2015 case report achieved greater than 80% pain relief in 2 patients with a TAP block injection of ropivacaine 0.375% and methylprednisolone 20 mg.[89] The postulated mechanism for the block's success was the proximity of the block to the rectus muscle, which theoretically allowed the injectate to diffuse to the adjacent site of nerve entrapment. Another group of investigators applied the same approach in the pediatric population in a case series of 3 pediatric patients with ACNES aged between 15 and 16 years. Although their injectate differed in that the investigators used 1% lidocaine 2 to 4 mL and triamcinolone 40 mg, they also saw improvement in pain relief and functional status in all 3 patients.[116] In 2016, a case report applied the TAP block in conjunction with an RSB and TAP block in a patient with bilateral ACNES. The investigators achieved significant pain relief with 0.5% mepivacaine, notably without the addition of corticosteroid.[117]

Complications and safety

USG abdominal cutaneous nerve block is a safe technique in the treatment of ACNES. In fact, blind injections have been associated with adverse events including unintended injection into the peritoneal cavity.[112] For this reason, USG treatment of ACNES is a preferred technique to blind injection for its favorable safety profile.[113] TAP blocks have a similar safety profile, with prior case reports not encountering adverse outcomes. Notably, in the pediatric population the injectate solution must be delivered at the minimum quantity possible to achieve symptomatic relief.[116]

Summary

Based on the available evidence, the authors' recommendation for USG ACN block for ACNES treatment is grade C, moderate level of certainty. Although one 2021 RCT has been performed in comparing US versus freehand technique, no significant differences were seen in technique. Additional RCTs with a larger sample size are needed

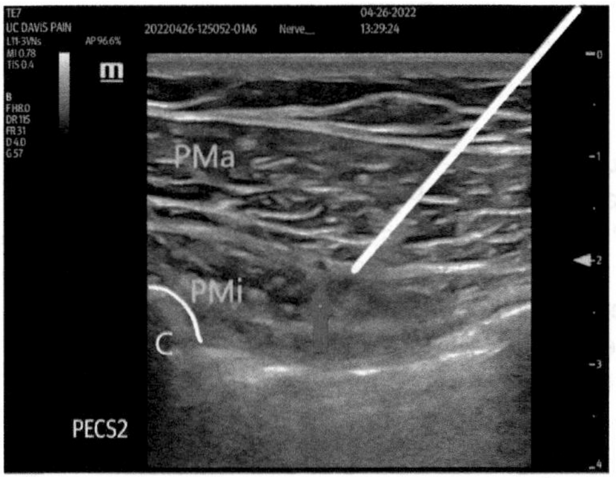

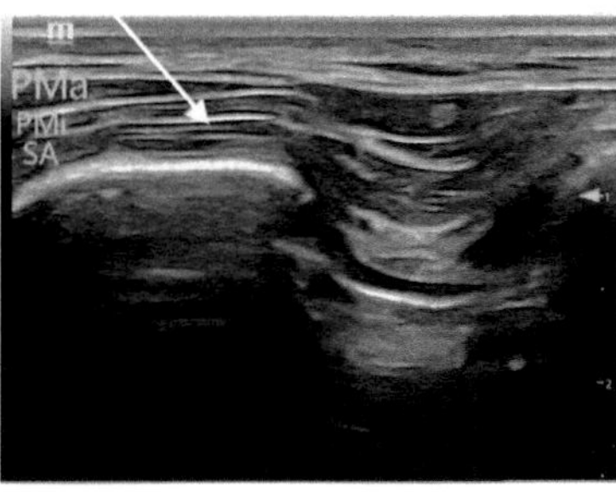

Fig. 13. PEC block and serratus anterior block. The patient should be in a supine position with the ipsilateral arm abducted to 90°. For PECS I block, a linear US transducer is placed in the parasagittal plane below the clavicle and pectoralis major and minor muscles are identified. The axillary vessels are also identified, as are the ribs and the underlying pleura. The lower end of the transducer is rotated toward the axilla and 10 to 20 mL LA is injected between the 2 pectoral muscles near the pectoral branch of the thoracoacromial artery (*red arrow*). For a PECS II block another 15 mL is injected deep to the pectoral minor muscle in the fascial plane between it and the serratus anterior muscle (*white arrow*). C, coracoid; PMa, pectoralis major; PMi, pectoralis minor; SA, serratus anterior.

to establish superiority of USG treatment of ACNES including USG abdominal cutaneous nerve block, TAP block, and RSB over other treatment modalities.

Pectoralis and Serratus plane nerve blocks

Anatomy and block technique

The technical challenges, adverse effects, and potential catastrophic complications of thoracic epidural and paravertebral blocks led to the development of a safer alternative for providing analgesia to the upper anterior chest wall. The first description of the PECS block by Blanco[118] in 2011 (later termed the *PECS1* block) described injection of LA in the plane between the pectoralis major and minor muscles and adjacent to the thoracoacromial artery. Although providing some analgesia for breast surgery, this approach did not offer complete cutaneous coverage of the axilla or chest wall and so was modified to involve a second injection more lateral to the first in the interfascial plane between the pectoralis minor and serratus anterior muscles, termed the *PECS2 block.*[119] After detailed evaluation of the spread of dye in this plane, Blanco and colleagues[120] further refined the optimal injection site to be superficial to the serratus anterior muscle, which produced intercostal spread and was referred to as the *serratus plane block* (SPB). In the initial characterization of these blocks the investigators reported good analgesia with both single-shot injections and continuous infusions. The utility of these blocks has subsequently been evaluated in several randomized controlled studies, most of which initially focused on breast surgery, but more recent studies have also investigated the use of PECS blocks for analgesia in cardiothoracic surgery, and chest wall trauma.

The PECS I block is an interpectoral injection of LA to target the medial and lateral pectoral nerves (**Fig. 13**), and the PECS II block is a combination of interpectoral (PECS I) and subpectoral injections that additionally target lateral cutaneous branches of intercostal nerves, long thoracic nerves, and thoracodorsal nerves (see **Fig. 11**B).

Thus, it is reasonable to perform PECS1 and either PECS2 or a serratus anterior plane block (see **Fig. 13**) whenever trying to achieve coverage of the entire anterolateral chest wall or axilla.

Evidence and indications for ultrasound

Most studies have used a combination of USG PECS1 and SPBs. Because the anatomic differences between the PECS2 and SPB is relatively small, most studies do not differentiate between these 2 approaches. In fact, Blanco and colleagues [118] recommended injection both deep and superficial to the serratus anterior muscle whenever performing these blocks, effectively performing a PECS2 and SPB with 1 needle pass. Although the nomenclature is not consistent, PECS1 with SPB is sometimes referred to as the *PECS block*. There is a lot of evidence on the use of PEC blocks for perioperative pain after breast and thoracic surgery and thoracic trauma.[121–130] The literature on PEC block for chronic pain is mostly in the setting of postmastectomy pain. The authors have found 5 papers[130–134] (see **Table 2**). In 1 RCT comparing PEC2 block versus SPB, more patients of the PEC 2 group had reduction of their moderate to severe pain compared with the serratus group (33% vs 10%, $P = .03$) and PEC2 block reduced the incidence of chronic pain at 6 months postoperatively compared with the comparator group.[130]

The rest of the literature spans 1 case series and 2 case reports with a total of 10 patients with postmastectomy pain and intercostal neuralgia receiving 1 or 2 SPBs with LA with or without steroid (see **Table 2**). All patients had significant pain relief, and the duration of effect ranged from 2 days to 11 months.[131–133] One patient had 70% pain relief and improved mobility up to 4 months after combined PEC I and II block and trigger points for postmastectomy pain.[134]

Complications and safety

There have been no studies directly addressing the complication rate of USG PECS blocks. In the meta-analysis by Lovett-Carter and colleagues,[127] 3 of the 458 patients had hematoma and/or bleeding following a USG PECS block, which suggests an incidence of 0.7% (0.1% to 2.0%). Another safety consideration for breast surgery is that a subpectoral block will potentially anesthetize the long thoracic nerve, which may

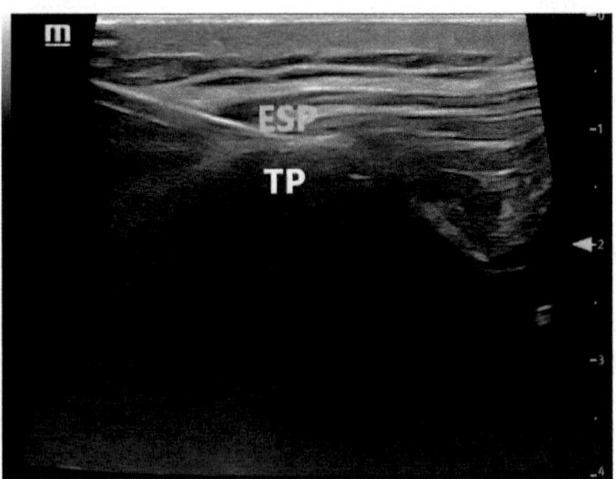

Fig. 14. Sonoanatomy of the ESPB. The probe is positioned 3 cm lateral to the T5 spinous process (TP). Needle is advanced in cephalad-to-caudad direction through trapezius, rhomboid major muscle, and erector spinae muscle (ESP) until contact with TP. Injection of LA results in spread beneath the ESP.

lead to increased incidence of nerve injury during axillary dissection if the surgeon is unable to locate the nerve (usually via electrical stimulation).[135] Finally, there has been 1 case report published of pneumothorax following US-guided serratus plane.[136]

Summary

Multiple 1b level RCTs suggest that USG PECS blocks offer excellent anterior chest wall coverage for a variety of breast surgeries. The evidence for use of PECs and SPBs for patients with posttraumatic neuropathies of the chest wall looks promising but is limited. The recommendation is grade C, moderate level of certainty.

Erector Spinae Plane Block

Anatomy and technique

The erector spinae plane block (ESPB) was initially described in 2016 as a treatment of thoracic neuropathic pain in 2 patients and for postoperative analgesia in 2 other patients undergoing video-assisted thoracoscopic surgery.[137] The investigators injected 20 mL LA in the plane between the erector spinae and rhomboid muscles 3 cm lateral to the T5 spinous process at the level of the transverse process. The injections resulted in multidermatomal spread with cutaneous coverage extending to the anterior chest wall and included the axilla and medial aspect of the inner arm. The injections also resulted in resolution of the patients' neuropathic pain and provided profound analgesia. Although these initial injections were performed superficial to the erector spinae muscle, the investigators concluded that the optimal injection site is deep to the muscle because an injection here would deposit the medicine closer to the dorsal and ventral rami of the spinal nerve roots. Furthermore, they suggested that using the transverse process as a backstop to the injection serves as an easily identifiable sonographic LM and provides additional safety during performance of the block. Since this first description of the ESPB there have been several studies that have explored the utility of this block for a variety of procedures; however, large RCTs are still lacking. The technique is described in **Fig. 14**.

Evidence and indications for ultrasound

The initial dye study performed in cadavers using 20 mL solution injected at the T5 level resulted in C7-T8 craniocaudal spread in what the investigators described as a paraspinous gutter bounded by the transverse process anteriorly and the erector spinae muscles posteriorly. Lateral spread was to the tips of the transverse processes at all levels, and dissection of the cadavers showed medial spread to the vicinity of the dorsal and ventral rami of the spinal nerve roots. A subsequent cadaver dye study by Ivanusic and colleagues[138] in 2018 confirmed extensive cephalocaudal spread; however, this study failed to show the same medial spread.

A handful of small RCTs has lent support that USG ESPB may offer good analgesia for wide scope of thoracic, cardiac, or spine surgeries.[139–147] The literature on chronic pain is limited to 2 case reports and 1 case series (total of 7 patients) with postmastectomy or thoracic spine tumor-related pain receiving single[148,149] or series[150] of ESPB with LA and steroid.[148–150] (see **Table 2**). Most patients had sustained pain relief that lasted 1 to 3 months with reduced analgesic intake.

Complications and safety

A pooled analysis examining 242 cases of ESPB revealed no adverse effects including no cases of hemodynamic effects.[151] Only 1 adverse outcome has been reported from ESPB—a pneumothorax after an ESPB single injection at T4 that required chest tube drainage.[152] No other adverse outcomes including bleeding have been reported. In fact, it is hypothesized that the position of the block lateral

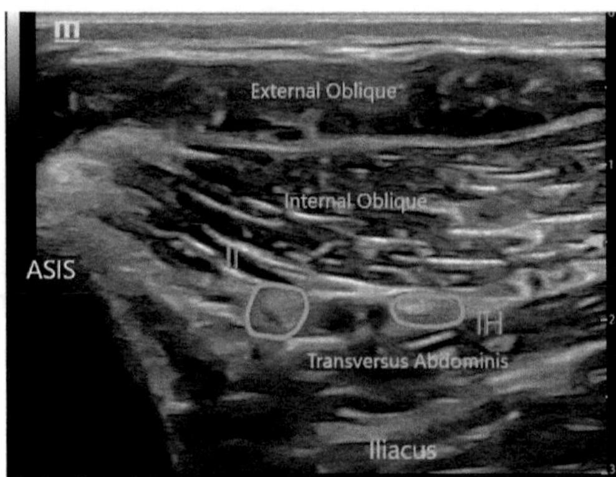

Fig. 15. Ultrasound image of the ilioinguinal (II) and iliohypogastric (IH) nerves between the internal oblique and transverse abdominis muscles at the anterior superior iliac spine. The IL and HN are the 2 blue circles. Block technique is similar to TAP technique.

to the paravertebral and epidural spaces and in a plane with a large capacity make it less susceptible to the risks of epidural hematoma or neuraxial injury. Thus, many propose that it is a potential "safe" alternative to epidural analgesia in patients with altered hemostasis; however, studies have been limited to case reports and case series. Galacho and colleagues[153] performed ESPB in 5 patients in the intensive care unit with coagulopathy (either elevated INR/PTT, thrombocytopenia, or anticoagulation) and none developed neurologic or hemorrhagic complications during a 5-day postblock surveillance.

Summary

The multidermatomal spread of dye seen in cadaver studies suggests that the ESPB has the potential to offer excellent pain for perioperative and chronic thoracic pain. The literature on chronic pain literature is limited but suggests analgesic effect. The recommendation is grade C, low level of certainty.

Ilioinguinal and Iliohypogastric Nerve Blocks

Anatomy and technique

The IHN innervates the transversus abdominis, rectus abdominis, pyramidal, and abdominal oblique muscles.[154] The branches of the IHN include the anterior cutaneous branch innervating the skin of the hypogastric region, the lateral cutaneous branch innervating the skin of the buttock area, and the genital branch innervating the skin over the pubic region and scrotum in males and labia majora in females. The ILN innervates the abdominal wall and branches into the anterior scrotal or labial nerve (innervating the skin over the anterior scrotum or labia majora), and cutaneous branches (innervating the skin over the medial thigh, hypogastric area, and buttock).[154] The IHN courses from the proximal and lateral border of the psoas major, and then crosses obliquely anterior to the quadratus lumborum toward the iliac crest. The IHN perforates the transversus abdominis muscle and ultimately branches between the transversus abdominis and internal oblique muscles.[154] The ILN traces a parallel course to the IHN from the proximal and lateral border of the psoas major muscle, exiting below the IHN, and perforating the transversus abdominis muscle closer to the iliac crest.[154] The ILN and IHN often communicate between the transversus abdominis and internal oblique muscles, which likely contributes to the overlapping sensory innervation between the 2 nerves. Even with LA volumes of 0.9 mL, LA spread

Table 3
Overview of literature of ultrasound-guided pelvic nerve blocks

First author, Year, Number of Patients, Type of Study	Pain Syndrome, Age (Mean + SD)	Ultrasound-Guided Intervention (Block/Neurolysis/RFA), Comparator, Injectate, Blocks (Single/Series), Outcomes Measured, FU Time Points	Outcomes
IL/IH block			
Bishoff et al,[157] 2012 (n = 24) RCT	Ilioinguinal postherniorrhaphy pain	• Nerve blocks • Healthy controls • LA 10 mL or 10 mL saline • Single • NRS & QST • 6 mo	• 1 Of 12 patients: lidocaine responder • 6 Of 12: nonresponder • 5 Of 12: placebo responder • No consistent QST changes observed after lidocaine block • Investigators concluded IHNB not useful for management
Gofeld & Christakis[158] 2006 (n = 8) CS	Ilioinguinal neuralgia	• Nerve block • N/A • LA 5 mL • Single • NRS • N/A	• All patients had sensory block at inguinal area postblock • In 63.5% of patients, diagnosis of ilioinguinal neuralgia was established, and achieved pain relief at several days • Others had no pain relief despite anesthesia of the corresponding area
Trainor et al,[159] 2015 (n = 36) R	Ilioinguinal postherniorrhaphy pain	• Nerve block • US vs LM • NP • Single • VAS • NP	• Mean baseline VAS: 7.08 of 10 vs 7 of 10 (LM vs US) • 50% pain reduction: 70% vs 77% (LM vs US) $P = 1.0$ • No significant VAS reduction between groups

(*continued on next page*)

Table 3
(continued)

First author, Year, Number of Patients, Type of Study	Pain Syndrome, Age (Mean + SD)	Ultrasound-Guided Intervention (Block/Neurolysis/RFA), Comparator, Injectate, Blocks (Single/Series), Outcomes Measured, FU Time Points	Outcomes
Thomassen et al,[160] 2013 (n = 43) R	Ilioinguinal postherniorrhaphy pain	• Nerve block • Nerve stimulator (NSG) • LA + steroid • Single • VAS, HADS, PDI • NP	• Median baseline VAS: 5 of 10 (rest), 7 of 10 (activity) • Postblock: Median VAS at rest: 3.2 vs 5.8 (NSG vs USG) $P = .005$ Median VAS activity: 4.8 vs 7.0 (NSG vs USG) $P = .033$
Suresh et al,[162] 2008 (n = 2) CR	Ilioinguinal neuralgia	• IINB • N/A • 3–5 mL bupivacaine 0.25% • 2 blocks (1 mo apart) • VAS • 6 mo	• Patient 1: pain reduction from VAS 8 of 10–2 of 10 for 3 mo. After second block, complete pain relief for > 6 mo • Patient 2: pain free after 1 block for > 6 mo
Lee et al,[164] 2019 (n = 10) CS	Ilioinguinal neuralgia	• Microwave ablation • N/A • N/A • Single • VAS • 12 mo	• Mean baseline pain 6.1 of 10 • Significantly reduced VAS at 1, 6, 12 mo • At 12 mo: 83% of patients had average of 69% ± 31% pain reduction • No complication
Cho et al,[161] 2017 (n = 1) CR	Ilioinguinal neuralgia postherniorrhaphy	• Nerve block • N/A • LA + TC • NRS • 60 d	• Pain relief for at least 60 d

Sivashanmugam et al,[163] 2013 (n = 1) CR	Ilioinguinal postherniorrhaphy pain	• Chemical neurolysis • N/A • Ethyl alcohol 1 mL at each nerve	• Complete pain relief for first week, only 25% pain relief thereafter until week 4. • Followed by surgical neurectomy
Thapa et al,[165] 2016 (n = 1) CR	Ilioinguinal postherniorrhaphy pain	• pRFA • N/A • 8 min at 42°C • Single • VAS	• Improved quality of life at 9 mo follow-up
Adler et al,[167] 2014 (n = 1) CR	Ilioinguinal neuralgia	• Cryoablation • N/A • N/A • Single • VAS • 4 wk	• Complete pain relief for 4 wk • Patient got referred for surgical excision of nerve
Carayannopoulos et al,[168] 2009 (n = 2) CR	Ilioinguinal neuralgia	• Trial of peripheral neurostimulation • N/A • N/A • N/A • VAS • 7 d	• Both patient had positive nerve block with LA • Both patient had positive trial: pain free at day 7 of trial
Elahi et al,[169] 2015 (n = 3) CS	Ilioinguinal postherniorrhaphy pain	• Peripheral neurostimulation • N/A • N/A • Single • NRS • 12 mo	• Signficant pain relief at 12 mo follow-up
Alici et al,[166] 2019 (n = 1) CR		• pRFA • N/A • 12 min at 42°C • Single • VAS • 6 mo	• Significant pain relief up to 6 mo

(*continued on next page*)

Table 3
(*continued*)

First author, Year, Number of Patients, Type of Study	Pain Syndrome, Age (Mean + SD)	Ultrasound-Guided Intervention (Block/Neurolysis/RFA), Comparator, Injectate, Blocks (Single/Series), Outcomes Measured, FU Time Points	Outcomes
GF block			
Hetta,[173] 2018 (n = 70) RCT	Chronic postsurgical orchialgia	• pRFA • Sham • N/A • single • VAS, GPE, reduction analgesics • 3 mo	• Reduction of analgesic intake: 50% vs 3.3% (PRF vs sham) • Significant reduction in mean VAS at 2,4, 6, 8,12 wk in PRF group compared with sham (P = .001) • Significant improvement GPE (PRF vs sham)
Shanthanna,[174] 2014 (n = 1) CS	Genitofemoral neuralgia	• Nerve block • N/A • LA + Depo medrol • blocks (1 mo apart) • NRS • 12 mo	• Baseline mean NRS 8 of 10 • After first block: NRS 4 of 10 for 3 mo • After second block: NRS 4 of 10 for 6 mo
Terkawi and Romdhane,[175] 2014 (n = 1) CR	Orchialgia	• pRFA • N/A • N/A • single • VAS • 7 mo	• At 7 mo: VAS 0 of 10 at rest and activity
Campos et al,[176] 2009 (n = 1) CR	Genitofemoral neuralgia	• Cryoablation • N/A • N/A • NRS • 2 mo	Pain-free at 2 mo follow-up

LFCN block			
Hurdle et al,[184] 2007 (n = 10) R	Meralgia paresthetica	• Nerve block • N/A • LA 2–10 • Series • Sensory • 30 min	• 100% success rate in US-guided blockage of the LFCN in all patients with all volumes of LA
Tagliafico et al,[185] 2011 (n = 20) CS	Lateral femoral cutaneous neuropathy	• Nerve block • N/A • LA + MP • Single • VAS • 2 mo	• Symptoms in 80% of patients diminished progressively after the first week. Remaining patients required a further perineural injection • VAS pain baseline: 8.1 ± 2.1, VAS QOL baseline: 6.9 ± 3.2 • VAS pain at 2 mo: 2.1 ± 0.5; t = 6.2; $P < .001$) VAS QOL at 2 mo: 2.3 ± 2.5 (t = 5.3; $P < .002$)
Khodair et al,[186] 2014 (n = 25) CS	Meralgia paresthetica	• Nerve block • N/A • LA + steroid • Series • VAS • NP	• Baseline VAS was mild in 3 patients, moderate in 10, severe in 12 • Successful pain relief was achieved in 24 of 25 patients in maximum 3 blocks • 3 of 25: 1 block, 6 of 25: 2 blocks, 16 of 24: 3 blocks

(*continued on next page*)

Table 3
(continued)

First author, Year, Number of Patients, Type of Study	Pain Syndrome, Age (Mean + SD)	Ultrasound-Guided Intervention (Block/Neurolysis/RFA), Comparator, Injectate, Blocks (Single/Series), Outcomes Measured, FU Time Points	Outcomes
Klauser[187] 2016 (n = 20) 12 mo 1b	Meralgia paresthestica	• Nerve block • LA + steroid • Series • VAS • 12 mo	• At 6 wk: 16 of 20 had residual pain and had repeated block • At 1 y: 15 of 20 still had significant pain relief: mean VAS reduction of 82 of 100 ($P < .0001$) with mean of 2 injections 5 of 20 had partial relief: mean VAS reduction of 50 of 100 with mean of 3 injections ($P < .01$)
Chen et al,[192] 2012 (n = 1) CR	Meralgia paresthetica	• Neurolysis • N/A • Alcohol • Single • VAS/functional activity • 6 mo	• Prolonged pain relief (VAS 1–2 of 10) at 6 mo follow-up • Return of ability to ambulate and perform daily activity
Kilic,[182] 2020 (n = 54) RCT	Meralgia paresthetica	• Nerve block • TENS vs sham-TENS • LA + steroid • Single • VAS • 1 mo	• Significant decrease in VAS at 1 mo compared with baseline in all groups • No significant difference in VAS between groups

Abbreviations: CR, case report; CS, case series; EMG, electromyography; FU; GF, genitofemoral; GPE, global perceived effect; HADS, Hospital Anxiety and Depression Scale; LFCN, lateral femoral cutaneous nerve; N/A, not applicable; NP, not provided; NSG, nerve stimulator guided; P, prospective observational study; PDI, pain disability index; QOL, quality of life; QST, quantitative sensory testing; R, retrospective observational study; TENS, transcutaneous electrical nerve stimulation.

from one nerve to the other can be directly visualized during 12% injections to the ILN or IHN, and the resulting skin anesthesia overlaps by 60.3%.[155] Thus, selective blockade of the ILN and IHN is not possible in the majority of cases.[139] The block technique is similar to the TAP block and described in **Fig. 15**.[31]

Evidence and indications for ultrasound

USG for iliohypogastric nerve blocks (ILHNB) likely improves efficacy through precision needle placement and deposition of LA. The traditional anatomic LM-based technique is limited by the variable course of the ILN and IHN in some individuals.

Compared with conventional USG, high-resolution USG (18 MHz vs 7–12 MHz) can identify the terminal branches of the ILN and IHN 60% of the time.[154] Also, distal-to-proximal scanning during high-resolution USG improves visualization of both the ILN and IHN.[154]

The use of USG for ILHNB has been studied in the context of patients undergoing open inguinal hernia repair, resulting in reduced intraoperative and postoperative analgesic requirements and a significant reduction of pain scores during hospital stay.[156]

Research pertaining specifically to the use of USG for the performance of ILHNB in the context of chronic pain is of moderate quality. The authors found 1 RCT, 2 retrospective chart reviews, 2 case series, and 1 case report (**Table 3**). Bischoff and colleagues[157] described a randomized, double-blind, placebo-controlled crossover study of 12 patients with chronic inguinal postherniorrhaphy pain and 12 healthy volunteers. All patients received USG ILHNB with 10 mL lidocaine or saline with administration of 5 mL around each nerve. Given the crossover, there was a washout period of 4 hours between the 2 blocks. Sensory mapping, functional pain tests, and quantitative sensory testing were completed immediately preceding each injection, and 20 minutes following each injection. The study was discontinued prematurely due to continued lack of analgesic efficacy. Only 1 of 12 patients demonstrated an increase in cool hypoesthesia after the lidocaine block compared with 10 of 12 healthy controls. Also, 6 patients were nonresponders to lidocaine and 5 patients were placebo responders. No consistent QST changes were noted among patients while the healthy volunteers demonstrated significantly decreased suprathreshold heat pain perception in the groin after lidocaine but not placebo nerve blocks. The investigators postulate the reasons for lack of analgesia among patients relating to communicating branches between nerves, more proximal nerve branches innervating the distal painful regions, and the GFN playing a greater role in postherniorrhaphy pain. Among the healthy controls, baseline quantitative sensory testing did not always include the areas of lidocaine-induced hypoesthesia implying that the ILN and IHN do not always innervate painful areas affected by postherniorrhaphy pain. Given these findings, the investigators did not recommend the use of US-guided lidocaine block of the ILN and IHN at the level of the ASIS for the diagnosis and management of postherniorrhaphy pain. The sequence of lidocaine and placebo administration may have potentially played a role in the lack of response to lidocaine. Initial administration of perineural saline may reduce the likelihood of subsequent lidocaine analgesia in an already edematous nerve. Without examination of administration order as a confounder, the implications of these study findings remain unclear. Gofeld and Christakis described a case series of successful USG ILNB in 8 patients with chronic inguinal pain and 1 patient scheduled for inguinal hernia repair. All patients demonstrated skin anesthesia in the corresponding inguinal area.[158] In contrast to the previously described RCT, Gofeld and colleagues report variations in anatomy with the IL nerve found between the external and internal oblique muscles, or lateral to the deep circumflex iliac artery. One patient required repeat injection due to a failed first attempt, with subsequent inguinal skin anesthesia. Future studies are needed to determine the incidence of skin anesthesia after USG ILNB and IHNB, and the optimal type and dose of LA needed for diagnosis.

In a retrospective chart review, Trainor and colleagues[159] compared 36 patients with chronic postherniorrhaphy groin pain receiving USG versus LMG ILHNB. Among 20 patients receiving the LM technique versus 16 patients receiving the US technique, no significant differences were found for reductions in VAS scores. Importantly, no complications were noted in either group. In contrast, a retrospective review of 43 adults with chronic inguinal postherniorrhaphy pain received either LM with nerve stimulator-guided ILHNB or USG ILHNB.[160] Interestingly, patients receiving USG blocks had significantly higher VAS scores (at rest and during activities), a higher proportion of moderate/severe pain, a higher proportion with daily pain, and higher incidence of depression and anxiety. Given this higher incidence of comorbid mood disorders, regression analyses are needed to account for these (and other) potential confounders. In addition, the analysis did not correct for multiple comparisons, and the results should be interpreted with caution.

The remaining literature spans case reports and small case series on USG blocks or (pulsed) RFA and peripheral neurostimulation and microwave nerve ablation with pain relief up to 12 months.[161–170]

Complications and safety

No major complications have been reported in the existing literature pertaining to these blocks.

Summary

There are insufficient data comparing the use of USG versus LMG ILNB and IHNB. There is uncertainty regarding the potential benefits and risks of USG, although research in patients undergoing surgery indicate the USG technique can be performed safely with minimal complications. The available evidence for recommending USG ILHNB for chronic pain is grade C, moderate level of certainty.

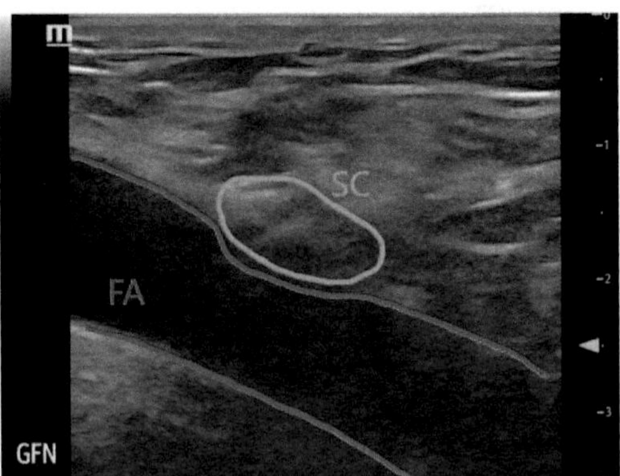

Fig. 16. Genital branch of the genitofemoral nerve. Probe position is perpendicular to the inguinal ligament and 1 finger breadth lateral to the pubic tubercle. The spermatic cord appears oval, and the testicular artery and artery to the vas deferens can be visualized through color Doppler. The vas deferens appears as a thick, noncompressible tubular structure within the spermatic cord. It is recommended to administer 5 mL LA inside and 5 mL outside of the spermatic cord. For females, start position is over infrainguinal region where femoral artery is visualized. Probe is then turned 90°, and the artery is traced cephalad until it dives deep where it transitions into the external iliac artery. At this point, the inguinal canal and its contents are seen superficially of the artery. FA, femoral artery; SC, spermatic cord.

Genitofemoral Nerve Block

Anatomy and technique

The GFN arises from the first and second lumbar nerves and has a long course running anterior to the psoas muscle continuing distally anterior to the common and external iliac arteries. Above the inguinal ligament, the nerve divides into the external spermatic (genital branch) and lumboinguinal (femoral branch) nerves.[171] The genital branch of the GFN passes through the inguinal ring terminating at the scrotum or labia majora. The femoral branch of the GFN passes underneath the inguinal ligament, enters the sheath of the femoral vasculature, and lies just superficial and lateral to the femoral artery. This branch supplies the anterior surface of the upper thigh.[171] Being prone to variations in anatomy, Rab and colleagues[171] describe 4 cutaneous branching patterns of the ILN and GFN. (1) The GFN may exclusively provide sensation to the scrotal/labial and ventromedial thigh regions; (2) the ILN may provide the majority of innervation to the region with only motor innervation of the cremaster muscle via the GFN; (3) the GFN may provide the majority of the innervation with sensory innervation of the mons pubis, inguinal crease, and anteroproximal root of the penis or labia majora provided by the ILN; or (4) innervation is split between the GFN and ILN.[171] Bellingham and Peng[172] initially reported the use of USG to block the genital branch of the GFN (**Fig. 16**).

Evidence and indications for ultrasound

The current literature on USG GFN block for chronic pain conditions is minimal (see **Table 3**). The authors found 1 relevant RCT, comparing USG pRFA of the ILN and genital branch of the GFN with a sham procedure among 70 patients with chronic postsurgical orchialgia.[173] Following the procedure, patients received variable doses of duloxetine, pregabalin, and tramadol. In the pRFA group, significantly more patients had greater than 50% pain reduction postprocedure and pain scores remained significantly lower up to 12 weeks. The administration of additional analgesics is a limitation to interpretation of the study findings. In addition, the investigators did not address any adverse effects in either treatment group.

The authors found additional 4 case reports. Shanthanna[174] described the case of USG selective ILN, IHN, and GFN blocks for managing groin pain after orchidectomy. Three case reports describe the use of pRFA of the genital branch of the GFN in an

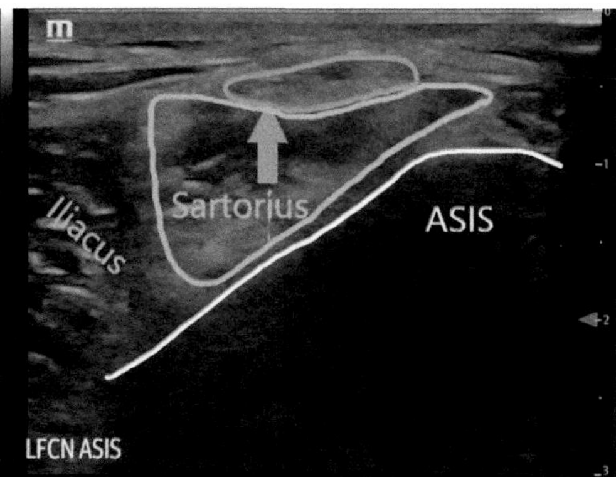

Fig. 17. Lateral femoral cutaneous nerve (LFCN).The probe is placed over the ASIS, and the sartorius muscle is identified as a triangular muscle coming off medial side of ASIS. The lateral femoral cutaneous nerve (*blue arrow*) indents and passes from medial to lateral over sartorius as it exits the inguinal ligament.

adolescent, US-guided cryoablation of the femoral branch of the GFN with good effect up to 7 months.[175–177]

Complications and safety

The limited number of studies did not identify any adverse events with USG GFN block. There is a theoretic risk of the needle entering the spermatic cord structures or peritoneum. It is recommended to use LA without epinephrine for this block if injected around the spermatic cord.

Summary

There are insufficient data comparing the use of USG versus LMG approach in the performance of GFN block to diagnose or treat chronic pain secondary to genitofemoral neuralgia. There is uncertainty regarding the optimal approach to US-guided GFN block among women.

Although 1 RCT and several case reports demonstrate promising results, more robust studies are needed to determine the utility of both femoral and genital branch of the GFN block, and additional nerve treatments including pRFA and cryoablation of the USG GFN block for the management of chronic pain. The current evidence for recommending USG GFN block for chronic pain is C, moderate level of certainty.

Lateral Femoral Cutaneous Nerve Block

Anatomy and technique

The LFCN is a sensory nerve originating from ventral rami of L2-L4 spinal nerves of the lumbar plexus, emerging at the lateral edge of the psoas major, and obliquely passes across the iliacus toward the ASIS. Various studies have demonstrated a variable course of the nerve at the ASIS in relation to the inguinal ligament.[178,179] Once distal to the inguinal ligament, the LFCN runs superficially in a fatty groove between the sartorius and tensor fascia lata, after which it divides into anterior and posterior divisions supplying the anterolateral thigh. LFCN blocks (LFCNBs) are commonly targeted at a location passing over, under, or through the inguinal ligament or distally in the fatty groove.[180] The technique is described in **Fig. 17**.

Evidence and indications for ultrasound

The current literature reporting USG for LFCNB for the management of chronic pain conditions is moderate (see **Table 3**). Traditionally, LMG blocks of the LFCN have been described; however, anatomic variations of the LFCN at the ASIS and block failure rates of 40% to 60% have prompted a need for more accurate visualization.[181] Ng and colleagues[182] investigated the accuracy of US imaging compared with LM, demonstrating that the rate of successful localization using USG resulted in higher rates of accurate contact with the LFCN.

In an RCT of Kiliç and colleagues,[183] patients diagnosed with meralgia paresthetica were randomized to USG LFCN injection, transcutaneous electrical nerve stimulation (TENS) (5 days per week for 2 weeks, 20 minutes per daily session), or sham TENS (same application frequency as the TENS group). Although there were no statistically significant differences in pain severity between groups, there was a significant decrease in pain severity after LFCN injection at 2 weeks and 1 month after treatment. Nociceptive pain improved in the injection and TENS groups, whereas neuropathic pain symptoms improved in all groups.[182] The authors found multiple case series of patients with meralgia paresthestica, receiving (series of) LFCNB with LA with or without steroid with prolonged relief up to from 2 months to 1 year.[184–187] The remaining literature spans case reports describing the use of USG LFCNB, pRFA, alcohol neurolysis, and cryoneurolysis for the treatment of chronic pain.[188–192]

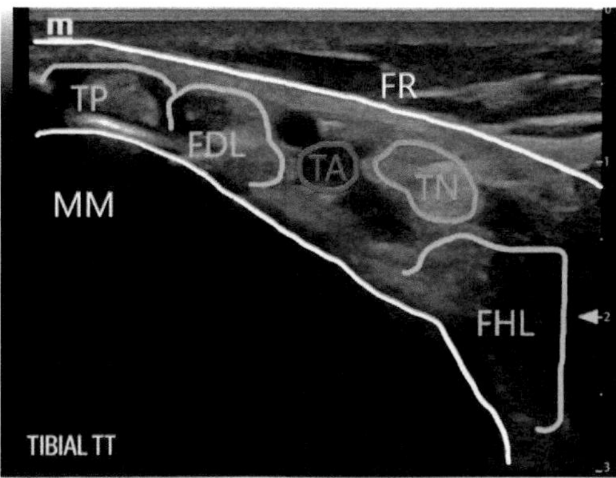

Fig. 18. Tibial nerve in tarsal tunnel. FR, flexor retinaculum; TP, tibialis posterior tendon and muscle; FDL, flexor digitorum longus tendon and muscle; TA, tibial artery; TN, tibial nerve; FHL, flexor hallucis longus muscle and tendon; MM, medial malleolus. The probe is placed immediately superior and slightly posterior to the medial malleolus, in the transverse plane, and the medial malleolus is visualized as a hyperechoic curvilinear shadow. From anterior to posterior, the following structures are visualized—tibialis posterior, flexor digitorum longus tendons, tibial artery and vein, tibial nerve, and the flexor hallucis tendon. An in-plane approach is most often used, but an out-of-plane approach is also acceptable. The goal of the injection is to ensure circumferential spread of LA around the nerve, and this usually requires a volume of around 5 mL.

Complications and safety

The limited number of studies did not identify any adverse events with USG LFCNB.

Summary

There are limited data showing superiority of USG versus LMG approach. There is moderate evidence of efficacy of USG LFCN procedures for meralgia paresthetica, but more robust studies are warranted. The available evidence for recommending USB LFCNB for chronic pain is I, insufficient.

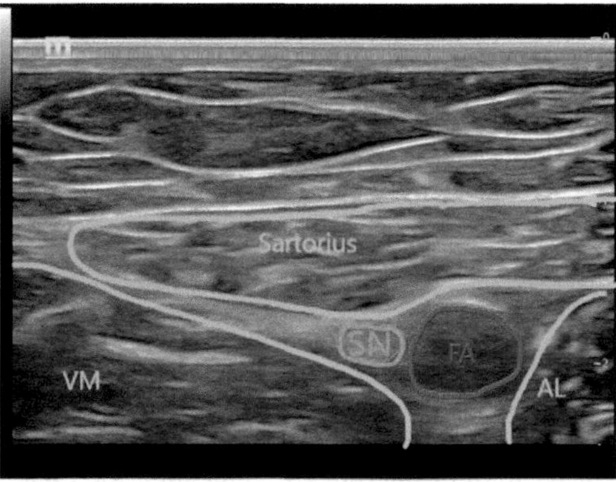

Fig. 19. Saphenous nerve. The saphenous nerve (SN) is usually located on the superomedial aspect of the femoral artery (FA) in the adductor canal. An in- or out-of-plane approach is used.AL, adductor longus; VM, vastus medialis.

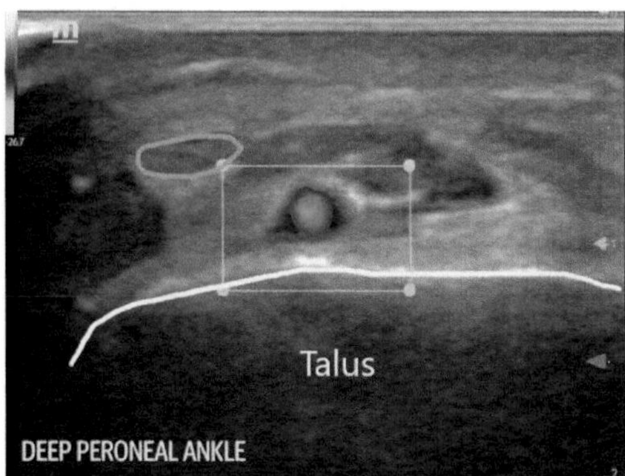

Fig. 20. Deep peroneal nerve. The nerve block is performed at the level of the intermalleolar line. The linear US probe is placed transversally just immediately proximal of the intermalleolar line. The key LM is the anterior tibial artery. The nerve can be seen a hyperechoic structure medial or lateral to the artery. An in- or out-of-plane approach can be used. Doppler: anterior tibial artery; blue circle, deep peroneal nerve.

Foot and Ankle Nerves

Anatomy and technique

The ankle nerve block is an excellent regional technique in providing anesthesia for foot surgery, but it can also be performed to treat chronic neuropathic pain in the foot in the distribution of each of the nerves. The ankle nerve block involves all 5 terminal nerves: tibial nerve, deep peroneal nerve, superficial peroneal nerve, sural nerve, and saphenous nerve. The sensory distribution of the individual nerves often overlaps and does not always follow textbook anatomic descriptions. Therefore, blockade of all 5 nerves is recommended for a complete sensory block of the foot.[193,194] It is important to be aware of the anatomic structures in the vicinity of each of these nerves to enhance the accuracy and safety of these injections.[195]

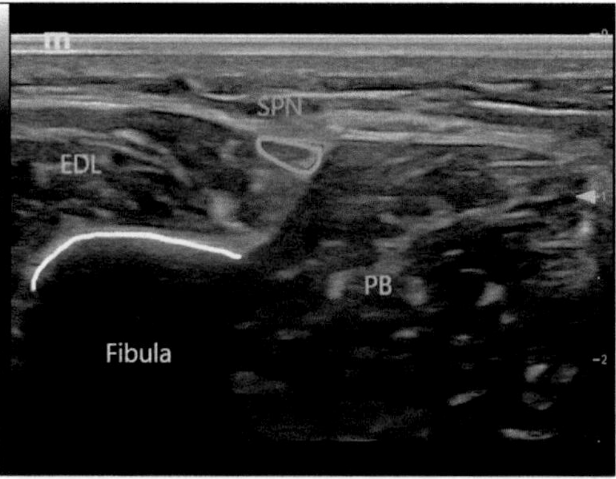

Fig. 21. Superficial peroneal nerve. The US probe is placed in a transverse orientation on the lateral aspect of the lower third of the calf. The chief LM is the fibula, with the superficial peroneal nerve lying as a small triangular structure above it and immediately deep to the crural fascia. An in- or out-of-plane technique is used. EDL, extensor digitorum longus; PB, peroneus brevis, SPN, superficial peroneal nerve.

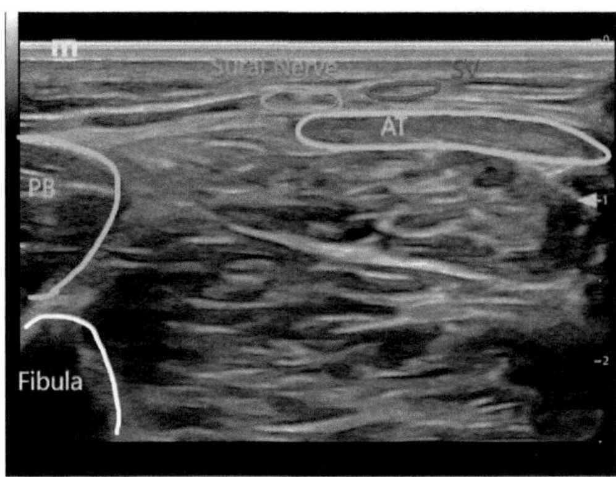

Fig. 22. Sural nerve. The probe is placed in a transverse orientation in the groove between the Achilles tendon and lateral malleolus. The sural nerve is a small hyperechoic round structure lateral to the lesser saphenous vein. An in- or out-of-plane technique is used. AT, Achilles tendon over triceps surae; PB, peroneus brevis; SV, lesser saphenous vein.

Tibial nerve: This nerve is a terminal branch of the sciatic nerve, and it supplies the deep plantar structures, the muscles, and sensory innervation to the sole of the foot through its 3 terminal branches—calcaneal, lateral, and medial plantar nerves. This nerve is blocked at the level of the medial malleolus where it lies in the tarsal tunnel formed by the flexor retinaculum. The contents of the tarsal tunnel include the tibial nerve, posterior tibial artery and vein, and 3 tendons—tibialis posterior, flexor digitorum longus, and flexor hallucis longus. A linear array US probe is used for the block because the nerve is usually quite superficial (**Fig. 18**).

Saphenous nerve: This nerve is a terminal branch of the femoral nerve, and it supplies the medial malleolus and medial side of the foot. Below the knee, it runs close to the great saphenous vein along the tibial surface. In the lower third of the leg, it runs posterior to the medial aspect of the tibia and divides into 2 terminal branches above the medial malleolus. This nerve block is performed just above the medial malleolus (**Fig. 19**).

Deep peroneal nerve: This nerve is 1 of the 2 terminal branches of the common peroneal nerve, and it supplies the deep dorsal structures and sensation to the web space between the first and second toes. This nerve arises at the level of the fibular neck; it passes inferomedially, deep to the extensor digitorum longus, then to the anterior surface of the interosseous membrane, and runs in close proximity to the anterior tibial artery. At the level of the intermalleolar line, where the nerve block is performed, the anterior tibial artery becomes the dorsalis pedis artery (**Fig. 20**).

Superficial peroneal nerve: This nerve is the other terminal branch of the common peroneal nerve, arising at the level of the fibular head, and it descends in the lateral compartment of the leg. In the distal part of the lower leg, the superficial peroneal nerve lies between the peroneus brevis and the extensor digitorum longus muscles, gradually becoming more superficial until it pierces the crural fascia. This nerve supplies sensation to the dorsum of the foot except for the area innervated by the deep peroneal nerve (**Fig. 21**).

Sural nerve: This nerve is a pure sensory nerve, formed by branches from the medial sural cutaneous nerve and the lateral sural cutaneous nerves at the level of the upper third of the calf. The nerve runs adjacent to the lesser saphenous vein in a joint

Table 4
Overview of literature of ultrasound-guided blocks of lower limb

First Author, Year, Number of Patients, Type of Study	Pain Syndrome	Ultrasound-Guided Intervention, Comparator, Outcome Tool	Outcomes
Ankle block			
Walter et al,[200] 2017 (n = 46) CS	Neuropathy in the foot and ankle	• Ankle blocks (DPN, MPN, SaN, SPN, SuN, TN) with LA + steroid (0.75-5 mL) • N/A • NRS, structural pathology	• 61% Of patients had therapeutic benefit: 12 patients < 30 d, 6 patients < 9 mo, 5 patients > 9 mo • US revealed structural abnormalities of nerve in 51% of patients: scar encasement (n = 14), thickening (n = 6), neuroma (n = 5), ganglion cyst (n = 5)
Sobey et al,[201] 2016 (n = 1) CR	Tarsal tunnel syndrome 11 y old	• Tibial nerve block • N/A • LA + MP • Series • NRS • NP	• Substantial relief after each block. Duration of effect not provided
Abd-Elsayed et al,[202] 2018 (n = 2) CS	Sural neuralgia 65 and 35 y old	• pRFA sural nerve • N/A • N/A • Single • NRS • 2 mo	• At 2 mo follow-up: both patients: 80% pain improvement
Genicular			
Ahmed, [219] 2018 (n = 4) CS	Knee OA	• Neurolysis of 6 genicular nerves • N/A • Alcohol 50% in bupivacaine 0.25% 0.5–0.75 mL • N/A • NRS, OKS, WOMAC, SF36 • 6 mo	• NRS at baseline 9 of 10, significantly lower up to 6 mo • OKS at baseline 7.75 ± 1.25–20.75 ± 1.70 (1 mo) and 18.25 ± 0.95 (6 mo). • WOMAC at baseline 77.75 ± 4.34–56.25 ± 3.09 (1 mo) and 52.00 ± 2.16 (6 mo)

Study	Condition	Intervention	Outcomes
			• SF36 physical health baseline 27.22 ± 6.95–47.12 ± 2.63 (1 mo) and 51.27 (6 mo) • SF36 mental health baseline 35.35 ± 3.30–52.45 ± 1.82 (1 mo) and 54.02 ± 2.59 (6 mo)
Kim et al,[216] 2018 (n = 48) RCT	Knee OA	• Nerve block of 3 nerves • Lidocaine vs lidocaine + triamcinolone • Single • VAS, OKS, GPE • 4 weeks	• VAS in LA group from 60.8 ± 7.2 (baseline) to 40.4 ± 9.1 (week 2). • VAS in LA + steroid group from 62.1 ± 9.8 (baseline) to 45.3 ± 19.8 (4 wk). • OKS in LA group from 37.1 ± 2.8 (baseline) to 30.1 ± 5.4 (2 wk). • OKS in LA + steroid from 37.6 ± 3.8 (baseline) to 31.8 ± 6.2 (4 wk)
Kim et al, [217] 2018 (n = 80) RCT	Knee OA	• US nerve blocks • Fluoro nerve blocks • 6 mL lidocaine 2% + triamcinolone 20 mL • ingle • NRS, WOMAC • 3 mo	• No significant differences between groups in terms in terms of NRS, WOMAC, and safety at 1 and 3 mo
Huang et al,[220] 2020 (n = 256) MA of 8 studies	Knee OA	• (p)RFA • N/A • N/A • Single • NRS, WOMAC • 1 year	• Significant pain relief (7 of 8 studies): pooled mean NRS difference compared with baseline: −4.196 (SE: 0.324; 95% CI: −4.832 to −3.560; $P < .001$) WOMAC (6 of 8 studies): significant improvement compared with baseline

Abbreviations: CI, confidence interval; DPN, deep peroneal nerve; GA, general anesthesia; GPE, global perceived effect; ILGN, inferior lateral genicular nerve; IMGN, inferior medial genicular nerve; MGN, middle genicular nerve; MPN, medial plantar nerve; NRS, numerical rating score; OA, osteoarthritis; OKS, osteoarthritis knee scale; PACU, postanesthesia care unit; PGNP, posterior genicular nerve plexus; PTN, posterior tibial nerve; R, retrospective observational study; RPN, recurrent peroneal nerve; SaN, saphenous nerve; SF36, 36-Item Short Form Survey; SLGN, superior lateral genicular nerve; SMGN, superior medial genicular nerve; SPN, superficial peroneal nerve; SuN, sural nerve; TKR, total knee replacement; TN, tibial nerve; USG, ultrasound guided; WOMAC, Western Ontario and McMaster Univerisities Osteoarthritis Index.

superficial fascial sheath. It runs on the anterolateral aspect of the lower leg toward the Achilles tendon, where it passes posterior to the lateral malleolus, on to the calcaneus and innervating lateral aspect of the foot (**Fig. 22**).

Evidence and indications for ultrasound

Three RCTs on healthy volunteers were found, comparing USG with LMG ankle nerve blocks. These studies showed that US improved success rates of tibial and sural nerve blocks compared with LMG, but success rates were equivalent for the deep peroneal nerve.[196–198] A large retrospective cohort study by Chin and colleagues[199] concluded that USG ankle blocks for perioperative analgesia resulted in statistically and clinically higher success rates and less conversion to unplanned general anesthesia.

The literature on ankle nerve blocks for chronic pain use is limited (**Table 4**). We only found 3 papers on foot and ankle nerve blocks (2 case series, 1 case report).[200–202]

Walter and colleagues[200] investigated the outcomes of injection of LA with steroid under USG for patients with chronic pain in a case series; 25% of the patients had short (up to 1 month) and another 25% had intermediate or long-term therapeutic benefit. US was also used as a diagnostic tool in this study through identification of structural pathologic condition (eg, scarring, neuroma formation) in over half of the patients. A case series of 2 patients reported on the use of pRFA for sural neuralgia with significant pain relief.[202]

Complications and safety

Overall, incidence of complications after USG and LMG blocks were low in these studies, but none of these studies were powered to detect differences in adverse outcomes between the 2 groups.

Summary

USG perioperative ankle blocks have demonstrated improved block quality and reduced postoperative opioid requirements with lower volume of injectates when compared with traditional LMG nerve blocks. However, for the indication of chronic pain, the evidence is grade I, insufficient.

Genicular Nerves

Anatomy and block technique

The innervation of the knee is complex. In 2011, Choi and colleagues[203] described a promising technique for GN RFA. Multiple cadaveric studies investigating this technique followed, reporting the anterior knee joint capsule to be innervated by articular branches that could be categorized into 4 quadrants based on their location and origin: superolateral (nerve to vastus lateralis, nerve to vastus intermedius, superior lateral genicular and common fibular nerves), inferolateral (inferior lateral GN and recurrent fibular nerves), superomedial (nerve to vastus medialis, nerve to vastus intermedius, and superior medial GN), and inferomedial (inferior medial GN and infrapatellar branch of saphenous nerve). No articular branches from the obturator nerve were found to supply the anterior knee joint capsule.[204]

These studies supported the methodology used by Choi and colleagues who targeted inferomedial, superomedial, and superolateral GN branches due to their proximity to bony structures (junction of the metaphysis and epiphysis of the femur and tibia).[186,205] However, mixed pain responses to these blocks were noted, spurring the continued search for the best anatomic targets. Recently, revised anatomic targets for GN blockade and RFA were proposed and will have to be further investigated.[206]

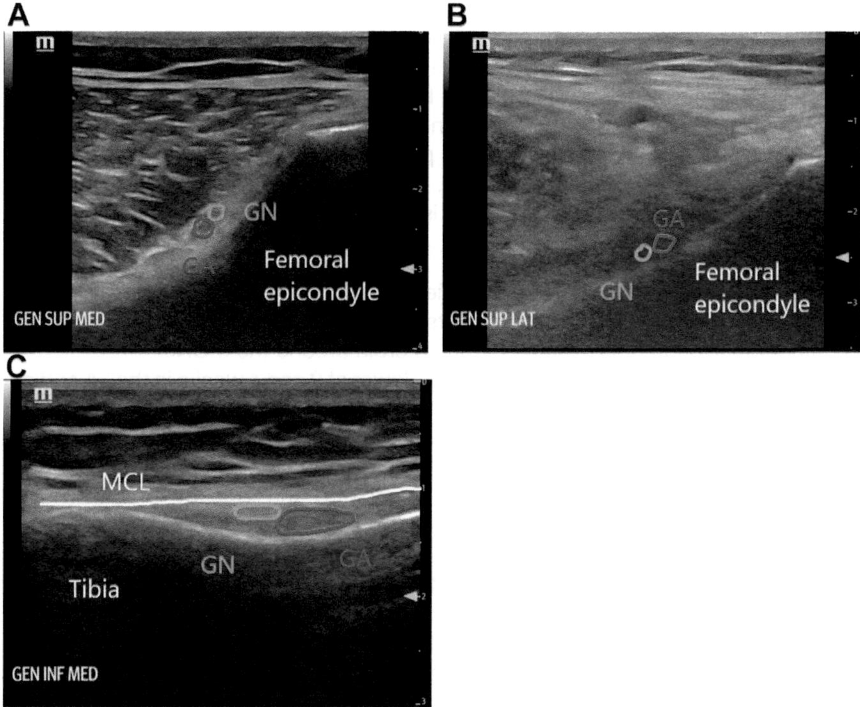

Fig. 23. Genicular nerves. Longitudinal image of the knee at level of the distal femoral condyle and medial tibial metaphysis. The superior medial (A), superior lateral (B), and inferior medial (C) genicular nerves (GN, *blue circle*) are each accompanied by a genicular artery (GA, *red circle*). MCC, medial collateral ligament. The US probe is placed along the medial or lateral aspect of long axis of the femur at the metaphysis, approximately 2 to 3 cm proximal to the knee. The neurovascular bundle is seen at the juncture of the femoral shaft and epicondyle. Approach can be in plane or out of plane. For the inferomedial articular branch, the US probe is placed over the medial aspect of the knee and then moved in caudal direction until the tibial metaphysis is seen. The medial collateral ligament (MCL) and the target, neurovascular bundle of the inferior medial genicular nerve (GN), are identified.

It has been proposed that the articular nerves of the knee form 2 groups, an anterior group and a posterior group. Branches of the femoral, common peroneal, and saphenous nerves innervate the anterior aspect of the knee, whereas the posterior aspect of the knee is innervated by branches of the obturator, tibial, and sciatic nerves.[207–209] The tibial nerve, after bifurcation of the sciatic nerve above the popliteal fossa, projects branches that innervate the articular capsule and follow the superior medial and superior lateral genicular vessels. The common peroneal nerve has 2 articular branches that innervate the inferolateral aspect of the articular capsule. An additional branch of the common peroneal nerve innervates the anterolateral side of the articular capsule and follows the inferior lateral genicular artery.[210,211] None of the publications included in this review targeted nerves at the inferolateral aspect of the knee; this is presumably due to concerns about inadvertent injury to the common peroneal nerve that lies in close proximity at the neck of the fibula. It has also been suggested that nerves innervating the capsule of the knee joint accompany small arteries supplying the joint, and that the latter can be used as an aid to identify the nerves sonographically.[212] Other sonoanatomic LMs include insertion of tendons (adductor magnus at the adductor tubercle) and ligaments (medial collateral ligament on tibia) on femur and tibia.[213] GN blocks (GNBs) are mostly performed in the context of chronic pain, to relieve chronic knee joint pain secondary to osteoarthritis. The anatomic targets in most clinical studies are the superior medial, superior lateral, middle genicular, inferomedial and inferolateral genicular, and recurrent peroneal nerves and the posterior GN plexus.[214] Nerve blocks, RFA, and neurolysis can be performed.[215] Both USG and fluoroscopic-guided techniques have been described. The USG block of the superomedial and superolateral, and inferomedial branches is described in **Fig. 23**.

Evidence and indications for ultrasound

The therapeutic effect of GNBs was studied in 2 RCTs by Kim and colleagues[216,217] (see **Table 4**). The first RCT of 48 patients with knee osteoarthritis (KOA) compared the effect of injection of LA versus LA and steroid around the 3 GNs.[216]

Pain and mobility scores were significantly lower at 2 and 4 weeks in the LA and steroid group, but the scores of all patients returned to baseline at 8 weeks after the procedures. Patients who had received LA and steroid felt significantly better at 4 weeks when compared with the LA group. No adverse events were noted in either group. The second RCT of Kim and colleagues[217] compared the efficacy of USG versus fluoroscopy-guided GNB in patients with KOA. No significant differences between groups in terms of NRS, Western Ontario and McMaster Universities Osteoarthritis Index (WOMAC), and safety were noted up to 3 months. The investigators commented that the US-guided procedure was quicker to perform. The comparable efficacy of both techniques was also confirmed by Sari and colleagues[218] (see **Table 4**).

The effect of neurolysis of the GN in patients with KOA was described by Ahmed and Arora[219] in a small case series of 4 patients who previously had failed to respond to the RFA procedure on GNs (see **Table 4**). All patients received chemical neurolysis with alcohol of the 6 GNs. This small study showed significant improvement in pain, mobility, and overall health scores up to 6 months after the procedures. Two of the 4 patients developed hypoesthesia and numbness in the knee that resolved by 6 months.

The evidence of the efficacy of (pulsed) RFA of the GN is summarized by a meta-analysis by Huang and colleagues,[220] including 3 RCTs, 3 prospective trials, and 2 retrospective studies.[197–206,216,217,221–226] (see **Table 4**). The studies had 256 patients with KOA in total, mean age ranging from 60 to 72.5 years. pRFA was used in 4 and RFA in 3 studies, and the combination in one study. The investigators compared VAS/NRS scores and WOMAC scores, with a follow-up up to half year. Significant pain relief was achieved in 7 of 8 studies and the pooled mean difference of pain score was −4.196 (SE, 0.324; 95% confidence interval, −4.832 to −3.560; $P < .001$) compared with baseline. Knee function was also significantly improved in 6 of 8 studies. Adverse events were uncommon (ecchymosis, hypoesthesia, numbness) and improved within 6 months.

Complications and safety

This limited number of studies showed an overall low risk for complications for USG GNB. However, temporary hypoesthesia and numbness have been described after RFA procedure on GNs, improving by 6 months postprocedure.[220]

Summary

USG GNB procedures have demonstrated to be effective and safe for patient with KOA. Long-lasting pain relief can be achieved by RFA and neurolysis procedures.

The available evidence for recommending USG GNB for chronic knee pain is A, high level of certainty.

Table 5
Overview of literature of ultrasound-guided pediatric blocks

First Author, Year, Number of Patients, Type of Study	Pain Syndrome, Age, Mean Baseline VAS	Ultrasound-Guided Intervention (Nerve Block/Neurolysis/RFA), Comparator, Injectate, Blocks (Single/Series), Outcomes Measured, FU Time Points	Outcomes
Franklin et al,[227] 2016 (n = 1) CR	Meralgia paresthetica, 9 y old, VAS 8 of 10	• LFCN block • N/A • 7.5 mL ropi 0.5% + BM 3 mg • 2 blocks (1 mo apart) • VAS • 4 mo	• At 1 mo after first block: VAS 4 of 10 • At 3 mo after second block: pain free
Suresh et al,[162] 2008 (n = 2) CS	Postoperative ilioinguinal neuralgia, 14 + 16 y old VAS 8 of 10	• IINB • N/A • 3–5 mL bupi 0.25% • 2 blocks (1 mo apart) • VAS • 6 mo	• Patient 1: pain reduction from VAS 8 of 10–2 of 10 for 3 mo. After second block, complete pain relief for > 6 mo • Patient 2: pain free after 1 block for > 6 mo
Simpson et al,[228] 2011 (n = 1) CR	Postoperative chronic abdominal wall pain (ACNES), 13 y, 5 of 10	• B/L TAP block • N/A • B/L 20 mLs bupi 0.25% • 2 blocks (1 mo apart) • VAS • 1 mo	• Reduction in pain to mean VAS 4 of 10 after first block, remained at 4 of 10 until 1 month after second block
Terkawi and Romdhane,[175] 2014 (n = 1) CR	Chronic orchialgia, 17 y old, VAS 10 of 10	• pRFA GFN block • N/A • N/A • Single • VAS • 7 mo	• At 7 mo FU: VAS at rest 0/10

(*continued on next page*)

Table 5
(*continued*)

First Author, Year, Number of Patients, Type of Study	Pain Syndrome, Age, Mean Baseline VAS	Ultrasound-Guided Intervention (Nerve Block/Neurolysis/RFA), Comparator, Injectate, Blocks (Single/Series), Outcomes Measured, FU Time Points	Outcomes
Martin et al,[229] 2013 (n = 1) CR	CRPS left arm, 10 y old, VAS 8 of 10	• SC catheter • N/A • Continuous infusion of ropi 0.1% for 5 d • N/A • VAS • NP	• Significant reduction of pain during infusion and after catheter removal. Duration of FU NP. Patient was concomitantly started on antineuropathics

*Abbreviations:*B/L, bilateral; BM, betamethasone; bupi, bupivacaine; CR, case report; CS, case series; FU; IIB, ilioinguinal block; N/A, not applicable; NP, not provided; ropi, ropivacaine; SC, supraclavicular.

Table 6
Grades of recommendation for use of ultrasound-guided block for chronic pain

Intervention	Grade	Level of Certainty	Suggestion for Practice
Greater occipital nerve	A	High	Offer or provide this service
Trigeminal nerve	I		If the service is offered, patients should understand the uncertainty about the balance of benefits and harms
Stellate ganglion	B	Moderate	Offer or provide this service
Suprascapular nerve	C	Moderate	Offer or provide this service for selected patients depending on individual circumstances
Median nerve	I		If the service is offered, patients should understand the uncertainty about the balance of benefits and harms
Radial nerve	I		If the service is offered, patients should understand the uncertainty about the balance of benefits and harms
Ulnar nerve	I		If the service is offered, patients should understand the uncertainty about the balance of benefits and harms
TAP	A	High	Offer or provide this service
QLB	I		If the service is offered, patients should understand the uncertainty about the balance of benefits and harms
RSB	I		If the service is offered, patients should understand the uncertainty about the balance of benefits and harms
ACNES	C	Moderate	Offer or provide this service for selected patients depending on individual circumstances
PECS	C	Moderate	Offer or provide this service for selected patients depending on individual circumstances
ESP	C	High	Offer or provide this service for selected patients depending on individual circumstances
IIHN	C	Moderate	Offer or provide this service for selected patients depending on individual circumstances

(*continued on next page*)

Table 6
(continued)

Intervention	Grade	Level of Certainty	Suggestion for Practice
GF	C	Moderate	Offer or provide this service for selected patients depending on individual circumstances
LFCN	C	Moderate	Offer or provide this service for selected patients depending on individual circumstances
Ankle	I		If the service is offered, patients should understand the uncertainty about the balance of benefits and harms
Genicular	A	High	Offer or provide this service

Definition of grades: A: The panel recommends the service. There is high certainty that the net benefit is substantial. B: The panel recommends the service. There is high certainty that the net benefit is moderate or there is moderate certainty that the net benefit is moderate to substantial. C: The panel recommends selectively offering or providing this service to individual patients based on professional judgment and patient preferences. There is at least moderate certainty that the net benefit is small. D: The panel recommends against the service. There is moderate or high certainty that the service has no net benefit or that the harms outweigh the benefits. I: The panel concludes that the current evidence is insufficient to assess the balance of benefits and harms of the service. Evidence is lacking, of poor quality, or conflicting, and the balance of benefits and harms cannot be determined.

Definition of level of certainty: High: The available evidence usually includes consistent results from well-designed, well-conducted studies in representative primary care populations. These studies assess the effects of the preventive service on health outcomes. This conclusion is therefore unlikely to be strongly affected by the results of future studies. Moderate: The available evidence is sufficient to determine the effects of the preventive service on health outcomes, but confidence in the estimate is constrained by such factors as the number, size, or quality of individual studies; inconsistency of findings across individual studies; limited generalizability of findings to routine primary care practice; and lack of coherence in the chain of evidence. As more information becomes available, the magnitude or direction of the observed effect could change, and this change may be large enough to alter the conclusion. Low: The available evidence is insufficient to assess effects on health outcomes. Evidence is insufficient because of the limited number or size of studies, important flaws in study design or methods; inconsistency of findings across individual studies, gaps in the chain of evidence, findings not generalizable to routine primary care practice, and lack of information on important health outcomes. More information may allow estimation of effects on health outcomes.

Pediatric Chronic Pain Blocks

Evidence and technique for ultrasound and safety

Although the popular use of US in adults has transferred to clinical use in pediatric procedures for chronic pain, literature search by the authors could only find 4 case reports (**Table 5**).

There is minimal published evidence validating the use of US for pediatric blocks.[162,175,227–229] These case reports, however, report promising and safe results. Pain interventionalists as in our pediatric pain practice in a major university hospital in the United States use US frequently for procedures including RFA of the hip for chronic joint pain, occipital nerve blocks for headache, and paravertebral/intercostal nerve blocks for chronic chest or abdominal pain. This list is not exhaustive or comprehensive in any manner but is an example of procedures in which the use of US is of value similar to adult pain procedures. USG procedures can offer new and expanded opportunities for targeted interventional pain treatment.

A significant barrier to more widespread use and third-party reimbursement of US is the paucity of evidence to authenticate the putative higher efficacy and safety of this modality when compared with traditional imaging techniques associated with significant radiation exposure in children. Future directions will be comparing imaging techniques of the various blocks that may use US to determine which block guidance methodology would be more effective in children.

DISCUSSION AND CONCLUSION

The use of US to guide procedures in the treatment of chronic pain is clinically well established in adult patients, and has gained popularity and applicability in the past decade. The increase in the use of US is attributed to its several advantages over other imaging techniques (fluoroscopy, CT) including portability, ease of performance, absence of ionizing radiation or need for use of contrast agents, better visualization of soft tissue (ie, muscle, ligament) and vascular structures, real-time visualization of needle advancement, and, at times, the ability to observe the spread of injectate.[230]

The goal of this review was to synthetize the available evidence for USG nerve and plane blocks for chronic pain management. The authors' literature search demonstrated that chronic pain management has undergone a significant boost thanks to the introduction of USG blocks, because they facilitate locating anatomically challenging nerves or fascial planes. USG blocks also allow for safe placement of a needle in the immediate vicinity of the nerve, which has opened the door for pRFA treatment of nerves, capable of extending the duration of analgesia of regular blocks with LA and steroid.[165,166,173,175,202,231] Similarly, several studies on USG-implanted peripheral nerve stimulators have indicated that peripheral nerve stimulation (PNS) is capable of providing sustained improvement of chronic pain.[232–234] Therefore, there is level 2 evidence supporting PNS in the treatment of refractory peripheral nerve neuropathic pain.[235] Similarly, the opportunity of real-time visualization of the injectate has made it possible to safely inject neurolytic products that have shown to provide sustained analgesia for certain indications such as cancer-related abdominal wall pain, inguinal neuralgia, meralgia paresthetica, and KOA.[85,86,163,190,192] Therefore, several previously intractable pain syndromes can now safely be treated interventionally.

This review also demonstrated that these USG nerve blocks can be useful for diagnostic purposes, as to differentiate between neuropathic pain and nociceptive pain, or to identify nerves for targets for other modalities like pRFA, RFA, cryoablation, or PNS. Although we understand that pain might not be cured by these nerve blocks, they can still be useful in the overall treatment process.

The authors aimed to gather evidence of the efficacy of USG blocks in the management of chronic pain. The recommendations for nerve or plane blocks are listed in **Table 6**. For the majority of the chronic pain blocks in this review, the current evidence indicates a positive effect on chronic pain. Unfortunately, the quality of these studies is low to moderate, because our search could only find high-quality evidence for USG pain blocks like GON blocks and GNBs. The paucity of high-quality evidence makes it hard to draw firm conclusions for recommendations at this time.

This review also aimed to gather evidence of the advantage of USG when performing chronic pain blocks. Although comparative studies of USG versus other types of imaging modalities and/or LMG is common in the perioperative setting, these comparative studies are scarce in the chronic pain literature. In the few comparative studies that the authors found, USG was proved to be superior to other modalities.

Further research in the form of prospective comparative effectiveness studies is required to further establish the efficacy of USG nerve and plane blocks for the indication of chronic pain and to demonstrate the advantage of using US to enhance safety and accuracy. It is hoped that this review can be a stimulus for more robust research.

CONFLICTS OF INTEREST

A.K. Aggarwal has no conflict of interest. E. Ottestad is a consultant for Bioness, SPR Therapeutics, Nalu Medical, Nine Continents Medical, Tulavi Medical, and WAPMU faculty. K.E. Pfaff has no conflict of interest. A.H.-Y. Li has no conflict of interest. L. Xu has no conflict of interest. R. Derby has no conflict of interest. D. Hecht has no conflict of interest. J. Hah is a consultant for SPR therapeutics, Nalu Medical, and WAPMU faculty. S. Pritzlaff is a consultant for Bioness, SPR therapeutics, Nalu Medical, and EBT Medical. N. Prabhakar has no conflict of interest. E. Krane has no conflict of interest. G. D'Souza has no conflict of interest. Y. Hoydonckx has no conflict of interest.

FUNDING

None.

ACKNOWLEDGMENTS

None.

REFERENCES

1. U.S. preventive services Task force. grade definitions. Available at: https://www.uspreventiveservicestaskforce.org/uspstf/grade-definitions. Accessed Sep 13 2020.
2. Cohen SP, Wallace MS, Rauck RL, et al. Unique aspects of clinical trials of invasive therapies for chronic pain: an ACTTION evidence-based review. Pain Rep 2019;4:e687.
3. Aggarwal A, Qian X. Destructive Procedures for Head and Neck. In: Deer T, Pope J, Lamer T, et al, editors. Deer's treatment of pain: an illustrated guide for practitioners. 1st edition. Cham: Springer; 2019. p. 321–33.
4. Shim JH, Ko SY, Bang MR, et al. Ultrasound-Guided Greater Occipital Nerve Block for Patients with Occipital Headache and Short Term Follow Up. Korean J Anesthesiol 2011;61(1):50–4.
5. Greher M, Moriggl B, Curatolo M, et al. Sonographic Visualization and Ultrasound-Guided Blockade of the Greater Occipital Nerve: A Comparison of

Two Selective Techniques Confirmed by Anatomical Dissection. Br J Anaesth 2010;104(5):637–42.

6. Flamer D, Alakkad H, Soneji N, et al. A Comparison of two ultrasound-guided techniques for greater occipital nerve injections in chronic migraine: a double-blind, randomized, controlled trial. Reg Anesth Pain Med 2019;44(5):595–603.
7. Ashkenazi A, Blumenfeld A, Napchan U, et al. Interventional Procedures Special Interest Section of the American. Peripheral nerve blocks and trigger point injections in headache management - a systematic review and suggestions for future research. Headache 2010;50(6):943–52.
8. Allen SM, Mookadam F, Cha SS, et al. Greater Occipital Nerve Block for Acute Treatment of Migraine Headache: A Large Retrospective Cohort Study. J Am Board Fam Med 2018;31(2):211–8.
9. Zhang H, Yang X, Lin Y, et al. The efficacy of greater occipital nerve block for the treatment of migraine: A systematic review and meta-analysis. Clin Neurol Neurosurg 2018;165:129–33.
10. Tang Y, Kang J, Zhang Y, et al. Influence of Greater Occipital Nerve Block on Pain Severity in Migraine Patients: A Systematic Review and Meta-analysis. AJEM (Am J Emerg Med) 2017;35(11):1750–4.
11. Chowdhury D, Mundra A. Role of greater occipital nerve block for preventive treatment of chronic migraine: A critical review. Cephalalgia Reports 2020;3. 251581632096440.
12. Lambru G, Abu Bakar N, Stahlhut L, et al. Greater Occipital Nerve Blocks in Chronic Cluster Headache: A Prospective Open-Label Study. Eur J Neurol 2013;21(2):338–43.
13. Gantenbein AR, Lutz NJ, Riederer F, et al. Efficacy and Safety of 121 Injections of the Greater Occipital Nerve in Episodic and Chronic Cluster Headache. Cephalalgia 2012;32(8):630–4.
14. VanderHoek MD, Hoang HT, Goff B. Ultrasound-Guided Greater Occipital Nerve Blocks and Pulsed Radiofrequency Ablation for Diagnosis and Treatment of Occipital Neuralgia. Anesthesiol Pain Med 2013;3(2):256–9.
15. Pingree MJ, Sole JS, O' Brien TG, et al. Clinical Efficacy of an Ultrasound-Guided Greater Occipital Nerve Block at the Level of C2. Reg Anesth Pain Med 2017;42(1):99–104.
16. Sahai-Srivastava S, Subhani D. Adverse Effect Profile of Lidocaine Injections for Occipital Nerve Block in Occipital Neuralgia. J Headache Pain 2010;11(6): 519–23.
17. Akyol F, Binici O, Kuyrukluyildiz U, et al. Ultrasound-guided bilateral greater occipital nerve block for the treatment of post-dural puncture headache. Pak J Med Sci 2015;31(1):111–5.
18. Go JL, Kim PE, Zee C-S. The Trigeminal Nerve. Seminars Ultrasound, CT MRI 2001;22(6):502–20.
19. Waldman SD. The trigeminal nerve—cranial nerve V. Pain review. New York, NY: Elsevier; 2009. p. 15–6.
20. Allam AE-S, Khalil AAF, Eltawab BA, et al. Ultrasound-Guided Intervention for Treatment of Trigeminal Neuralgia: An Updated Review of Anatomy and Techniques. Pain Res Manag 2018;2018:5480728.
21. Chang K-V, Lin C-S, Lin C-P, et al. Recognition of the Lateral Pterygoid Muscle and Plate during Ultrasound-Guided Trigeminal Nerve Block. J Clin Diagn Res : J Clin Diagn Res 2017;11(5):UL01–2.

22. Nader A, Kendall MC, De Oliveria GS, et al. Ultrasound-Guided Trigeminal Nerve Block via the Pterygopalatine Fossa: An Effective Treatment for Trigeminal Neuralgia and Atypical Facial Pain. Pain Physician 2013;16(5):E537–45.
23. Anugerah A, Nguyen K, Nader A. Technical considerations for approaches to the ultrasound-guided maxillary nerve block via the pterygopalatine fossa: a literature review. Reg Anesth Pain Med 2020 Apr;45(4):301–5.
24. Kampitak W, Tansatit T, Shibata Y. A Cadaveric Study of Ultrasound-Guided Maxillary Nerve Block Via the Pterygopalatine Fossa. Reg Anesth Pain Med 2018;43(6):625–30.
25. Nader A, Schittek H, Kendall MC. Lateral Pterygoid Muscle and Maxillary Artery Are Key Anatomical Landmarks for Ultrasound-guided Trigeminal Nerve Block. Anesthesiology 2013;118(4):957.
26. Nader A, Bendok BR, Prine JJ, et al. Ultrasound-Guided Pulsed Radiofrequency Application via the Pterygopalatine Fossa: A Practical Approach to Treat Refractory Trigeminal Neuralgia. Pain Physician 2015;18(3):E411–5.
27. Gupta N, Dattatri R, Bharati SJ, et al. Ultrasound-Guided Real-Time Pterygopalatine Block for Analgesia in an Oral Cancer Patient. Indian J Palliat Care 2018; 24(1):112–4.
28. Gofeld M, Bhatia A, Abbas S, et al. Development and Validation of a New Technique for Ultrasound-Guided Stellate Ganglion Block. Reg Anesth Pain Med 2009;34(5):475–9.
29. Chang K-V, Lin C-P, Hung C-Y, et al. Sonographic Nerve Tracking in the Cervical Region. Am J Phys Med Rehabil 2016;95(11):862–70.
30. Ramsaroop L, Partab P, Singh B, et al. Thoracic origin of a sympathetic supply to the upper limb: the 'nerve of Kuntz' revisited. J Anat 2001;199(Pt 6):675–82.
31. Soneji N, Peng PW. Ultrasound-guided pain interventions - a review of techniques for peripheral nerves. Korean J Pain 2013;26(2):111–24.
32. Wang D. Image Guidance Technologies for Interventional Pain Procedures: Ultrasound, Fluoroscopy, and CT. Curr Pain Headache Rep 2018;22(1):6.
33. Duong S, Bravo D, Todd KJ, et al. Treatment of Complex Regional Pain Syndrome: An Updated Systematic Review and Narrative Synthesis. Canadian Journal of Anesthesia/Journal canadien d'anesthésie. 2018;65(6):658–84.
34. Makharita MY, Amr YM, El-Bayoumy Y. Effect of Early Stellate Ganglion Blockade for Facial Pain from Acute Herpes Zoster and Incidence of Postherpetic Neuralgia. Pain Physician 2012;15(6):467–74.
35. Wu CL, Marsh A, Dworkin RH. The Role of Sympathetic Nerve Blocks in Herpes Zoster and Postherpetic Neuralgia. Pain 2000;87(2):121–9.
36. Rae Olmsted KL, Bartoszek M, Mulvaney S, et al. Effect of Stellate Ganglion Block Treatment on Posttraumatic Stress Disorder Symptoms: A Randomized Clinical Trial [published correction appears in JAMA Psychiatry. JAMA Psychiatr 2020;77(2):130–8. https://doi.org/10.1001/jamapsychiatry.2019.3474, published correction appears in JAMA Psychiatry. 2020 Sep 1;77(9):982.
37. Aleanakian R, Chung B, Feldmann RE, et al. Effectiveness, Safety, and Predictive Potential in Ultrasound-Guided Stellate Ganglion Blockades for the Treatment of Sympathetically Maintained Pain. Pain Pract 2020;20:626–38.
38. Wei K, Feldmann RE, Brascher A-K, et al. Ultrasound-Guided Stellate Ganglion Blocks Combined with Pharmacological and Occupational Therapy in Complex Regional Pain Syndrome (CRPS): A Pilot Case SeriesAd Interim. Pain Med 2014; 15(12):2120–7.

39. Yoo SD, Jung SS, Kim HS, et al. Efficacy of ultrasonography guided stellate ganglion blockade in the stroke patients with complex regional pain syndrome. Ann Rehabil Med 2012;36(5):633–9.
40. Ghai A, Kaushik T, Kundu ZS, et al. Evaluation of new approach to ultrasound guided stellate ganglion block. Saudi J Anaesth 2016;10(2):161–7.
41. Messina C, Banfi G, Orlandi D, et al. Ultrasound-guided interventional procedures around the shoulder. Br J Radiol 2016;89(1057). https://doi.org/10.1259/BJR.20150372.
42. Aydın T, Şen Eİ, Merve, et al. Efficacy of ultrasound-guided suprascapular nerve block treatment in patients with painful hemiplegic shoulder. Neurol Sci 2019. https://doi.org/10.1007/s10072-019-03749-y.
43. Wu YT, Ho CW, Chen YL, et al. Ultrasound-guided pulsed radiofrequency stimulation of the suprascapular nerve for adhesive capsulitis: A prospective, randomized, controlled trial. Anesth Analg 2014;119(3):686–92.
44. Abdelshafi ME, Yosry M, Elmulla AF. Relief of Chronic Shoulder Pain: a Comparative Study of Three Approaches. J Anesth 2011;21(1):83–92.
45. Sá Malheiro N, Afonso NR, Pereira D, et al. Efficacy of ultrasound guided suprascapular block in patients with chronic shoulder pain: retrospective observational study. Brazilian J Anesthesiol 2020;70(1):15–21.
46. Thompson WL, Malchow RJ. Peripheral Nerve Blocks and Anesthesia of the Hand. Mil Med 2002;167(6):478–82.
47. Jackson SA, Derr C, De Lucia A, et al. Sonographic Identification of Peripheral Nerves in the Forearm. J Emerg Trauma Shock 2016;9(4):146–50.
48. Boeckstyns MEH, SØRensen AI. Does Endoscopic Carpal Tunnel Release have a Higher Rate of Complications than Open Carpal Tunnel Release? J Hand Surg Am 1999;24(1):9–15.
49. Macaire P, Singelyn F, Narchi P, et al. Ultrasound- or Nerve Stimulation-Guided Wrist Blocks for Carpal Tunnel Release. Reg Anesth Pain Med 2008;33(4): 363–8.
50. Liebmann O. Feasibility of Forearm Ultrasound-Guided Nerve Blocks of the Radial, Ulnar, and Median Nerves for Hand Procedures in the Emergency Department (The FUN Block Study). Acad Emerg Med 2006;14(1):e14–.
51. Wu YT, Wu CH, Lin JA, et al. Efficacy of 5% Dextrose Water Injection for Peripheral Entrapment Neuropathy: A Narrative Review. Int J Mol Sci 2021;22(22): 12358.
52. To P, McClary KN, Sinclair MK, et al. The Accuracy of Common Hand Injections With and Without Ultrasound: An Anatomical Study. Hand 2017;12(6):591–6.
53. Amini R, Patricia Javedani P, Amini A, et al. Ultrasound-Guided Forearm Nerve Blocks: A Novel Application for Pain Control in Adult Patients with Digit Injuries. Case reports in emergency medicine 2016;2016:2518596.
54. Frenkel O, Liebmann O, Fischer JW. Ultrasound-Guided Forearm Nerve Blocks in Kids. Pediatr Emerg Care 2015;31(4):255–9.
55. Kalava A, Colon BC. Ultrasound-guided median and ulnar nerve blocks in the forearm to facilitate onabotulinum toxin A injection for palmar hyperhidrosis. J Am Acad Dermatol 2020 Oct;83(4):e277–8. https://doi.org/10.1016/j.jaad.2020.01.033.
56. Chen LC, Ho CW, Sun CH, et al. Ultrasound-guided pulsed radiofrequency for carpal tunnel syndrome: A single-blinded randomized controlled study. PLoS One 2015;10. https://doi.org/10.1371/journal.pone.0129918.

57. Anagnostopoulou S, Saranteas T, Chantzi C, et al. Ultrasound Identification of the Radial Nerve and its Divisions. Is Rescue Nerve Block at or Below the Elbow Possible? Anaesth Intensive Care 2008;36(3):457–9.
58. Guo S, Mansour R, and Henderson Slater D. Ultrasound-Guided Continuous Radiofrequency Ablation of Painful Residual Limb Neuroma in Individuals with Limb Amputation: A Retrospetic Case Series, Canadian Prosthetics & Orthotics J, 2019;2(1):4.
59. Zhang X, Xu Y, Zhou J, et al. Ultrasound-guided Alcohol Neurolysis and Radiofrequency Ablation of Painful Stump Neuroma: Effective Treatments for Post-Amputation Pain. J Pain Res 2017;10:295–302.
60. Oh DS, Kang TH, Kim HJ. Pulsed Radiofrequency on Radial Nerve under Ultrasound Guidance for Treatment of Intractable Lateral Epicondylitis. J Anesth 2016;30(3):498–502.
61. Waldman SD. Radial Nerve Block at the Humerus. Atlas of pain management injection techniques. New York, NY: Elsevier; 2013. p. 144–7.
62. Varshney R, Sharma N, Malik S, et al. A Cadaveric Study Comparing the Three Approaches for Ulnar Nerve Block at Wrist. Saudi J Anaesth 2014;8(Suppl 1): S25–8.
63. Prithishkumar IJ, Joy P, Satyanandan C. Comparison of the Volar and Medial Approach in Peripheral Block of Ulnar Nerve at the Wrist - a Cadaveric Study. J Clin Diagn Res : J Clin Diagn Res 2014;8(11):AC01–4.
64. Eichenberger U, Stöckli S, Marhofer P, et al. Minimal Local Anesthetic Volume for Peripheral Nerve Block. Reg Anesth Pain Med 2009;34(3):242–6.
65. Ponrouch M, Bouic N, Bringuier S, et al. Estimation and Pharmacodynamic Consequences of the Minimum Effective Anesthetic Volumes for Median and Ulnar Nerve Blocks: A Randomized, Double-Blind, Controlled Comparison Between Ultrasound and Nerve Stimulation Guidance. Anesth Analg 2010;111(4): 1059–64.
66. Mizuno J, Sugimoto S, Ikeda M, et al. Treatment with Stellate Ganglion Block, Continuous Epidural Block and Ulnar Nerve Block of a Patient with Postherpetic Neuralgia who Developed Complex Regional Pain Syndrome (CRPS). Masui 2001;50(5):548–51.
67. Yadav N, Philip FA, Gogia V, et al. Radio Frequency Ablation in Drug Resistant Chemotherapy-induced Peripheral Neuropathy: A Case Report and Review of Literature. Indian J Palliat Care 2010;16(1):48–51.
68. Kwak S, Jeong D, Choo YJ, et al. Management of neuropathic pain induced by cubital tunnel syndrome using pulsed radiofrequency: Two case reports. Medicine (Baltim) 2019;98:e15599.
69. Vlassakov KV, Narang S, Kissin I. Local Anesthetic Blockade of Peripheral Nerves for Treatment of Neuralgias. Anesth Analg 2011;112(6):1487–93.
70. Rozen WM, Tran TMN, Ashton MW, et al. Refining the Course of the Thoracolumbar Nerves: A New Understanding of the Innervation of the Anterior Abdominal Wall. Clin Anat 2008;21(4):325–33.
71. Barrington MJ, Ivanusic JJ, Rozen WM, Hebbard P. Spread of injectate after ultrasound-guided subcostal transversus abdominis plane block: a cadaveric study. Anaesthesia 2009;64(7):745–50.
72. Barrington MJ, Ivanusic JJ, Rozen WM, et al. Spread of Injectate after Ultrasound-Guided Subcostal Transversus Abdominis Plane Block: A Cadaveric Study. Anaesthesia 2009;64(7):745–50.
73. Blanco R. TAP Block under Ultrasound Guidance: The Description of a "No Pops" Technique. Reg Anesth Pain Med 2007;32(5):130.

74. Tran TMN, Ivanusic JJ, Hebbard P, et al. Determination of Spread of Injectate after Ultrasound-guided Transversus Abdominis Plane Block: A Cadaveric Study. Br J Anaesth 2009;102(1):123–7.
75. Lee THW, Barrington MJ, Tran TMN, et al. Comparison of Extent of Sensory Block following Posterior and Subcostal Approaches to Ultrasound-Guided Transversus Abdominis Plane Block. Anaesth Intensive Care 2010;38(3): 452–60.
76. Støving K, Rothe C, Rosenstock CV, et al. Cutaneous Sensory Block Area, Muscle-Relaxing Effect, and Block Duration of the Transversus Abdominis Plane Block. Reg Anesth Pain Med 2015;40(4):355–62.
77. Jankovic ZB. Du Feu F. M., McConnell P. An anatomical study of the transversus abdominis plane block: Location of the lumbar triangle of petit and adjacent nerves. Anesth Analg 2009;109(3):981–5.
78. Zietek Z, Starczewski K, Sulikowski T, et al. Useful points of geometry and topography of the lumbar triangle for transversus abdominis plane block. Med Sci Mon Int Med J Exp Clin Res 2015;21:4096–101.
79. Hopkins PM. Ultrasound guidance as a gold standard in regional anaesthesia. Br J Anaesth 2007;98(3):299–301.
80. Covotta M, Claroni C, Costantini M, et al. The effects of ultrasound-guided transversus abdominis plane block on acute and chronic postsurgical pain after robotic partial nephrectomy: A prospective randomized clinical trial. Pain Med 2020;21:378–86.
81. Moeschler SM, Pollard EM, Pingree MJ, et al. Ultrasound-guided transversus abdominis plane block vs. trigger point injections for chronic abdominal wall pain: a randomized clinical trial. Pain 2021;162(6):1800–5.
82. Niraj G, Kamel Y. Ultrasound-guided subcostal tap block with depot steroids in the management of chronic abdominal pain secondary to chronic pancreatitis: A three-year prospective audit in 54 patients. Pain Med 2020;21:118–24.
83. Baciarello M, Migliavacca G, Marchesini M, et al. Transversus Abdominis Plane Block for the Diagnosis and Treatment of Chronic Abdominal Wall Pain Following Surgery: A Case Series. Pain Pract 2018;18:109–17.
84. Abd-Elsayed A, Luo S, Falls C. Transversus Abdominis Plane Block as a Treatment Modality for Chronic Abdominal Pain. Pain Physician 2020;23:405–12.
85. Gebhardt R, Wu K. Transversus abdominis plane neurolysis with phenol in abdominal wall cancer pain palliation. Pain Physician 2013;16:E325–30.
86. Restrepo-Garces CE, Asenjo JF, Gomez CM, et al. Subcostal Transversus Abdominis Plane Phenol Injection for Abdominal Wall Cancer Pain. Pain Pract 2014;14:278–82.
87. Sakamoto B, Kuber S, Gwirtz K, et al. Neurolytic transversus abdominis plane block in the palliative treatment of intractable abdominal wall pain. J Clin Anesth 2012;24:58–61.
88. Lee KH, Kim DH, Kim YH, et al. Neurolytic abdominal wall blocks with alcohol for intractable gastrostomy site pain in a cancer patient-a case report-. Korean J Anesthesiol 2020;73:247–51.
89. Sahoo RK, Nair AS. Ultrasound guided transversus abdominis plane block for anterior cutaneous nerve entrapment syndrome. Korean J Pain 2015;28:284–6.
90. Johns N, O'Neill S, Ventham NT, et al. Clinical Effectiveness of Transversus Abdominis Plane (TAP) Block in Abdominal Surgery: A Systematic Review and Meta-Analysis. Colorectal Dis 2012;14(10):e635–42.

91. Farooq M, Carey M. A Case of Liver Trauma With a Blunt Regional Anesthesia Needle While Performing Transversus Abdominis Plane Block. Reg Anesth Pain Med 2008;33(3):274–5.
92. Abrahams M, Derby R, Horn J-L. Update on Ultrasound for Truncal Blocks. Reg Anesth Pain Med 2016;41(2):275–88.
93. Tsai HC, Yoshida T, Chuang TY, et al. Transversus Abdominis Plane Block: An Updated Review of Anatomy and Techniques. BioMed Res Int 2017;2017: 8284363.
94. Blanco R, Ansari T, Riad W, et al. Quadratus Lumborum Block Versus Transversus Abdominis Plane Block for Postoperative Pain After Cesarean Delivery. Obstet Anesth Digest 2017;37(3):164–5.
95. El-Boghdadly K, Elsharkawy H, Short A, et al. Quadratus Lumborum Block Nomenclature and Anatomical Considerations. Reg Anesth Pain Med 2016; 41(4):548–9.
96. Carney J, Finnerty O, Rauf J, et al. Studies on the Spread of Local Anaesthetic Solution in Transversus Abdominis Plane Blocks. Anaesthesia 2011;66(11): 1023–30.
97. Irwin R, Stanescu S, Buzaianu C, et al. Quadratus Lumborum Block for Analgesia after Caesarean Section: A Randomised Controlled Trial. Anaesthesia 2019;75(1):89–95.
98. Öksüz G, Bilal B, Gürkan Y, et al. Quadratus Lumborum Block Versus Transversus Abdominis Plane Block in Children Undergoing Low Abdominal Surgery. Reg Anesth Pain Med 2017;42(5):674–9.
99. Liu X, Song T, Chen X, et al. Quadratus Lumborum Block versus Transversus Abdominis Plane Block for Postoperative Analgesia in Patients undergoing Abdominal Surgeries: A Systematic Review and Meta-Analysis of Randomized Controlled Trials. BMC Anesthesiol 2020;20(1):53.
100. Ökmen K, Metin Ökmen B, Topal S. Ultrasound-Guided Posterior Quadratus Lumborum Block for Postoperative Pain after Laparoscopic Cholecystectomy: A Randomized Controlled Double Blind Study. J Clin Anesth 2018;49:112–7.
101. Dewinter G, Coppens S, Van de Velde M, et al. Quadratus Lumborum Block Versus Perioperative Intravenous Lidocaine for Postoperative Pain Control in Patients Undergoing Laparoscopic Colorectal Surgery. Ann Surg 2018;268(5): 769–75.
102. Kukreja P, MacBeth L, Sturdivant A, et al. Anterior Quadratus Lumborum Block Analgesia for Total Hip Arthroplasty: A Randomized, Controlled Study. Reg Anesth Pain Med 2019;rapm(2019):100804.
103. Fernandez Martín MT, López Álvarez S, Ortigosa Solorzano E. Quadratus lumborum block. New approach for a chronic hip pain. Cases report. Rev Esp Anestesiol Reanim 2020;67:44–8.
104. Carvalho R, Segura E, Loureiro M, do C, et al. Quadratus lumborum block in chronic pain after abdominal hernia repair: case report. Brazilian J Anesthesiol (English 2017;67:107–9.
105. Visoiu M, Pan S. Quadratus Lumborum Blocks: Two Cases of Associated Hematoma. Pediatric Anesthesia 2019;29(3):286–8.
106. Gurnaney HG, Maxwell LG, Kraemer FW, et al. Prospective Randomized Observer-Blinded Study Comparing the Analgesic Efficacy of Ultrasound-Guided Rectus Sheath Block and Local Anaesthetic Infiltration for Umbilical Hernia Repair. Br J Anaesth 2011;107(5):790–5.

107. Hamill JK, Rahiri J-L, Liley A, et al. Rectus Sheath and Transversus Abdominis Plane Blocks in Children: A Systematic Review and Meta-Analysis of Randomized Trials. Pediatric Anesthesia 2016;26(4):363–71.
108. Hong S, Kim H, Park J. Analgesic Effectiveness of Rectus Sheath Block during Open Gastrectomy: A Prospective Double-Blinded Randomized Controlled Clinical Trial. Medicine 2019;98(15):e15159.
109. Bakshi SG, Mapari A, Shylasree TS. Rectus Sheath Block for Postoperative Analgesia in Gynecological Oncology Surgery (RESONS): A Randomized-Controlled Trial. Canadian Journal of Anesthesia/Journal canadien d'anesthésie. 2016;63(12):1335–44.
110. Van Der Graaf T, Verhagen PCMS, Kerver ALA, et al. Surgical anatomy of the 10th and 11th intercostal, and subcostal nerves: prevention of damage during lumbotomy. J Urol 2011;186(2):579–83.
111. Jacobs MLYE, van den Dungen-Roelofsen R, Heemskerk J, et al. Ultrasound-guided abdominal wall infiltration versus freehand technique in anterior cutaneous nerve entrapment syndrome (ACNES): randomized clinical trial. BJS open 2021;5(6):zrab124.
112. Applegate WV. Abdominal Cutaneous Nerve Entrapment Syndrome (ACNES): A Commonly Overlooked Cause of Abdominal Pain. Pain Physician 2014;17(5): E623–7.
113. Chrona E, Kostopanagiotou G, Damigos D, et al. Anterior cutaneous nerve entrapment syndrome: management challenges. J Pain Res 2017;10:145.
114. Chrysanthi B, Theodosios S, Areti AKG. Ultrasound-Guided Anterior Abdominal Cutaneous Nerve Block for the Management of Bilateral Abdominal Cutaneous Nerve Entrapment Syndrome (ACNES). Pain Physician 2013;16(6):E799–801.
115. Kanakarajan S, High K, Nagaraja R. Chronic abdominal wall pain and ultrasound-guided abdominal cutaneous nerve infiltration: a case series. Pain Med 2011;12(3):382–6.
116. Gulur P, Nizamuddin SL, Koury KM, et al. Use of Targeted Transversus Abdominus Plane Blocks in Pediatric Patients with Anterior Cutaneous Nerve Entrapment Syndrome. Pain Physician 2014;17:E623–6.
117. Imajo Y, Komasawa N, Fujiwara S, et al. Transversus abdominal plane and rectus sheath block combination for intractable anterior cutaneous nerve entrapment syndrome after severe cholecystitis. J Clin Anesth 2016;31:119.
118. Blanco R. The 'Pecs Block': A Novel Technique for Providing Analgesia after Breast Surgery. Anaesthesia 2011;66(9):847–8.
119. Blanco R, Fajardo M, Parras Maldonado T. Ultrasound Description of Pecs II (Modified Pecs I): A Novel Approach to Breast Surgery. Rev Esp Anestesiol Reanim 2012;59(9):470–5.
120. Blanco R, Parras T, McDonnell JG, et al. Serratus Plane Block: A Novel Ultrasound-Guided Thoracic Wall Nerve Block. Anaesthesia 2013;68(11): 1107–13.
121. Cros J, Sengès P, Kaprelian S, et al. Pectoral I Block Does Not Improve Postoperative Analgesia After Breast Cancer Surgery. Reg Anesth Pain Med 2018; 43(6):596–604.
122. Versyck B, van Geffen G-J, Van Houwe P. Prospective Double Blind Randomized Placebo-controlled Clinical Trial of the Pectoral Nerves (Pecs) Block Type II. J Clin Anesth 2017;40:46–50.
123. Wang K, Zhang X, Zhang T, et al. The Efficacy of Ultrasound-guided Type II Pectoral Nerve Blocks in Perioperative Pain Management for Immediate

Reconstruction after Modified Radical Mastectomy. A Prospective, Randomized Study. Clin J Pain 2017;34(3):231–6.
124. Karaca O, Pınar HU, Arpacı E, et al. The Efficacy of Ultrasound-Guided Type-I and Type-II Pectoral Nerve Blocks for Postoperative Analgesia after Breast Augmentation: A Prospective, Randomised Study. Anaesthesia Critical Care & Pain Medicine 2019;38(1):47–52.
125. O'Scanaill P, Keane S, Wall V, et al. Single-Shot Pectoral Plane (PECs I and PECs II) Blocks versus Continuous Local Anaesthetic Infusion Analgesia or Both after Non-Ambulatory Breast-Cancer Surgery: A Prospective, Randomised, Double-Blind Trial. Br J Anaesth 2018;120(4):846–53.
126. Kulhari S, Bharti N, Bala I, et al. Efficacy of Pectoral Nerve Block versus Thoracic Paravertebral Block for Postoperative Analgesia after Radical Mastectomy: A Randomized Controlled Trial. Br J Anaesth 2016;117(3):382–6.
127. Lovett-Carter D, Kendall MC, McCormick ZL, et al. Pectoral Nerve Blocks and Postoperative Pain Outcomes after Mastectomy: A Meta-Analysis of Randomized Controlled Trials. Reg Anesth Pain Med 2019;44(10):923–8.
128. De Cassai A, Bonanno C, Sandei L, et al. PECS II Block is Associated with Lower Incidence of Chronic Pain after Breast Surgery. The Korean journal of pain 2019;32(4):286–91.
129. Viti A, Bertoglio P, Zamperini M, et al. Serratus Plane Block for Video-Assisted Thoracoscopic Surgery Major Lung Resection: A Randomized Controlled Trial. Interact Cardiovasc Thorac Surg 2019;30(3):366–72.
130. Fujii T, Shibata Y, Akane A, et al. A randomised controlled trial of pectoral nerve-2 (PECS 2) block vs. serratus plane block for chronic pain after mastectomy. Anaesthesia 2019;74:1558–62.
131. Zocca JA, Chen GH, Puttanniah VG, et al. Ultrasound-Guided Serratus Plane Block for Treatment of Postmastectomy Pain Syndromes in Breast Cancer Patients: A Case Series. Pain Pract 2017;17:141–6.
132. Sir E, Eksert S, Ince ME, et al. A Novel Technique: Ultrasound-Guided Serratus Anterior Plane Block for the Treatment of Posttraumatic Intercostal Neuralgia. Am J Phys Med Rehabil 2019;98:e132–5.
133. Takimoto K, Nishijima K, Ono M. Serratus Plane Block for Persistent Pain after Partial Mastectomy and Axillary Node Dissection. Pain Physician 2016;19: E481–6.
134. Bawany MH, Oswald J. Pecs Blocks for Chronic Pain: A Case Report of Successful Postmastectomy Pain Syndrome Management. A&A Pract 2020;14: e01299.
135. Miller B, Pawa A, Mariano E. Problem with the Pecs II Block: The Long Thoracic Nerve is Collateral Damage. Reg Anesth Pain Med 2019;44(8):817–8.
136. Desai M, Narayanan MK, Venkataraju A. Pneumothorax Following Serratus Anterior Plane Block. Anaesthesia reports 2020;8(1):14–6.
137. Forero M, Adhikary SD, Lopez H, et al. The Erector Spinae Plane Block. Reg Anesth Pain Med 2016;41(5):621–7.
138. Ivanusic J, Konishi Y, Barrington MJ. A Cadaveric Study Investigating the Mechanism of Action of Erector Spinae Blockade. Reg Anesth Pain Med 2018;43(6): 567–71.
139. Yao Y, Fu S, Dai S, et al. Impact of Ultrasound-guided Erector Spinae Plane Block on Postoperative Quality of Recovery in Video-assisted Thoracic Surgery: A Prospective, Randomized, Controlled Trial. J Clin Anesth 2020;63:109783.
140. Yao Y, Li H, He Q, et al. Efficacy of Ultrasound-guided Erector Spinae Plane Block on Postoperative Quality of Recovery and Analgesia after Modified

Radical Mastectomy: Randomized Controlled Trial. Reg Anesth Pain Med 2019; 45(1):5–9.
141. Krishna SN, Chauhan S, Bhoi D, et al. Bilateral Erector Spinae Plane Block for Acute Post-Surgical Pain in Adult Cardiac Surgical Patients: A Randomized Controlled Trial. J Cardiothorac Vasc Anesth 2019;33(2):368–75.
142. Adhikary SD, Liu WM, Fuller E, et al. The Effect of Erector Spinae Plane Block on Respiratory and Analgesic Outcomes in Multiple Rib Fractures: A Retrospective Cohort Study. Anaesthesia 2019;74(5):585–93.
143. Singh S, Choudhary NK, Lalin D, et al. Bilateral Ultrasound-guided Erector Spinae Plane Block for Postoperative Analgesia in Lumbar Spine Surgery. J Neurosurg Anesthesiol 2019;32(4):330–4.
144. Diwan SM, Yamak Altinpulluk E, Khurjekar K, et al. Bilateral Erector Spinae Plane Block for Scoliosis Surgery: Case Series. Rev Esp Anestesiol Reanim 2020; 67(3):153–8.
145. Tulgar S, Selvi O, Ozer Z. Clinical experience of ultrasound-guided single and bi-level erector spinae plane block for postoperative analgesia in patients undergoing thoracotomy. J Clin Anesth 2018;50:22–3.
146. Bugada D, Zarcone AG, Manini M, et al. Continuous Erector Spinae Block at Lumbar Level (L4) for Prolonged Postoperative Analgesia after Hip Surgery. J Clin Anesth 2019;52:24–5.
147. Tsui BCH, Mohler D, Caruso TJ, et al. Cervical Erector Spinae Plane Block Catheter Using a Thoracic Approach: An Alternative to Brachial Plexus Blockade for Forequarter Amputation. Canadian Journal of Anesthesia/Journal canadien d'anesthésie. 2018;66(1):119–20.
148. Hasoon J, Urits I, Viswanath O, et al. Erector Spinae Plane Block for the Treatment of Post Mastectomy Pain Syndrome. Cureus 2021;13. https://doi.org/10.7759/cureus.12656.
149. Rispoli L, Rakesh N, Shah R, et al. Interventional Pain Treatments in the Management of Oncologic Patients With Thoracic Spinal Tumor–Related Pain: A Case Series. Pain Pract 2019;19:866–74.
150. Piraccini E, Calli M, Taddei S, et al. Erector spinae plane block and rhomboid intercostal block for the treatment of post-mastectomy pain syndrome. Saudi J Anaesth 2020;14:517–9.
151. Tsui BCH, Fonseca A, Munshey F, et al. The Erector Spinae Plane (ESP) Block: A Pooled Review of 242 Cases. J Clin Anesth 2019;53:29–34.
152. Hamilton DL. Pneumothorax Following Erector Spinae Plane Block. J Clin Anesth 2019;52:17.
153. Galacho J, Veiga M, Ormonde L. Erector Spinae Plane Block and Altered Hemostasis: Is it a Safe Option? A Case Series. Korean J Anesthesiol. 2020;73(5): 445–9.
154. Tagliafico A, Bignotti B, Cadoni A, et al. Anatomical Study of the Iliohypogastric, Ilioinguinal, and Genitofemoral Nerves Using High-resolution Ultrasound. Muscle Nerve 2014;51(1):42–8.
155. Schmutz M, Schumacher PM, Luyet C, et al. Ilioinguinal and Iliohypogastric Nerves Cannot Be Selectively Blocked by Using Ultrasound Guidance: A Volunteer Study. Br J Anaesth 2013;111(2):264–70.
156. Wang Y, Wu T, Terry MJ, et al. Improved Perioperative Analgesia with Ultrasound-guided Ilioinguinal/iliohypogastric Nerve or Transversus Abdominis Plane Block for Open Inguinal Surgery: A Systematic Review and Meta-analysis of Randomized Controlled Trials. J Phys Ther Sci 2016;28(3):1055–60.

157. Bischoff JM, Koscielniak-Nielsen ZJ, Kehlet H, et al. Ultrasound-Guided Ilioinguinal/Iliohypogastric Nerve Blocks for Persistent Inguinal Postherniorrhaphy Pain. Anesth Analg 2012;114(6):1323–9.
158. Gofeld M, Christakis M. Sonographically Guided Ilioinguinal Nerve Block. J Ultrasound Med 2006;25(12):1571–5.
159. Trainor D, Moeschler S, Pingree M, et al. Landmark-based versus Ultrasound-guided Ilioinguinal/iliohypogastric Nerve Blocks in the Treatment of Chronic Postherniorrhaphy Groin Pain: A Retrospective Study. J Pain Res 2015;8: 767–70.
160. Thomassen I, van Suijlekom JA, van de Gaag A, et al. Ultrasound-guided Ilioinguinal/iliohypogastric Nerve Blocks for Chronic Pain after Inguinal Hernia Repair. Hernia 2012;17(3):329–32.
161. Cho H-M, Park D-S, Kim DH, et al. Diagnosis of Ilioinguinal Nerve Injury Based on Electromyography and Ultrasonography: A Case Report. Annals of rehabilitation medicine 2017;41(4):705–8.
162. Suresh S, Patel A, Porfyris S, et al. Ultrasound-guided Serial Ilioinguinal Nerve Blocks for Management of Chronic Groin Pain Secondary to Ilioinguinal Neuralgia in Adolescents. Pediatric Anesthesia 2008;18(8):775–8.
163. Sivashanmugam T, Saraogi A, Smiles SR, et al. Ultrasound Guided Percutaneous Electro-coagulation of Iilioinguinal and Iliohypogastric Nerves for Treatment of Chronic Groin Pain. Indian J Anaesth 2013;57(6):610–2.
164. Lee KS, Sin JM, Patil PP, et al. Ultrasound-Guided Microwave Ablation for the Management of Inguinal Neuralgia: A Preliminary Study with 1-Year Follow-up. J Vasc Interv Radiol 2019;30(2):242–8.
165. Thapa D, Ahuja V, Verma P, et al. Successful Management of a Refractory Case of Postoperative Herniorrhaphy Pain with Extended Duration Pulsed Radiofrequency. Saudi J Anaesth 2016;10(1):107–9.
166. Alici HA, Ahiskalioglu A, Celik M, et al. Ultrasound-Guided Pulsed Radiofrequency to the Ilio-Inguinal/Iliohypogastric Nerves to Manage Chronic Pain after Caesarean Delivery in a Breast-Feeding Woman. Int J Obstet Anesth 2019;40: 157–9.
167. Adler AC, Smith DI, Parikh PM. Chronic Pain Localized to the Iliohypogastric Nerve. Plast Reconstr Surg 2014;134(1):182e–3e.
168. Carayannopoulos A, Beasley R, Sites B. Facilitation of Percutaneous Trial Lead Placement with Ultrasound Guidance for Peripheral Nerve Stimulation Trial of Ilioinguinal Neuralgia: A Technical Note. Neuromodulation: Technology at the Neural Interface 2009;12(4):296–301.
169. Elahi F, Reddy C, Ho D. Ultrasound Guided Peripheral Nerve Stimulation Implant for Management of Intractable Pain after Inguinal Herniorrhaphy. Pain Physician 2015;18(1):E31–8.
170. Khedkar SM, Bhalerao PM, Yemul-Golhar SR, et al. Ultrasound-Guided Ilioinguinal and Iliohypogastric Nerve Block, a Comparison with the Conventional Technique: An Observational Study. Saudi J Anaesth 2015;9(3):293–7.
171. Rab M, Ebmer J, Dellon LA. Anatomic Variability of the Ilioinguinal and Genitofemoral Nerve: Implications for the Treatment of Groin Pain. Plast Reconstr Surg 2001;108(6):1618–23.
172. Bellingham GA, Peng PWH. Ultrasound-Guided Interventional Procedures for Chronic Pelvic Pain. Tech Reg Anesth Pain Manag 2009;13(3):171–8.
173. Hetta DF. Pulsed Radiofrequency Treatment for Chronic Post-Surgical Orchialgia: A Double-Blind, Sham-Controlled, Randomized Trial: Three Month Results. American Society of Interventional Pain Physicians 2018;1(21):199–205.

174. Shanthanna H. Successful Treatment of Genitofemoral Neuralgia Using Ultrasound Guided Injection: A Case Report and Short Review of Literature. Case reports in anesthesiology 2014;2014:371703.
175. Terkawi AS, Romdhane K. Ultrasound-guided Pulsed Radiofrequency Ablation of the Genital Branch of the Genitofemoral Nerve for Treatment of Intractable Orchalgia. Saudi J Anaesth 2014;8(2):294–8.
176. Campos NA, Chiles JH, Plunkett AR. Ultrasound-guided cryoablation of genitofemoral nerve for chronic inguinal pain. Pain Physician 2009;12(6):997–1000.
177. Thottungal AR, Peng P. Genitofemoral nerve. Ultrasound for interventional pain management. NY, USA: Springer International Publishing; 2019. p. 83–92.
178. Aszmann OC, Dellon ES, Dellon AL. Anatomical Course of the Lateral Femoral Cutaneous Nerve and Its Susceptibility to Compression and Injury. Plast Reconstr Surg 1997;100(3):600–4.
179. Dimitropoulos G, Schaepkens van Riempst J, Schertenleib P. Anatomical Variation of the Lateral Femoral Cutaneous Nerve: A Case Report and Review of the Literature. J Plast Reconstr Aesthet Surg 2011;64(7):961–2.
180. Joshi A, Kostakis GC. An investigation of post-operative morbidity following iliac crest graft harvesting. Br Dent J 2004 Feb 14;196(3):167–71 [discussion: 155].
181. Kim JE, Lee SG, Kim EJ, et al. Ultrasound-guided Lateral Femoral Cutaneous Nerve Block in Meralgia Paresthetica. The Korean journal of pain 2011;24(2): 115–8.
182. Ng I, Vaghadia H, Choi PT, et al. Ultrasound Imaging Accurately Identifies the Lateral Femoral Cutaneous Nerve. Anesth Analg 2008;107(3):1070–4.
183. Kiliç S, Özkan FÜ, Külcü DG, et al. Conservative Treatment Versus Ultrasound-Guided Injection in the Management of Meralgia Paresthetica: A Randomized Controlled Trial. Pain Physician 2020;23:253–62.
184. Hurdle MF, Weingarten TN, Crisostomo RA, et al. Ultrasound-Guided Blockade of the Lateral Femoral Cutaneous Nerve: Technical Description and Review of 10 Cases. Arch Phys Med Rehabil 2007;88(10):1362–4.
185. Tagliafico A, Serafini G, Lacelli F, et al. Ultrasound-Guided Treatment of Meralgia Paresthetica (Lateral Femoral Cutaneous Neuropathy). J Ultrasound Med 2011; 30(10):1341–6.
186. Khodair S, Elshafey R. Ultrasound Guided Lateral Femoral Cutaneous Nerve Block in Meralgia Paresthesia; Review of 25 Cases. The Egyptian Journal of Radiology and Nuclear Medicine 2014;45(4):1127–31.
187. Klauser AS, Abd Ellah MMH, Halpern EJ, et al. Meralgia Paraesthetica: Ultrasound-Guided Injection at Multiple Levels with 12-Month Follow-Up. Eur Radiol 2015;26(3):764–70.
188. Philip CN, Candido KD, Joseph NJ, et al. Successful Treatment of Meralgia Paresthetica with Pulsed Radiofrequency of the Lateral Femoral Cutaneous Nerve. Pain Physician 2009;12(5):881–5.
189. Mulvaney SW. Ultrasound-Guided Percutaneous Neuroplasty of the Lateral Femoral Cutaneous Nerve for the Treatment of Meralgia Paresthetica. Curr Sports Med Rep 2011;10(2):99–104.
190. Ahmed A, Arora D, Kochhar AK. Ultrasound-Guided Alcohol Neurolysis of Lateral Femoral Cutaneous Nerve for Intractable Meralgia Paresthetica: A Case Series. British journal of pain 2016;10(4):232–7.
191. Johnson C, Sisante JF, Alm J, et al. Cryoneurolysis for the Treatment of Lateral Femoral Cutaneous Nerve Pain: A Case Report. Pharm Manag PM R 2020;12(4): 423–4.

192. Chen CK, Phui VE, Saman MA. Alcohol neurolysis of lateral femoral cutaneous nerve for recurrent meralgia paresthetica. Agri 2012;24:42–4.
193. López AM, Sala-Blanch X, Magaldi M, et al. Ultrasound-Guided Ankle Block for Forefoot Surgery. Reg Anesth Pain Med 2012;37(5):554–7.
194. Madhavi C, Isaac B, Antoniswamy B, et al. Anatomical Variations of the Cutaneous Innervation Patterns of the Sural Nerve on the Dorsum of the Foot. Clin Anat 2005;18(3):206–9.
195. Soneji N, Peng P. Ankle joint and nerves. Ultrasound for interventional pain management. NY, USA: Springer International Publishing; 2019. p. 301–16.
196. Redborg KE, Antonakakis JG, Beach ML, et al. Ultrasound Improves the Success Rate of a Tibial Nerve Block at the Ankle. Reg Anesth Pain Med 2009;34(3):256–60.
197. Antonakakis JG, Scalzo DC, Jorgenson AS, et al. Ultrasound Does Not Improve the Success Rate of a Deep Peroneal Nerve Block at the Ankle. Reg Anesth Pain Med 2010;35(2):217–21.
198. Fredrickson MJ, White R, Danesh-Clough TK. Low-Volume Ultrasound-Guided Nerve Block Provides Inferior Postoperative Analgesia Compared to a Higher-Volume Landmark Technique. Reg Anesth Pain Med 2011;36(4):393–8.
199. Chin KJ, Wong NWY, Macfarlane AJR, et al. Ultrasound-Guided Versus Anatomic Landmark-Guided Ankle Blocks. Reg Anesth Pain Med 2011;36(6):611–8.
200. Walter WR, Burke CJ, Adler RS. Ultrasound-guided Therapeutic Injections for Neural Pathology about the Foot and Ankle: A 4 year Retrospective Review. Skeletal Radiol 2017;46(6):795–803.
201. Sobey JH, Franklin A. Ultrasound-guided tibial nerve block for definitive treatment of tarsal tunnel syndrome in a pediatric patient. Reg Anesth Pain Med 2016;41:415–6.
202. Abd-Elsayed A, Jackson M, Plovanich E. Pulsed Radiofrequency Ablation for Treating Sural Neuralgia. Ochsner J 2018;18:88–90.
203. Choi W-J, Hwang S-J, Song J-G, et al. Radiofrequency treatment relieves chronic knee osteoarthritis pain: a double-blind randomized controlled trial. Pain 2011;152:481–7.
204. Tran J, Peng PWH, Lam K, et al. Anatomical Study of the Innervation of Anterior Knee Joint Capsule. Reg Anesth Pain Med 2018;43(4):407–14.
205. Franco CD, Buvanendran A, Petersohn JD, et al. Innervation of the Anterior Capsule of the Human Knee. Reg Anesth Pain Med 2015;40(4):363–8.
206. Fonkoue L, Behets CW, Steyaert A, et al. Current versus revised anatomical targets for genicular nerve blockade and radiofrequency ablation: evidence from a cadaveric model. Reg Anesth Pain Med 2020;45(8):603–9.
207. Choi W-J. Ultrasound-Guided Genicular Nerve Block for Knee Osteoarthritis: A Double-Blind, Randomized Controlled Trial of Local Anesthetic Alone or in Combination with Corticosteroid. Pain Physician 2018;1(21):41–51.
208. Horner G, Dellon AL. Innervation of the Human Knee Joint and Implications for Surgery. Clin Orthop Relat Res 1994;301:221–6.
209. Kennedy JC, Alexander IJ, Hayes KC. Nerve Supply of the Human Knee and its Functional Importance. Am J Sports Med 1982;10(6):329–35.
210. Tran J, Peng PWH, Gofeld M, et al. Anatomical Study of the Innervation of Posterior Knee Joint Capsule: Implication for Image-guided Intervention. Reg Anesth Pain Med 2019;44(2):234–8.

211. Sluijter ME, Teixeira A, Serra V, et al. Intra-articular Application of Pulsed Radiofrequency for Arthrogenic Pain—Report of Six Cases. Pain Pract 2008;8(1):57–61.
212. Hirasawa Y, Okajima S, Ohta M, et al. Nerve Distribution to the Human Knee Joint: Anatomical and Immunohistochemical Study. Int Orthop 2000;24(1):1–4.
213. Protzman NM, Gyi J, Malhotra AD, et al. Examining the Feasibility of Radiofrequency Treatment for Chronic Knee Pain After Total Knee Arthroplasty. Pharm Manag PM R 2014;6(4):373–6.
214. Adiguzel E, Uran A, Kesikburun S, et al. Knee Pain Relief with Genicular Nerve Blockage in Two Brain Injured Patients with Heterotopic Ossification. Brain Inj 2015;29(13–14):1736–9.
215. Bhatia A, Peng P, Cohen SP. Radiofrequency Procedures to Relieve Chronic Knee Pain. Reg Anesth Pain Med 2016;41(4):501–10.
216. Kim DH, Choi SS, Yoon SH, et al. Ultrasound-guided genicular nerve block for knee osteoarthritis: a double-blind, randomized controlled trial of local anesthetic alone or in combination with corticosteroid. Pain Physician 2018;21(1):41–52.
217. Kim DH, Lee MS, Lee S, et al. A Prospective Randomized Comparison of the Efficacy of Ultrasound- vs Fluoroscopy-Guided Genicular Nerve Block for Chronic Knee Osteoarthritis. Pain Physician 2019;22(2):139–46.
218. Sari S, Aydin ON, Turan Y, et al. Which imaging method should be used for genicular nerve radio frequency thermocoagulation in chronic knee osteoarthritis? J Clin Monit Comput 2017;31:797–803.
219. Ahmed A, Arora D. Ultrasound-Guided Neurolysis of Six Genicular Nerves for Intractable Pain from Knee Osteoarthritis: A Case Series. Pain Pract 2018;19(1):16–26.
220. Huang Y, Deng Q, Yang L, et al. Efficacy and Safety of Ultrasound-Guided Radiofrequency Treatment for Chronic Pain in Patients with Knee Osteoarthritis: A Systematic Review and Meta-Analysis. Pain Res Manag 2020;2020:2537075.
221. Monerris Tabasco MM, Roca Amatria G, Ríos Márquez N, et al. Assessment of the effectiveness and safety of two radiofrequency techniques for the treatment of knee pain secondary to gonarthrosis. Prospective randomized double blind study. Rev Esp Anestesiol Reanim 2019 Aug-Sep;66(7):362–9. English, Spanish.
222. E Djibilian Fucci R, Pascual-Ramírez J, Martínez-Marcos A, et al. Ultrasound-guided sciatic nerve pulsed radiofrequency for chronic knee pain treatment: a novel approach. J Anesth 2013;27(6):935–8.
223. Aly I, El- Karadawy S, Ahmed Gab, et al. Ultrasound guided intra-articular pulsed radiofrequency in patients with primary chronic knee osteoarthritis. ARC Journal of Anesthesiology 2018;3:25–34.
224. Santana Pineda MM, Vanlinthout LE, Moreno Martín A, et al. Analgesic Effect and Functional Improvement Caused by Radiofrequency Treatment of Genicular Nerves in Patients With Advanced Osteoarthritis of the Knee Until 1 Year Following Treatment. Reg Anesth Pain Med 2017;42(1):62–8.
225. Erdem Y, Sir E. The Efficacy of Ultrasound-Guided Pulsed Radiofrequency of Genicular Nerves in the Treatment of Chronic Knee Pain Due to Severe Degenerative Disease or Previous Total Knee Arthroplasty. Med Sci Monit 2019;25:1857–63.
226. Ahmed A, Arora D. Ultrasound-guided radiofrequency ablation of genicular nerves of knee for relief of intractable pain from knee osteoarthritis: a case series. Br J Pain 2018;12(3):145–54.

227. Franklin AD, Cierny GB, Luckett TR. Interventional and Multimodal Pain Rehabilitation in a Child with Meralgia Paresthetica. J Clin Anesth 2016;33:456–9.
228. Simpson DM, Tyrrell J, De Ruiter J, et al. Use of Ultrasound-Guided Subcostal Transversus Abdominis Plane Blocks in a Pediatric Patient with Chronic Abdominal Wall Pain. Paediatr Anaesth 2011;21(1):88–90.
229. Martin DP, Bhalla T, Rehman S, et al. Successive Multisite Peripheral Nerve Catheters for Treatment of Complex Regional Pain Syndrome Type I. Pediatrics 2013;131(1):e323–6.
230. Bhatia A, Brull R. Is Ultrasound Guidance Advantageous for Interventional Pain Management. A Systematic Review of Chronic Pain Outcomes. Anesth Analg 2013;117(1):236–51.
231. Chang MC. Efficacy of Pulsed Radiofrequency Stimulation in Patients with Peripheral Neuropathic Pain: A Narrative Review. Pain Physician 2018;21(3): E225–34.
232. Deer TR, Esposito MF, McRoberts WP, et al. A Systematic Literature Review of Peripheral Nerve Stimulation Therapies for the Treatment of Pain. Pain Med 2020;21(8):1590–603.
233. Xu J, Sun Z, Wu J, et al. Peripheral Nerve Stimulation in Pain Management: A Systematic Review. Pain Physician 2021;24(2):E131–52.
234. Strand N, D'Souza RS, Hagedorn JM, et al. Evidence-Based Clinical Guidelines from the American Society of Pain and Neuroscience for the Use of Implantable Peripheral Nerve Stimulation in the Treatment of Chronic Pain. J Pain Res 2022; 15:2483–504.
235. Helm S, Shirsat N, Calodney A, et al. Peripheral Nerve Stimulation for Chronic Pain: A Systematic Review of Effectiveness and Safety. Pain Ther 2021;10(2): 985–1002.

Disparities in Pain Management

Lee Huynh Nguyen, MD[a], Jessica Esther Dawson, MD, MPH[a], Meredith Brooks, MD, MPH[b], James S. Khan, MD, MSc[c], Natacha Telusca, MD, MPH[a,*]

KEYWORDS

- Chronic pain • Disparities • Ethnicity • Race • Acute pain • Pediatric • Cancer
- Gender • Obstetric • Socioeconomic • Diversity • Geography
- Advanced pain procedure • Rural • Veteran • Elderly

KEY POINTS

- Disparities in pain management have remained pervasive for decades.
- These disparities are observed in all aspects of pain management from acute pain, chronic pain, pediatric pain, obstetric pain, and advanced pain procedures.
- Disparities are not limited to race and ethnicity, because they have been identified in multiple less-studied vulnerable populations.
- Plans of action must focus on research, advocacy, policy changes, structural changes, and targeted interventions to patients and clinicians.

INTRODUCTION

Chronic pain is highly prevalent in the United States affecting an estimated 50 million adults.[1] It is a cause of significant morbidity, mortality, and disability, and is costly to society in terms of treatment expenses and lost productivity. It is a universal problem, and racial minorities and vulnerable populations experience additional suffering because of inadequate pain care resulting from disparities in access and treatment. The large body of research, patient reports, and other sources that form the basis of the Institute of Medicine (IOM) report "Relieving Pain in America"[2] indicate that racial disparities in the incidence, assessment, treatment, and outcomes of pain are common. Racial disparities in pain care are complex because of multiple contributing

[a] Department of Anesthesiology, Perioperative and Pain Medicine, Stanford University, Stanford, CA, USA; [b] Department of Anesthesiology, Cook Children's Health Care System, Texas Christian University School of Medicine, Fort Worth, TX, USA; [c] Department of Anesthesia and Pain Medicine, Mount Sinai Hospital, University of Toronto, Toronto, Ontario, Canada
* Corresponding author. Department Anesthesiology, Perioperative and Pain Medicine, Stanford University School of Medicine, 450 Broadway Street, Pavilion A, MC5340, Redwood City, CA 94063.
E-mail address: ntelusca@stanford.edu

Anesthesiology Clin 41 (2023) 471–488
https://doi.org/10.1016/j.anclin.2023.03.008
anesthesiology.theclinics.com
1932-2275/23/

factors within and outside the health care sector. Most notably, socioeconomic status compounds these disparities, and its impact on vulnerable populations is profound.

The Health and Human Services National Pain Strategy[3] summarized the problem of disparities in pain management with the following statement:

> *The Problem:* A significant problem facing vulnerable populations arises from conscious and unconscious biases and negative attitudes, beliefs, perceptions, and misconceptions about higher-risk population groups (eg, gender or racial bias) or about pain itself. If held by clinicians, social service program administrators, or other decision-makers, these attitudes can negatively affect the care and services they provide. For example, inappropriate or inadequate treatment may result if clinicians fail to understand or accept that individuals differ in pain sensitivity and treatment response due to various factors. People with pain who encounter these biases can feel stigmatized, which may decrease their willingness to report pain timely, participate in decisions about their care, adhere to a recommended treatment plan, or follow a self-care protocol. This perception also may negatively affect their psychological state.
>
> An additional barrier to eliminating pain disparities is the lack of sufficient knowledge of behavioral and biological issues (eg, genomic variability, pharmacokinetic and pharmacodynamic differences) that affect pain onset and management and data to understand pain patterns and its treatment in higher risk and vulnerable populations.

Harmful and inaccurate stereotypes ascribed to Black and White people have been prevalent throughout American history to justify slavery, segregation, and inhumane treatment of Black people and racial minorities in medical research.[4,5] Messaging, such as Black people have thicker skulls, are less sensitive to pain, and have a lower need for analgesia and anesthesia, were promoted by scientists, physicians, and community leaders until well into the twentieth century.[5] The assumption that Black people experience pain differently fueled unethical experimentation, such as exposing Black soldiers to mustard gas during World War II and the experiments conducted by the US Public Health Service in Tuskegee, Alabama, which left syphilis untreated in Black men and recorded the results in Black families over the four decades from 1932 to 1972.[5] These and other historic atrocities contributed to a pervasive culture of mistrust among many Black and indigenous communities, resulting in mistrust of medical institutions, leading to reluctance to seek care or participate in medical research.

The causes of health care disparities are multifactorial and include societal, systems, provider, community, and individual components. Socioeconomic status includes education level, family income, and occupation.[6] Additional factors contributing to health disparities include health insurance status, health literacy, and individual beliefs. Access to health care, childcare, shelter, green spaces, transportation, clean air, and so forth all have the power to affect health. Policy changes are needed on local, state, and national levels to promote equity. This review specifically targets health care disparities in the management of pain, with a focus on steps health care providers and organizations can take to promote health care equity.

RACIAL AND ETHNIC DISPARITIES IN HEALTH CARE

Racial and ethnic health care disparities in America present a long-standing issue. In 2003 the IOM (now National Academy of Medicine) published a special report entitled "Unequal Treatment: Confronting Racial and Ethnic Disparities in Health Care."[7] This report produced the following major findings[7]:

1. Racial and ethnic disparities in health care exist, are associated with worse health outcomes, and are therefore unacceptable.

2. Racial and ethnic disparities in health care occur in the context of broader historic and contemporary social and economic inequalities, and there is evidence of persistent racial and ethnic discrimination in many sectors of American life.
3. Many sources, including clinicians, patients, and utilization managers, may contribute to racial and ethnic disparities in health care.
4. Bias, stereotyping, prejudice, and clinical uncertainty on the part of clinicians may contribute to racial and ethnic disparities in health care.
5. Certain patients may be more likely to refuse treatment; however, these refusal rates are generally small and do not fully explain health care disparities.

Ample evidence exists in the current literature describing racially discrepant care. In a recent systematic review spanning 20 years, Morales and Yong[8] demonstate disparities in chronic pain management, particularly among Black and Hispanic patients. An overwhelming body of evidence reveals Black and Hispanic patients were consistently prescribed fewer opioids and other prescription analgesics.[8] Additionally, when compared with White patients, Black patients were more likely to be subjected to long-term monitoring for opioid misuse even though rates of opioid misuse were highest in White patients.[8] Another large, systematic review noted a striking difference in pain treatment in Black and Hispanic Americans compared with White Americans.[9] Black and Hispanic patients were consistently prescribed fewer analgesics and opioids, regardless of their type of pain. There is abundant confirmation that Black Americans and other ethnic minorities are treated differently from their White counterparts.

The preponderance of racial disparities research focuses on Black versus White, although a recent study reveals that less-studied racial groups are also affected.[10] An examination of pain prevalence in Asian, Hispanic, Native American, and multiracial individuals found that Native American and multiracial patients reported the highest pain prevalence of all racial subgroups.[10] This difference was attributable to socioeconomic status, a widespread systemic disparity. This work is incredibly important because the United States population is only becoming more diverse, with the number of multiracial patients expected to double between 2020 and 2050.[10] Additionally, there is a paucity of studies on chronic pain in Native Americans, although they cite high pain prevalence and poor patient-provider communications.[11,12] More attention needs to be focused on other racial subgroups in the United States, including but not limited to, those of Asian, Hispanic, and Middle Eastern descent. Eventually, data disaggregation should be examined because there is significant variability within subgroups, such as the Hispanic and Asian categories.[10,13]

OTHER VULNERABLE POPULATIONS

LGBTQ+

The number of individuals who identify as lesbian, gay, bisexual, transgender, queer, and others (LGBTQ+) in the United States increased from 4% in 2016 to 7% in 2022.[14,15] Despite this growing population, only a minimal number of studies exist on chronic pain in gender-diverse adults. Studies that exist suggest disparities in pain and care experienced by these minorities.

Sexual minority women were more likely to experience pain and pain impairment. One cross-sectional study found that sexual minority women (lesbian, bisexual, and primarily heterosexual defined as those who did not identify as entirely heterosexual) were more likely to report headaches and muscle aches.[16] Another cross-sectional study of more than 6000 women found that sexual minority women had a greater lifetime risk of experiencing chronic pelvic pain.[17] Additionally, women who identified as bisexual were more likely to experience chronic pelvic pain that interfered with their quality of life. This result is echoed by a prospective cohort study of more than 100,000 nurses, which found that bisexual women are more likely to experience pain with functional impairment.[18] These results highlight the importance of screening for chronic pain and pelvic pain in sexual minority women.

A limited number of transgender community studies also suggest an increase in pain prevalence pain in this population. A retrospective cohort study in Israel reported that 19.4% of transgender men and 7% of transgender women met the criteria for fibromyalgia, which is six times that of the general Israeli population.[19] A retrospective cohort study of transgender men undergoing hysterectomy reported that only 32% of patients with pelvic pain preoperatively were found with pathologic evidence of endometriosis.[20] Accordingly, there are possibly alternative causes of pelvic pain or pain perception in this population. The authors posited that the higher prevalence may be caused by increased psychiatric comorbidity and changes in pain perception in transgender patients undergoing hormone therapy.[21] Furthermore, a study that explored pain responses found that transgender women and cisgender women responded to pain similarly when compared with cisgender men, suggesting that there are alternative determinants to pain response other than simply genetic sex.[22]

A literature search revealed even less information regarding chronic pain in other LGBTQ+ populations, although a handful of studies exist that focus on chronic pain in sexual minority men concurrently diagnosed with HIV.[23,24] More assessment is necessary to understand the complex needs of those who identify as a sexual minority.

Military Veterans

Chronic pain is common in military veterans because of combat injuries and psychiatric comorbidities, such as posttraumatic stress disorder.[25] Examinations of the veteran population reveal persistent racial disparities and challenges unique to this population. A large, national, retrospective cohort study comparing more than 99,000 veterans diagnosed with chronic noncancer pain found that Black veterans younger than the age of 65 were less likely than their White counterparts to receive opioid prescriptions for moderate to severe pain.[26] This finding remained after controlling for confounders, such as substance use and psychiatric comorbidities. This study likely underestimates this effect because White patients are more likely to obtain opioid prescriptions from sources outside of the Veterans Administration Health System.[26] A cross-sectional analysis of more than 250,000 veterans similarly found that Black men were less likely than White men to report effective treatment of their pain.[27] An examination of interviews with military women about chronic pain revealed disparities in health care based on perceived racial and gender biases.[25] Military women are particularly vulnerable, given their increased risk of military and sexual trauma. A study of more than 2 million veterans found that female veterans were less likely to be prescribed opioids and more likely to be prescribed serotonin-norepinephrine reuptake inhibitors and muscle relaxants compared with their male counterparts, even when controlling for type of pain (eg, headache, fibromyalgia).[28]

Socioeconomic Status

Multiple longitudinal cross-sectional studies have connected pain disparities to socioeconomic status. In 2016, the Centers for Disease Control and Prevention conducted the National Health Interview Survey, which estimated that 20% of Americans (50 million) suffer from chronic pain and 8% (nearly 20 million) from high-impact chronic pain. The authors defined high-impact pain as pain affecting life or work on most days over 6 months. The prevalence of high-impact pain was greater among individuals who were unemployed, in or near poverty, less educated, from rural areas, and uninsured or with public health care coverage.[1] Similarly, Janevic and colleagues[29] found that patients in the lowest wealth quartile had increased rates of high-impact pain. Both lower family income and not attending college were associated with a 40% increase in the odds of having chronic pain.[30] This finding was echoed in another longitudinal cross-sectional study of 20,000 older adults, which found that those in the lowest quartile of wealth or who did not graduate from high school were the most likely to report severe pain.[31]

Elderly

A large, national, cross-sectional study of more than 400,000 adults over 16 years found that patients aged 65 to 84 had steeper increases in their pain scores compared with younger patients.[30] Additionally, adults older than 80 years were more likely to have severe pain compared with their wealthier counterparts.[31] The Centers for Disease Control and Prevention survey in 2016 also reported a statistically significant increased prevalence of high-impact pain with advancing age.[1] Despite this increase in chronic pain and high-impact pain in the aging population, adults older than the age of 65 were less likely to receive opioids than those who were younger.[8]

Other marginalized populations not discussed, although deserving full attention, include the homeless, refugees, indigenous populations, and patients with HIV.[32]

Pediatric Populations

Well into the twentieth century, neonates and infants were thought incapable of perceiving pain, so they were seldom given analgesics for surgery.[33] Various reasons have been promulgated for this decreased administration of analgesia for children, including misconceptions,[34–36] concerns about safety,[37,38] and practice variability.[39,40] Despite evidence that children do experience pain,[34] children with pain from fractures,[41,42] burns,[41] appendicitis,[43,44] and sickle cell crises[41] still receive less analgesia than adults.

Compared with adult pain research, fewer studies document racial and ethnic disparities in pain management for children,[45] but as with adults, the extant studies indicate that racial and ethnic disparities have been reported. In managing children suffering from acute abdominal pain in the emergency department (ED), including those with appendicitis,[43,46] Black and Hispanic patients were less likely than White patients to receive analgesics for abdominal pain.[43,46,47]

A small retrospective study of 94 children found that Hispanic patients received 30% fewer opioid analgesics than White patients postoperatively.[48] Subsequent larger prospective observational studies found that minority children experienced more postoperative pain and received more opioid analgesics than their White counterparts.[49,50] In a prospective, observational study of 194 children undergoing tonsillectomy, Sadhasivam and colleagues[50] found White children had a higher incidence of opioid-related adverse events. In a follow-up study, they observed that Black patients had greater morphine clearance compared with White patients.[51] These studies underscore that a child's race is important in personalizing analgesia care, which may help decrease postoperative complications.

There is evidence that pain sensitivity also differs among ethnicities and races. Specifically, minorities tend to be more sensitive to pain.[52,53] An experimental pain study in children found that coping ability was a moderating effect in the relationship between pain sensitivity and race.[54] Thus, it is possible for Black and White children receiving similar doses of opioids for the same procedure to have completely different pain experiences postoperatively.[50]

Unconscious pro-White bias on the part of pediatricians was found to negatively impact opioid medication prescribing practices for Black children but not for White children.[45] Development of educational programs that target improved provider-patient communication and clinical behavior and the creation of standard protocols may help address implicit bias and contribute to decreasing disparities in pain management.[45] Clinicians caring for children should be aware of the existing inequalities in analgesic administration and consciously make efforts to consider race and ethnicity to optimize pain control.

Acute Pain

Numerous reports have documented the disparities in pain management between racial and ethnic groups seeking care for acute pain. An analysis of a national database of 6710 ED visits between 2006 and 2010 found that, compared with non-Hispanic White patients, non-Hispanic Black patients and patients of other races and ethnicities had 22% to 30% lower risk-adjusted odds of receiving any analgesic and 17% and 30% lower risk-adjusted odds of receiving an opioid analgesic for non-traumatic abdominal pain ($P < .05$).[55] Moreover, studies of racial-ethnic disparities in the ED for pain-related complaints often associated with drug-seeking behaviors (eg, toothache, back pain, and abdominal pain) found that compared with non-Hispanic Whites, non-Hispanic Blacks were less likely to receive an opioid prescription.[56]

These findings remain significant despite adjustments for covariates that could potentially explain differences in care and support the notion that some disparities may be caused by inherent and unconscious biases that influence changes in practice behaviors.

To evaluate pain care disparities in the ED, in 2019 investigators conducted a systematic review and meta-analysis of opioid prescribing practices. They found a total of 14 articles that included more than 11,000 patients.[57] In their meta-analysis, Black patients were 40% less likely to receive any analgesia than White patients (odds ratio, 0.60; 95% confidence interval, 0.43–0.83; random effects model). Hispanic patients were also less likely to receive analgesic medications than non-Hispanic White patients. However, only their fixed-effect-model meta-analysis was statistically significant.

Racial and ethnic disparities in acute pain management have also been demonstrated in pediatric populations. Compared with White non-Hispanic children, Black non-Hispanic and Hispanic children were less likely to receive opioid analgesia after limb fracture and in cases of suspected appendicitis.[58] Moreover, differences in acute pain management begin to occur even before arrival in the ED. A retrospective analysis of 25,732 patient encounters with emergency medical services in Oregon between 2015 and 2017 found that all racial and ethnic patients were less likely to receive pain medication compared with White patients, and that Hispanic and Asian patients were less likely than White and Black patients to have any assessment for pain.[59]

Cancer Pain

Pain can arise during or after treatment of cancer and pain control is a key part of comprehensive cancer management, particularly in patients receiving palliative care. Management of cancer pain tends to include ample use of opioid analgesics, which contrasts with noncancer pain management. Although several reports have indicated differences in cancer management between ethnic groups,[60,61] few reports have categorized those differences. A cross-sectional study in 2018 examining more than 340,000 patients with cancer newly admitted to a nursing home indicated that

Black patients were less likely to be assessed for pain and, subsequently, less likely to receive either pharmacologic or nonpharmacologic pain intervention compared with Whites.[62] This is consistent with a prospective study of outpatients in a clinic that manages pain for patients with recurrent or metastatic cancer. The study found that 65% of the minority patients did not receive guideline-recommended analgesic prescriptions compared with 50% of nonminority patients ($P < .001$).[63]

To further compound the issue, when analgesics are prescribed, they are often done so with less consideration for potential adverse effects. Morphine administration produces 3- and 6-glucuronide metabolites, which are neurotoxic and can accumulate in patients with chronic kidney disease. Therefore, the use of morphine is avoided in patients with chronic kidney disease. An analysis of patients with cancer attending an academic-affiliated oncology clinic found that Black patients with chronic kidney disease were disproportionately prescribed morphine more often than safer options (oxycodone), which was associated with a greater incidence of analgesic-related adverse effects.[64] Other reports have found differences in racial groups obtaining nonopioid analgesic agents, such as antidepressants, and anxiolytics and sleep agents for other cancer-related symptom management.[65]

These studies documenting disparities in cancer pain management are unfortunate, particularly considering that racial and ethnic populations tend to suffer greater pain during and after cancer treatment. An analysis of patients receiving active cancer treatment found that Black patients reported significantly greater pain intensity, more pain-related distress, and more pain-related interference with functioning compared with White patients.[66] Furthermore, Black women are more likely to report pain, skin irritation, and decreased physical functioning during breast cancer treatment than White women.[67,68] Unsurprisingly, Black patients with breast cancer commonly report greater unmet symptom management than their White counterparts.

OBSTETRIC ANESTHESIA

Racial and ethnic disparities in obstetric anesthesia have been studied in neuraxial labor analgesia, general anesthesia use for cesarean, and postpartum pain management.

Neuraxial Labor Analgesia

Neuraxial labor analgesia includes epidural, spinal, and combined spinal-epidural analgesia.[69] Neuraxial analgesia is the preferred form of analgesia in vaginal and cesarean deliveries because of its effectiveness and safety profile for mother and baby. Neuraxial analgesia causes local vasodilation, improves blood flow, and decreases the risk for venous thromboembolism when compared with general anesthesia.[70] A large, multistate study of 6,872,588 births found that Black women were significantly more likely than White women to receive no analgesia for vaginal deliveries.[71] A qualitative study in which 82 postpartum women were interviewed suggested that minority women with low levels of education were more likely to feel pressured to get an epidural and experience epidural failure than White women with higher levels of education.[72] Disparities in analgesia administration for vaginal deliveries should be further explored to understand and address the system, provider, and patient factors contributing to these disparities.

General Anesthesia Use in Cesarean Delivery

Cesarean sections are the most common surgical procedure for women in the United States, accounting for one-third of all births.[73] Black, Hispanic, and Asian women are more likely to undergo cesarean delivery than non-Hispanic White women.[74,75]

Multiple studies that adjusted for obstetric and nonobstetric covariates also found that Black and Hispanic women are more likely than White women to receive general anesthesia for term and preterm cesarean deliveries.[70,76–78] Although general anesthesia is more likely to be used in emergency cesarean sections in all racial and ethnic groups, it continues to be used more often in nonemergency and potentially avoidable settings for minority women when compared with White women.[70] General anesthesia is associated with worse outcomes for mother and baby, including increased risk of aspiration, surgical site infections, venous thromboembolism/pulmonary embolism, significant maternal pain, and postpartum depression.[79]

Postpartum Pain Management

Timely recognition and treatment of postpartum pain is critical to avoid long-term sequelae. A multicenter longitudinal study of 1288 women found that women with severe acute postpartum pain had a 2.5-fold increased risk of persistent pain and a 3.0-fold increased risk of postpartum depression when compared with patients with mild postpartum pain, independent of the type of delivery.[80]

After adjusting for potential confounding covariates, another study of 9900 postpartum patients demonstrated that Hispanic women and non-Hispanic black women were significantly more likely than non-Hispanic white women to report postpartum pain scores of at least 5, receive less inpatient morphine milligram equivalents, and be discharged without an opioid prescription.[81] A single-institution study noted that Hispanic women and non-English-speaking patients had the lowest administered oxycodone therapeutic equivalents at 25 to 48 hours after delivery and the lowest number of pain assessments throughout their hospital stays.[82] Another single-institution study of 1701 postpartum women noted similar results, with minority women less likely to undergo pain assessment during their hospital stay and receive fewer oxycodone tablet equivalents on discharge.[83] Implicit bias, language barriers, patient medical beliefs, provider prescribing habits, and frequency of quality pain assessments can all contribute to disparities in postpartum pain management.

Delays in Epidural Patches for Postdural Puncture Headaches

Postdural puncture headaches (PDPH) are a common and debilitating complication of neuraxial procedures. PDPH is a severe positional headache that can prolong hospital stays and hinder the ability of mothers to care for and bond with their newborns. If left untreated, PDPH is associated with chronic headaches, cerebral venous thrombosis, subdural hematoma, and postpartum depression.[84] Epidural blood patches (EBP) are the standard treatment of severe PDPH. A cross-sectional study of 8921 obstetric patients with PDPH in New York hospitals found that Black and other minority patients were significantly less likely to receive an EBP than White patients.[84] The study also noted that minority women who did receive an EBP for PDPH management did so a median of 1 day later than their White counterparts.[84]

GEOGRAPHIC DISPARITIES IN PAIN MANAGEMENT

Chronic pain is not distributed equitably across the United States. Adults living in rural areas are more likely to experience chronic pain than those living in urban areas.[85–87] Possible causes for higher rates of chronic pain in rural areas include older populations and higher employment rates in agriculture, mining, or manufacturing, which may increase the risk of chronic pain.[88] Rural residents are more likely to be uninsured and to report higher levels of disability and more depression and sadness.[89] They are also less likely to receive specialty care for low back pain when compared with urban residents.[89] A recent covariate analysis comparing rural, suburban, and urban residents of North Carolina showed 60% lower use of nonmedication pain treatments, such as physical therapy, acupuncture, or yoga, in rural and suburban areas as compared with urban areas.[89]

Suburban and rural residents were less likely to report using multiple treatments for chronic pain, suggesting a disparity in chronic pain treatment as compared with residents in more populated communities. Multimodal, interdisciplinary treatments that target comprehensive pain management are recommended over single-modal treatments, which often fail.[2,3] Accessibility of nonmedication treatment is an issue because rural areas have fewer specialists and principally rely on primary care providers for pain treatment.[90] Primary care providers often have little education in chronic pain.[91] Research has shown that rural residents are more likely to be prescribed an opioid analgesic than urban residents.[90,92] The opioid epidemic has significantly affected rural communities across the United States.[93] An October 2017 survey by the National Farmers Union and the American Farm Bureau Federation found that three out of four farmers have been directly impacted by the opioid crisis.[94] Chronic pain is a substantial public health problem that may contribute to significant morbidity, mortality, disability, poor quality of life, and increased health care costs in the United States.[2,95–97] Public health interventions emphasizing multimodal treatments and provider education are needed to target rural and suburban patients, which may help decrease geographic disparities in the United States.

ADVANCED PAIN PROCEDURES

Only a few studies exist examining disparities in advanced pain procedures, particularly neuromodulation devices. A large retrospective study of more than 1.2 million Medicare patients found that minorities were significantly less likely to receive spinal cord stimulators (SCS) for either postlaminectomy syndrome or chronic pain syndrome; 90% of those recipients were White.[98] Another study found that among 40,000 hospitalized patients, minority patients were more likely than White patients to receive an SCS for inpatient admissions for complex regional pain syndrome I and failed back surgery syndrome.[99] Although the reasons are unclear, the authors posit that it may be that minority patients present later with more severe disease. Comorbidities may limit surgical intervention. Additionally, there exists a disparity in SCS costs. One study found that Hispanic patients were more likely to have higher charges for an inpatient SCS, whereas there was no difference between the charges for Black and White patients.[100] An income disparity was also observed in counties where neuromodulation devices were implanted.[101] With the increasing popularity of advanced pain procedures, we expect to see increasing disparity in access. Further research is needed to evaluate for disparities among those receiving other advanced pain procedures, such as peripheral nerve stimulators, intrathecal pumps, radiofrequency ablation, Vertiflex (Boston Scientific, Marlborough, MA), minimally invasive lumbar decompression, etc.

WHAT HEALTH CARE PROVIDERS AND ORGANIZATIONS CAN DO

Decades have lapsed since the IOM report was issued yet chronic pain persists as a public health crisis. Because pain levels in themselves are predictive of death, disparities in pain management put marginalized groups in danger of their lives.[31] Since disparities in chronic pain have not only persisted but have grown, action must be taken. In 2012, Meghani and coworkers[9] identified five domains of action: (1) structural, (2) policy and advocacy, (3) workforce, (4) provider, and (5) research. Similarly, Campbell and coworkers[102] indicate that improvement is needed in research, advocacy, and policy. We agree with a comprehensive plan of action that includes the previously mentioned areas for improvement and the addition of the improvements described in the following sections.

Clinician Education

There is a gap in clinician education. In a national survey of clinicians who manage chronic pain, nearly 90% of respondents agreed that chronic pain is a public health issue, but fewer than 40% believed that undertreated pain is most common in minorities.[103] Interventions that target clinician education can effect change throughout a clinician's career, because one clinician can treat many patients with chronic pain over the life of that career. Recent interventions have targeted physicians who treated chronic pain, although efficacy is variable. One effective intervention comes from a randomized controlled trial of more than 400 resident physicians and fellows, which demonstrated a clear benefit of individualized feedback on perspective-taking.[104] In this study, physicians were presented with virtual patient encounters and were tasked to treat either Black or White patients with chronic pain. Participants who showed a treatment bias were then randomized to an intervention where they were given individual feedback on their biases and videos highlighting how pain affected their patients' lives. As a result, the treatment group showed 85% lower odds of treatment bias in treating Black patients and 76% lower odds of exhibiting treatment bias in patients with low socioeconomic statue.[104] Indeed, perspective-taking in itself seems to be an effective means of reducing the incidence of treatment bias, according to the results of a prior study that showed a reduction in treatment bias by more than 50% in an intervention group coached in perspective-taking.[105] However, varying success was seen in a virtual continuing medical education–certified educational publication targeted toward clinicians who treated chronic pain. Postsurvey questions showed improved confidence in identifying barriers when managing chronic pain in minorities. Unfortunately, improvement in knowledge was seen in only one of the three postsurvey questions.[103] A more effective means of educating providers includes incorporating pain management training early in graduate medical education and longitudinally through continuing medical education focused on perspective-taking.[7]

Clinician Diversity

Diversity among pain medicine providers is critical to providing care for an increasingly diverse patient population. Racial concordance is defined as a shared racial identity between a patient and physician. A systematic review of racial concordance on the effects of patient-physician communication in Black versus White patients found that racial concordance consistently improved communication, whereas racial discordance was consistently associated with poorer communication.[106] To improve concordance, it is important to increase diversity among medical school matriculants, including residency specialties that feed into pain medicine. A cross-sectional analysis of pain fellowship training noted that despite an increased number of pain fellowship positions, males consistently outnumbered females at a ratio of 4:1 to 5:1.[107] Additionally, nearly 40% of pain fellows identified as non-Hispanic White and 22% identified as Asian/Pacific Islander.[107] It is important to have providers who reflect the diversity of patients, because concordance has been shown to improve patient quality of care.[108,109]

Patient-Centeredness

Patient-centeredness also remains a key to improving health disparities. Digitally recorded interviews of patients who identified as transgender underscored a particular need for patient-centered communication, including "active listening, affirming language, and clear explanations about their healthcare"; asking patients for their preferred pronouns; and incorporating interdisciplinary care teams that include psychologists.[110]

Interpreters

A randomized controlled trial in an inner-city pain clinic found that reminder telephone calls in the patient's preferred language increased adherence to their scheduled appointments.[111,112] This study was conducted using certified Spanish speakers. The authors intend to continue language-based interventions focused on the appointment-making process. Altogether, these results are promising and invite continued research on improving access to pain services for non-English speakers.

Telehealth

One Veterans Administration successfully launched comprehensive telehealth pain services to address the needs of rural veterans. Their program included classes on pain education, cognitive behavior therapy, opioid safety, and acupuncture, which reduced in-person visits while allowing for regional expansion of this program.[113]

Patient-Tailored Intervention

Patient-targeted interventions have been attempted to address racial disparities in pain management, with varying degrees of success. A randomized controlled trial attempted to reduce chronic musculoskeletal pain in Black veterans by tailoring interventions using evidence-based literature and focus groups. A total of 380 patients were randomized to either usual care or telephone motivational interviewing and action planning to encourage walking. Although the primary outcome of improved pain-related physical functioning was not achieved, intervention participants did report a reduction in pain intensity and interference.[114,115] The authors noted that more intense intervention is needed to reach this population. It is important to continue exploring tailored, evidence-based interventions.

Research

There is a large health care disparity research gap. Campbell and coworkers[102] discuss the challenges in recruiting minority groups, including mistrust, low participation, and access to research sites. Additionally, much research is conducted with studies in English, making it difficult to assess pain in the non-English-speaking population.[8] Outreach targeting these barriers is essential in continuing research for those who may benefit the most. Currently, only a small number of interventions have been implemented, with varying degrees of success. It is crucial to continue focusing on targeted interventions and examine the causes of these growing disparities.

SUMMARY

The IOM reports from 2003 and 2011 provided several recommendations for improving existing disparities in health care.[2,7] However, since the first report's release almost 20 years ago, minimal progress has been made to reduce health care disparities in the United States. In this article, we discuss areas in pain medicine with significant disparities and make recommendations for promoting health care equity. To reduce health care disparities and foster health care equity in an increasingly diverse population, it is crucial that health care providers and organizations proactively institute the steps and actions outlined in this article.

CLINICS CARE POINTS

- Despite a dire call to action in by the IOM in 2003, racial and ethnic disparities persist in pain management.
- Disparities exist in all aspects of pain medicine: acute pain, pediatric pain, cancer pain, obstetric pain management, and advanced pain procedures.
- Evidence of disparities is emerging in vulnerable populations, including the LGBTQ+, socioeconomic, military veterans, elderly, and rural communities.
- Plans of action must focus on structural change, workforce diversity, policy and advocacy, research, and targeted interventions to patients and health care clinicians.
- Continued research is critical and must remain inclusive and accessible to ensure accurate representation of these vulnerable populations.

DISCLOSURE

The authors have nothing to disclose.

REFERENCES

1. CDC. Prevalence of chronic pain and high-impact chronic pain among adults — United States, 2016. MMWR Morb Mortal Wkly Rep 2018;67:1001–6.
2. IOM (Institute of Medicine). Relieving pain in America: a Blueprint for Transforming Prevention, care, education, and research. Washington, DC: The National Academies Press; 2011.
3. Committee IPRC. National Pain Strategy: a comprehensive population health-level strategy for pain. Washington, DC: Department of Health and Human Services; 2015.
4. Chapman EN, Kaatz A, Carnes M. Physicians and implicit bias: how doctors may unwittingly perpetuate health care disparities. J Gen Intern Med 2013;28(11):1504–10.
5. Hoffman KM, Trawalter S, Axt JR, et al. Racial bias in pain assessment and treatment recommendations, and false beliefs about biological differences between blacks and whites. Proc Natl Acad Sci U S A 2016;113(16):4296–301.
6. Adler NE, Ostrove JM. Socioeconomic status and health: what we know and what we don't. Ann N Y Acad Sci 1999;896:3–15.
7. Institute of Medicine (US) Committee on Understanding and Eliminating Racial and Ethnic Disparities in Health Care, Smedley BD, Stith AY, Nelson AR, eds. Unequal Treatment: Confronting Racial and Ethnic Disparities in Health Care. Washington (DC): National Academies Press (US); 2003.
8. Morales ME, Yong RJ. Racial and ethnic disparities in the treatment of chronic pain. Pain Med 2021;22(1):75–90.
9. Meghani SH, Byun E, Gallagher RM. Time to take stock: a meta-analysis and systematic review of analgesic treatment disparities for pain in the United States. Pain Med 2012;13(2):150–74.
10. Zajacova A, Grol-Prokopczyk H, Fillingim R. Beyond Black vs White: racial/ethnic disparities in chronic pain including Hispanic, Asian, Native American, and multiracial US adults. Pain 2022;163(9):1688–99.
11. Huber FA, Kell PA, Kuhn BL, et al. The association between adverse life events, psychological stress, and pain-promoting affect and cognitions in Native

Americans: results from the Oklahoma Study of Native American Pain Risk. J Racial Ethn Health Disparities 2022;9(1):215–26.

12. Jimenez N, Garroutte E, Kundu A, et al. A review of the experience, epidemiology, and management of pain among American Indian, Alaska Native, and Aboriginal Canadian peoples. J Pain 2011;12(5):511–22.
13. Nahin RL. Pain prevalence, chronicity and impact within subpopulations based on both Hispanic ancestry and race: United States, 2010-2017. J Pain 2021; 22(7):826–51.
14. Gates G. In U.S., More Adults Identifying as LGBT. Accessed August 25, 2022. Available at: https://news.gallup.com/poll/201731/lgbt-identification-rises.aspx.
15. Jones J. LGBT Identification in U.S. Ticks Up to 7.1%. Accessed September 4, 2022. Available at: https://news.gallup.com/poll/389792/lgbt-identification-ticks-up.aspx.
16. Katz-Wise SL, Everett B, Scherer EA, et al. Factors associated with sexual orientation and gender disparities in chronic pain among U.S. adolescents and young adults. Prev Med Rep 2015;2:765–72.
17. Tabaac AR, Chwa C, Sutter ME, et al. Prevalence of chronic pelvic pain by sexual orientation in a large cohort of young women in the United States. J Sex Med 2022;19(6):1012–23.
18. Case P, Austin SB, Hunter DJ, et al. Sexual orientation, health risk factors, and physical functioning in the Nurses' Health Study II. J Womens Health (Larchmt) 2004;13(9):1033–47.
19. Levit D, Yaish I, Shtrozberg S, et al. Pain and transition: evaluating fibromyalgia in transgender individuals. Clin Exp Rheumatol 2021;39(Suppl 130):27–32.
20. Ferrando CA, Chapman G, Pollard R. Preoperative pain symptoms and the incidence of endometriosis in transgender men undergoing hysterectomy for gender affirmation. J Minim Invasive Gynecol 2021;28(9):1579–84.
21. Schertzinger M, Wesson-Sides K, Parkitny L, et al. Daily fluctuations of progesterone and testosterone are associated with fibromyalgia pain severity. J Pain 2018;410–7.
22. Strath LJ, Sorge RE, Owens MA, et al. Sex and gender are not the same: why identity is important for people living with HIV and chronic pain. J Pain Res 2020;13:829–35.
23. McKetchnie SM, Beaugard C, Taylor SW, et al. Perspectives on pain, engagement in HIV care, and behavioral interventions for chronic pain among older sexual minority men living with HIV and chronic pain: a qualitative analysis. Pain Med 2021;22(3):577–84.
24. Taylor SW, McKetchnie SM, Batchelder AW, et al. Chronic pain and substance use disorders among older sexual minority men living with HIV: implications for HIV disease management across the HIV care continuum. AIDS Care 2022;1–10.
25. Peppard SW, Burkard J, Georges J, et al. The lived experience of military women with chronic pain: a phenomenological study. Mil Med 2022. https://doi.org/10.1093/milmed/usac134.
26. Burgess DJ, Nelson DB, Gravely AA, et al. Racial differences in prescription of opioid analgesics for chronic noncancer pain in a national sample of veterans. J Pain 2014;15(4):447–55.
27. Dobscha SK, Soleck GD, Dickinson KC, et al. Associations between race and ethnicity and treatment for chronic pain in the VA. J Pain 2009;10(10):1078–87.

28. Hadlandsmyth K, Driscoll MA, Mares JG, et al. Rurality impacts pain care for female veterans similarly to male veterans. J Rural Health 2022. https://doi.org/10.1111/jrh.12646.
29. Janevic MR, McLaughlin SJ, Heapy AA, et al. Racial and socioeconomic disparities in disabling chronic pain: findings from the Health and Retirement Study. J Pain 2017;18(12):1459–67.
30. Zajacova A, Grol-Prokopczyk H, Zimmer Z. Pain trends among American adults, 2002-2018: patterns, disparities, and correlates. Demography 2021;58(2):711–38.
31. Grol-Prokopczyk H. Sociodemographic disparities in chronic pain, based on 12-year longitudinal data. Pain 2017;158(2):313–22.
32. Craig KD, Holmes C, Hudspith M, et al. Pain in persons who are marginalized by social conditions. Pain 2020;161(2):261–5.
33. Beyer JE, DeGood DE, Ashley LC, et al. Patterns of postoperative analgesic use with adults and children following cardiac surgery. Pain 1983;17(1):71–81.
34. Truog R, Anand KJ. Management of pain in the postoperative neonate. *Clin Perinatol.* Mar 1989;16(1):61–78.
35. Purcell-Jones G, Dormon F, Sumner E. Paediatric anaesthetists' perceptions of neonatal and infant pain. Pain 1988;33(2):181–7.
36. Kim MK, Strait RT, Sato TT, et al. A randomized clinical trial of analgesia in children with acute abdominal pain. Acad Emerg Med 2002;9(4):281–7.
37. Beasley SW, Tibballs J. Efficacy and safety of continuous morphine infusion for postoperative analgesia in the paediatric surgical ward. Aust N Z J Surg 1987;57(4):233–7.
38. Murat I, Delleur MM, Esteve C, et al. Continuous extradural anaesthesia in children. Clinical and haemodynamic implications. Br J Anaesth 1987;59(11):1441–50.
39. Mather L, Mackie J. The incidence of postoperative pain in children. Pain 1983;15(3):271–82.
40. Kost-Byerly S, Chalkiadis G. Developing a pediatric pain service. Paediatr Anaesth 2012;22(10):1016–24.
41. Selbst SM, Clark M. Analgesic use in the emergency department. Ann Emerg Med 1990;19(9):1010–3.
42. Brown JC, Klein EJ, Lewis CW, et al. Emergency department analgesia for fracture pain. Ann Emerg Med 2003;42(2):197–205.
43. Goyal MK, Kuppermann N, Cleary SD, et al. Racial disparities in pain management of children with appendicitis in emergency departments. JAMA Pediatr 2015;169(11):996–1002.
44. Furyk J, Sumner M. Pain score documentation and analgesia: a comparison of children and adults with appendicitis. Emerg Med Australas 2008;20(6):482–7.
45. Sabin JA, Greenwald AG. The influence of implicit bias on treatment recommendations for 4 common pediatric conditions: pain, urinary tract infection, attention deficit hyperactivity disorder, and asthma. Am J Public Health 2012;102(5):988–95.
46. Johnson TJ, Weaver MD, Borrero S, et al. Association of race and ethnicity with management of abdominal pain in the emergency department. Pediatrics 2013;132(4):e851–8.
47. Pletcher MJ, Kertesz SG, Kohn MA, et al. Trends in opioid prescribing by race/ethnicity for patients seeking care in US emergency departments. JAMA 2008;299(1):70–8.

48. Jimenez N, Seidel K, Martin LD, et al. Perioperative analgesic treatment in Latino and non-Latino pediatric patients. J Health Care Poor Underserved 2010;21(1): 229–36.
49. Nafiu OO, Chimbira WT, Stewart M, et al. Racial differences in the pain management of children recovering from anesthesia. Paediatr Anaesth 2017;27(7): 760–7.
50. Sadhasivam S, Chidambaran V, Ngamprasertwong P, et al. Race and unequal burden of perioperative pain and opioid related adverse effects in children. Pediatrics 2012;129(5):832–8.
51. Sadhasivam S, Krekels EH, Chidambaran V, et al. Morphine clearance in children: does race or genetics matter? J Opioid Manag 2012;8(4):217–26.
52. Edwards RR, Moric M, Husfeldt B, et al. Ethnic similarities and differences in the chronic pain experience: a comparison of African American, Hispanic, and white patients. Pain Med 2005;6(1):88–98.
53. Rahim-Williams FB, Riley JL, Herrera D, et al. Ethnic identity predicts experimental pain sensitivity in African Americans and Hispanics. Pain 2007; 129(1–2):177–84.
54. Evans S, Lu Q, Tsao JC, et al. The role of coping and race in healthy children's experimental pain responses. J Pain Manag 2008;1(2):151–62.
55. Shah AA, Zogg CK, Zafar SN, et al. Analgesic access for acute abdominal pain in the emergency department among racial/ethnic minority patients: a nationwide examination. Med Care 2015;53(12):1000–9.
56. Singhal A, Tien YY, Hsia RY. Racial-ethnic disparities in opioid prescriptions at emergency department visits for conditions commonly associated with prescription drug abuse. PLoS One 2016;11(8):e0159224.
57. Lee P, Le Saux M, Siegel R, et al. Racial and ethnic disparities in the management of acute pain in US emergency departments: meta-analysis and systematic review. Am J Emerg Med 2019;37(9):1770–7.
58. Guedj R, Marini M, Kossowsky J, et al. Racial and ethnic disparities in pain management of children with limb fractures or suspected appendicitis: a retrospective cross-sectional study. Front Pediatr 2021;9:652854.
59. Kennel J, Withers E, Parsons N, et al. Racial/ethnic disparities in pain treatment: evidence from Oregon Emergency Medical Services Agencies. Med Care 2019; 57(12):924–9.
60. Janz NK, Mujahid MS, Hawley ST, et al. Racial/ethnic differences in adequacy of information and support for women with breast cancer. Cancer 2008;113(5): 1058–67.
61. Samuel CA, Schaal J, Robertson L, et al. Racial differences in symptom management experiences during breast cancer treatment. Support Care Cancer 2018;26(5):1425–35.
62. Mack DS, Hunnicutt JN, Jesdale BM, et al. Non-Hispanic Black-White disparities in pain and pain management among newly admitted nursing home residents with cancer. J Pain Res 2018;11:753–61.
63. Cleeland CS, Gonin R, Baez L, et al. Pain and treatment of pain in minority patients with cancer. The Eastern Cooperative Oncology Group Minority Outpatient Pain Study. Ann Intern Med 1997;127(9):813–6.
64. Meghani SH, Kang Y, Chittams J, et al. African Americans with cancer pain are more likely to receive an analgesic with toxic metabolite despite clinical risks: a mediation analysis study. J Clin Oncol 2014;32(25):2773–9.

65. Check DK, Samuel CA, Rosenstein DL, et al. Investigation of racial disparities in early supportive medication use and end-of-life care among Medicare beneficiaries with stage IV breast cancer. J Clin Oncol 2016;34(19):2265–70.
66. Vallerand AH, Hasenau S, Templin T, et al. Disparities between black and white patients with cancer pain: the effect of perception of control over pain. Pain Med 2005;6(3):242–50.
67. Eversley R, Estrin D, Dibble S, et al. Post-treatment symptoms among ethnic minority breast cancer survivors. Oncol Nurs Forum 2005;32(2):250–6.
68. Wright JL, Takita C, Reis IM, et al. Racial variations in radiation-induced skin toxicity severity: data from a prospective cohort receiving postmastectomy radiation. Int J Radiat Oncol Biol Phys 2014;90(2):335–43.
69. Lange EMS, Rao S, Toledo P. Racial and ethnic disparities in obstetric anesthesia. Article. Semin Perinatol 2017;41(5):293–8.
70. Guglielminotti J, Landau R, Li G. Adverse events and factors associated with potentially avoidable use of general anesthesia in cesarean deliveries. Anesthesiology 2019;130(6):912–22.
71. Tangel V, White RS, Nachamie AS, et al. Racial and ethnic disparities in maternal outcomes and the disadvantage of peripartum Black women: a multistate analysis, 2007-2014. Am J Perinatol 2019;36(8):835–48.
72. Morris T, Schulman M. Race inequality in epidural use and regional anesthesia failure in labor and birth: an examination of women's experience. Sexual & Reproductive Healthcare 2014;5(4):188–94.
73. Osterman M, Hamilton B, Martin J, Driscoll A, Valenzuela C. Births: Final Data for 2020. Vol. 70. 2022. National Vital Statistics Reports. Available at: https://www.cdc.gov/nchs/data/nvsr/nvsr70/nvsr70-17.pdf.
74. Edmonds JK, Yehezkel R, Liao X, et al. Racial and ethnic differences in primary, unscheduled cesarean deliveries among low-risk primiparous women at an academic medical center: a retrospective cohort study. BMC Pregnancy Childbirth 2013;13(1):168.
75. Lange EMS, Rao S, Toledo P. Racial and ethnic disparities in obstetric anesthesia. Semin Perinatol 2017;41(5):293–8.
76. Butwick AJ, Blumenfeld YJ, Brookfield KF, et al. Racial and ethnic disparities in mode of anesthesia for cesarean delivery. Anesth Analg 2016;122(2):472–9.
77. Butwick AJ, El-Sayed YY, Blumenfeld YJ, et al. Mode of anaesthesia for preterm caesarean delivery: secondary analysis from the Maternal-Fetal Medicine Units Network Caesarean Registry. Br J Anaesth 2015;115(2):267–74.
78. Tangel VE, Matthews KC, Abramovitz SE, et al. Racial and ethnic disparities in severe maternal morbidity and anesthetic techniques for obstetric deliveries: a multi-state analysis, 2007-2014. J Clin Anesth 2020;65:109821.
79. Ring L, Landau R, Delgado C. The current role of general anesthesia for cesarean delivery. Curr Anesthesiol Rep 2021;24:1–10.
80. Eisenach JC, Pan PH, Smiley R, et al. Severity of acute pain after childbirth, but not type of delivery, predicts persistent pain and postpartum depression. Pain 2008;140(1):87–94.
81. Badreldin N, Grobman WA, Yee LM. Racial disparities in postpartum pain management. Obstet Gynecol 2019;134(6):1147–53.
82. Wiles A, Korn E, Dinglas C, et al. Disparities in post cesarean section pain management. Journal of Clinical Gynecology and Obstetrics 2022;11(2).
83. Johnson JD, Asiodu IV, McKenzie CP, et al. Racial and ethnic inequities in postpartum pain evaluation and management. Obstet Gynecol 2019;134(6):1155–62.

84. Lee A, Guglielminotti J, Janvier AS, et al. Racial and ethnic disparities in the management of postdural puncture headache with epidural blood patch for obstetric patients in New York State. JAMA Netw Open 2022;5(4):e228520.
85. Rafferty AP, Luo H, Egan KL, et al. Rural, suburban, and urban differences in chronic pain and coping among adults in North Carolina: 2018 Behavioral Risk Factor Surveillance System. Prev Chronic Dis 2021;18:E13.
86. Dahlhamer J, Lucas J, Zelaya C, et al. Prevalence of chronic pain and high-impact chronic pain among adults—United States, 2016. MMWR Morb Mortal Wkly Rep 2018;67(36):1001–6.
87. Hoffman PK, Meier BP, Council JR. A comparison of chronic pain between an urban and rural population. J Community Health Nurs 2002;19(4):213–24.
88. Kusmin L. Rural America at a Glance. 2016. Available at: https://www.ers.usda.gov/publications/pub-details/?pubid=80893.
89. Goode AP, Freburger JK, Carey TS. The influence of rural versus urban residence on utilization and receipt of care for chronic low back pain. J Rural Health 2013;29(2):205–14.
90. Eaton LH, Langford DJ, Meins AR, et al. Use of self-management interventions for chronic pain management: a comparison between rural and nonrural residents. Pain Manag Nurs 2018;19(1):8–13.
91. Mezei L, Murinson BB, Team JHPCD. Pain education in North American medical schools. J Pain 2011;12(12):1199–208.
92. Prunuske JP, St Hill CA, Hager KD, et al. Opioid prescribing patterns for non-malignant chronic pain for rural versus non-rural US adults: a population-based study using 2010 NAMCS data. BMC Health Serv Res 2014;14:563.
93. US Department of Agriculture. Opioid Misuse in Rural America. Available at: https://www.usda.gov/topics/opioids.
94. American Farm Bureau Federation. National Farmers Union. The opioid crisis in Farm Country. Available at: https://1vix7b4f3jvk2x4eqy1byl1n-wpengine.netdna-ssl.com/wp-content/uploads/sites/13/2017/12/171015-AFB-Opioids-LE.pdf.
95. Schappert SM, Burt CW. Ambulatory care visits to physician offices, hospital outpatient departments, and emergency departments: United States, 2001-02. Vital Health Stat 13 2006;(159):1–66.
96. Pitcher MH, Von Korff M, Bushnell MC, et al. Prevalence and profile of high-impact chronic pain in the United States. J Pain 2019;20(2):146–60.
97. Gaskin DJ, Richard P. The economic costs of pain in the United States. J Pain 2012;13(8):715–24.
98. Jones MR, Orhurhu V, O'Gara B, et al. Racial and socioeconomic disparities in spinal cord stimulation among the Medicare population. Neuromodulation 2021;24(3):434–40.
99. Orhurhu V, Gao C, Agudile E, et al. Socioeconomic disparities in the utilization of spinal cord stimulation therapy in patients with chronic pain. Pain Pract 2021;21(1):75–82.
100. Ovrom E, Hagedorn JM, Bhandarkar A, et al. Racial disparities in the cost of inpatient spinal cord stimulator surgery among patients in the 2016-2018 National Inpatient Sample. J Clin Neurosci 2022;98:189–93.
101. Leiphart J, Barrett M, Shenai MB. Economic inequities in the application of neuromodulation devices. Cureus 2019;11(9):e5685.
102. Campbell LC, Robinson K, Meghani SH, et al. Challenges and opportunities in pain management disparities research: implications for clinical practice, advocacy, and policy. J Pain 2012;13(7):611–9.

103. Bekanich SJ, Wanner N, Junkins S, et al. A multifaceted initiative to improve clinician awareness of pain management disparities. Am J Med Qual 2014; 29(5):388–96.
104. Hirsh AT, Miller MM, Hollingshead NA, et al. A randomized controlled trial testing a virtual perspective-taking intervention to reduce race and socioeconomic status disparities in pain care. Pain 2019;160(10):2229–40.
105. Drwecki BB, Moore CF, Ward SE, et al. Reducing racial disparities in pain treatment: the role of empathy and perspective-taking. Pain 2011;152(5):1001–6.
106. Shen MJ, Peterson EB, Costas-Muñiz R, et al. The effects of race and racial concordance on patient-physician communication: a systematic review of the literature. J Racial Ethn Health Disparities 2018;5(1):117–40.
107. Odonkor CA, Leitner B, Taraben S, et al. Diversity of pain medicine trainees and faculty in the United States: a cross-sectional analysis of fellowship training from 2009-2019. Pain Med 2021;22(4):819–28.
108. Heins A, Homel P, Safdar B, et al. Physician race/ethnicity predicts successful emergency department analgesia. J Pain 2010;11(7):692–7.
109. Saha S, Komaromy M, Koepsell TD, et al. Patient-physician racial concordance and the perceived quality and use of health care. Arch Intern Med 1999;159(9): 997–1004.
110. Pratt-Chapman ML, Murphy J, Hines D, et al. When the pain is so acute or if I think that I'm going to die": Health care seeking behaviors and experiences of transgender and gender diverse people in an urban area. PLoS One 2021; 16(2):e0246883.
111. Andreae MH, White RS, Chen KY, et al. The effect of initiatives to overcome language barriers and improve attendance: a cross-sectional analysis of adherence in an inner city chronic pain clinic. Pain Med 2017;18(2):265–74.
112. Andreae MH, Nair S, Gabry JS, et al. A pragmatic trial to improve adherence with scheduled appointments in an inner-city pain clinic by human phone calls in the patient's preferred language. J Clin Anesth 2017;42:77–83.
113. Glynn LH, Chen JA, Dawson TC, et al. Bringing chronic-pain care to rural veterans: a telehealth pilot program description. Psychol Serv 2021;18(3):310–8.
114. Burgess DJ, Hagel Campbell E, Hammett P, et al. Taking ACTION to reduce pain: a randomized clinical trial of a walking-focused, proactive coaching intervention for Black patients with chronic musculoskeletal pain. J Gen Intern Med 2022. https://doi.org/10.1007/s11606-021-07376-2.
115. Bhimani RH, Cross LJ, Taylor BC, et al. Taking ACTION to reduce pain: ACTION study rationale, design and protocol of a randomized trial of a proactive telephone-based coaching intervention for chronic musculoskeletal pain among African Americans. BMC Musculoskelet Disord 2017;18(1):15.

Clinical Approach to Chronic Pain due to Perioperative Nerve Injury

Abdullah Sulieman Terkawi, MD, MS(Epi)*,
Omar Khalid Altirkawi, MD[1], Vafi Salmasi, MD, MS(Epi)[2],
Einar Ottestad, MD[3]

KEYWORDS

• Acute • Chronic • Postsurgical • Pain • Nerve injury • Nerve management

KEY POINTS

- Perioperative nerve injuries are common and can be prevented.
- The estimated incidence of perioperative nerve injury is 10% to 50%. However, most of these injuries are minor and self-recovering. Severe injuries account for up to 10%.
- Early diagnosis and management are the key to prevent chronic intractable pain.

Iatrogenic perioperative nerve injuries are more common than we would like, and if promptly and appropriately managed, long-term disability can be prevented. The estimated incidence of perioperative nerve injury is 10% to 50%.[1] However, most of those injuries are minor and self-recovering, with severe injuries accounting for up to 10%.[2] In general, obesity, hypertension, smoking, diabetes mellitus, open versus laparoscopic surgery, positioning during surgery, and longer duration are all potential risk factors for perioperative nerve injury.[2,3] Proper positioning during surgery, careful surgical dissection and retraction, as well as controlling patient's comorbidities may help reduce the incidence and severity of perioperative nerve injury.

MECHANISMS OF INJURY

Mechanisms of peripheral nerve injury can include stretch (retractors and poor positioning), compression (tourniquet, tight belts, and poor positioning), hypoperfusion (vascular injury), direct trauma (complete or partial laceration), and injury during vessel

Department of Anesthesiology, Perioperative and Pain Medicine, Stanford University School of Medicine, Palo Alto, CA, USA
[1] Present address: 280 West California Avenue, Apartment 107, Sunnyvale, CA 94086.
[2] Present address: 1070 Arastradero Road Suite 200, Palo Alto, CA 94304.
[3] Present address: 127 Elliott Drive, Menlo Park, CA 94025.
* Corresponding author. 1070 Arastradero Road Suite 200, Palo Alto, CA 94304.
E-mail address: aterkawi@stanford.edu

Anesthesiology Clin 41 (2023) 489–502
https://doi.org/10.1016/j.anclin.2023.03.009 anesthesiology.theclinics.com
1932-2275/23/

cannulation (eg, blind femoral vessels cannulation). Peripheral nerve injury due to regional analgesia is rare but possible.[4] Fortunately, ultrasound has increased safety by reducing direct nerve trauma secondary to perioperative blocks. Nerve hypoperfusion and consequent ischemia can be secondary to physical disruption of the vasa nervorum, intraneural hemorrhage, or endoneural edema.[5] The severity and duration of the ischemia can determine whether temporal or permanent disruption to nerve impulse transmission occurs.[6] **Fig. 1** summarizes 2 commonly used classification systems for nerve injury and their clinical presentation.

CAUSES

Fig. 2 summarizes the most injured nerves with specific surgeries. As discussed earlier, nerve injury may not be necessary because of direct injury. For example, a patient after total knee arthroplasty may present with posterior femoral cutaneous neuralgia because of prolonged and tight tourniquet time.

CLINICAL PRESENTATION

Nerve injury pain usually presents as neuropathic pain that ranges from mild to severe mononeuropathy and extends to complex regional pain syndrome (CRPS type 2). Neuropathic pain is typically described as burning, shooting, electric shocks associated with numbness and tingling but can include almost any sensation,

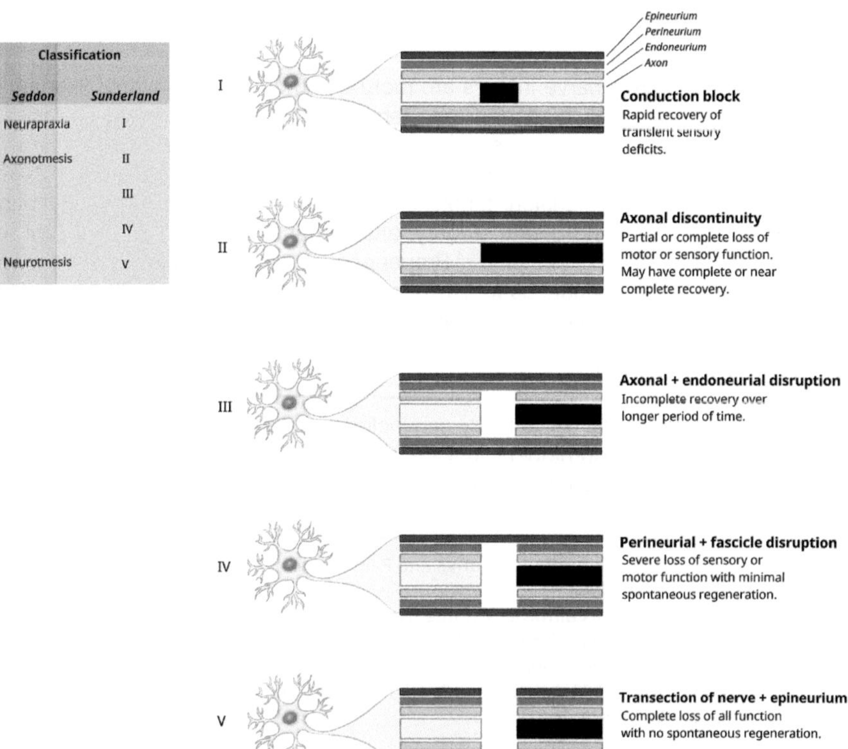

Fig. 1. Classification of severity of nerve injuries. (*Courtesy of* Omar Khalid Altirkawi.)

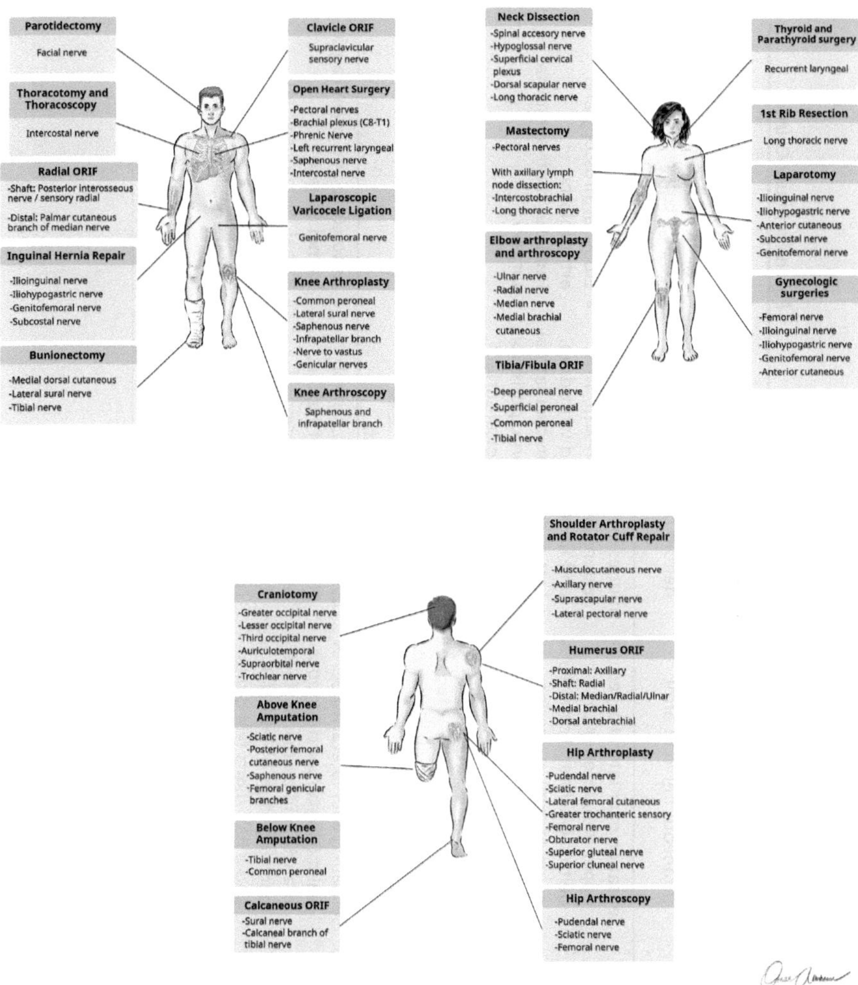

Fig. 2. Summary of commonly potential nerves injury with different surgeries. ORIF, open reduction and internal fixation. (*Courtesy of* Omar Khalid Altirkawi.)

including dull ache and itch. Common descriptors include allodynia, primary and secondary hyperalgesia, and hyperpathia, with hypoesthesia to touch and pinprick.[7] CRPS manifest as severe and continuous neuropathic pain with sensory, vasomotor (temperature asymmetry), sudomotor (edema), and motor (and atrophic) changes.[8] **Table 1** summarizes common nerve injury presentations. Injury to any of these nerves may present as pain concomitant with the sensory distribution of the nerve. Secondary myofascial pain is also common, as overactive nerves cause overactive muscles, and history and physical examination should guide the physician on whether further workup (eg, MRI and nerve conduction studies) is needed. It is essential not to miss other causes of peripheral neuropathy while evaluating those patients. Common causes of peripheral neuropathy that should be evaluated as possible contributing factors include diabetes, vitamin B12 deficiency, chronic alcohol abuse, toxin exposure, hereditary diseases, and unrelated neural compression.[9]

Table 1
Commonly injured nerves: function, presentation, and potential causes[10–20]

Nerve	Motor Function	Sensory Function	Clinical Presentation	Potential Injury Causes
Upper extremities				
Axillary	Innervates deltoid (abduction of arm) and teres minor (adduction and external rotation)	Sensation over deltoid and lateral arm (via upper lateral cutaneous nerve of arm)	Loss of arm abduction above 15°, loss of sensation over deltoid (regimental badge)	• Poor axilla positioning • Shoulder arthroplasty • Rotator cuff repair • Proximal humerus surgery
Radial	Innervates triceps brachii and extensor muscles of hand (elbow, wrist, and finger extension, forearm pronation)	Sensation over lateral aspect of upper arm, inferior to deltoid (via lateral cutaneous nerve of arm), posterior surface of arm and part of posterior forearm (via dorsal antebrachial cutaneous nerve), and dorsal surface of lateral 3 and a half digits (via superficial branch)	Injuries in axilla lead to loss of extension at forearm, wrist and fingers, and wrist drop. Loss of sensation over lateral and posterior arm, posterior forearm, and dorsal surface of lateral 3 and a half digits. Injuries below elbow cause distal paresthesias without wrist drop unless deep branch is affected.	• Radial artery cannulation • Elbow arthroscopy and arthroplasty • Humerus shaft and distal surgery
Median	Innervates flexor and pronator muscles in anterior compartment of forearm (except flexor carpi ulnaris and part of flexor digitorum profundus)	Sensation over lateral aspect of palm (via palmar cutaneous branch) and palmar surface and fingertips of lateral 3 and a half digits (via digital cutaneous branch)	Loss of wrist flexion, thumb flexion, MCP joint flexion, and IP joint extension of index and middle fingers. Loss of sensation over lateral aspect of palm and palmar surface of lateral 3 and a half digits. "Ape hand" and "hand of benediction."	• Endoscopic and open carpal tunnel release • Radial fracture surgery • Elbow arthroscopy and arthroplasty • Distal humerus surgery

Ulnar	Innervates flexor carpi ulnaris (flexion and abduction of hand at wrist), medial half of flexor digitorum profundus (ring and little finger extension), and most intrinsic hand muscles (via deep branch of ulnar nerve)	Sensation over medial half of palm (palmar cutaneous branch), dorsal surface of medial one and a half fingers (dorsal cutaneous branch), and palmar surface of medial one and a half fingers (superficial branch)	Decreased flexion, abduction, and adduction of ulnar fingers. Loss of sensation over ulnar one and a half fingers. "Ulnar claw" on digit extension and positive "Froment's sign"—muscle weakness of the pinch grip.	• Poor elbow positioning • Displaced supracondylar fracture surgery (eg, lateral, and cross pinning) • Elbow arthroscopy and arthroplasty
Musculocutaneous	Innervates biceps brachii, brachialis, and coracobrachialis (flexion of upper arm and supination of forearm)	Sensation over anterolateral aspect of forearm (via lateral cutaneous nerve of forearm)	Decreased biceps reflex, loss of forearm flexion and supination. Loss of sensation over radial and dorsal forearm.	• Shoulder arthroplasty • Rotator cuff repair
Trunk				
Ilioinguinal	Innervates internal abdominal oblique and transversus abdominis muscles	Sensation over upper anteromedial thigh and part of external genitalia (via anterior labial/scrotal nerve branch)	Weakening of internal oblique and transversus abdominal muscles (may lead to development of inguinal hernia). Pain in the sensory distribution.	• Inguinal hernia repair • Emergency laparotomy with lateral extension
Iliohypo-gastric	Innervates internal abdominal oblique and transversus abdominis muscles	Sensation over suprapubic region. Also supplies sensory fibers to external oblique, transversus abdominis, and internal oblique muscles	Burning pain in suprapubic and inguinal regions. Damage to iliohypogastric nerve is rarely isolated.	• Similar to ilioinguinal nerve
Anterior cutaneous	Rectus abdominis muscle	Sensation from anterior midabdominal wall	Anterior cutaneous nerve entrapment syndrome (ACNES): severe, chronic pain due to entrapment of cutaneous branches of thoracoabdominal nerves	• Abdominal surgeries

(*continued on next page*)

Table 1
(continued)

Nerve	Motor Function	Sensory Function	Clinical Presentation	Potential Injury Causes
Genitofemoral	Innervates the cremaster muscle (genital branch)	Sensation over medial thigh (femoral branch) and scrotum/labia majora and mons pubis (genital branch)	Genitofemoral neuralgia, absent cremasteric reflex, and decreased sensation over upper, medial thigh	• Laparoscopic and open varicocele ligation • Laparoscopic and open inguinal hernia repair
Pectoral nerves	Innervates pectoralis minor and major muscles (arm extension and forced inspiration)	No cutaneous sensory function	Anterior chest wall pain. Patient may have weakness in elevating shoulder, which may eventually manifest as myofascial pain.	• Open heart surgery with sternotomy • Mastectomy • Shoulder arthroplasty • Rotator cuff repair
Intercostobrachial	Pierces serratus anterior and intercostal muscles but does not provide motor function (pure sensory nerve)	Sensation over skin of axilla, lateral chest, and upper, medial aspect of the arm	Intercostobrachial neuralgia: constant paresthesias and dull, aching, or burning pain over the sensory distribution	• Axillary lymph node dissection • Transaxillary breast augmentation
Suprascapular	Innervates supraspinatus (arm abduction, before deltoid) and infraspinatus (external rotation) muscles	Sensory innervation for glenohumeral and acromioclavicular joints	Suprascapular neuropathy: pain and weakness in abduction and external rotation of the shoulder	• Shoulder arthroplasty • Rotator cuff repair
Long thoracic	Innervates serratus anterior (pulls scapula anteriorly and elevates ribs)	No cutaneous sensory function	Winged scapula	• Axillary lymph node dissection • First rib resection • Neck dissection
Dorsal scapular	Innervates levator scapulae, rhomboid major, and rhomboid minor muscles. Retract and elevate the scapula.	No cutaneous sensory function	Neck and/or shoulder pain. Possible weakness	• Neck dissection

Intercostal	Intercostal muscles that help in respiration (accessory muscles).	Sensory innervation of the back, trunk, and upper abdomen that follow dermatomal pattern	Intercostal neuralgia: pain that is distributed along the affected dermatome or in a band-like pattern, often perceived as pain, tightness, stabbing, aching, and/or burning along the rib, chest and/or back and/or upper abdomen.	• Thoracotomy and thoracoscopy • Rib fractures surgery • Abdominal surgery • Breast surgery
Lower extremities				
Femoral	Innervates the anterior thigh muscles: pectineus, iliacus, sartorius (hip flexion). Also innervates the quadriceps femoris muscles: rectus femoris, vastus lateralis, vastus intermedius, and vastus medialis (knee extension)	Sensation over anterior thigh (anterior cutaneous branch of femoral nerve) and medial leg (saphenous nerve)	Pain (mostly throbbing) and altered sensation. Decreased leg extension and patellar reflex	• Open hysterectomy • Cesarean section • Tight femoral belt • During blind femoral vessels cannulation • Hip arthroplasty and arthroscopy
Obturator	Innervates medial thigh muscles: obturator externus, adductor longus, adductor brevis, adductor magnus, gracilis, and pectineus (collectively work to adduct hip)	Sensation over skin of medial thigh (via cutaneous branches of obturator nerve)	Pain and altered sensation with possible thigh adduction weakness	• Hip arthroplasty
Sciatic	Innervates posterior thigh muscles: biceps femoris, semitendinosus, semimembranosus. Also innervates hamstring portion of adductor magnus	No direct sensory function before branching. Indirect sensory innervation by terminal branches (tibial and common fibular nerves)	Pain along the distribution of sciatic nerve (sciatica), numbness, and muscle weakness	• Periacetabular osteotomy • Acetabular fracture surgery • Hip arthroplasty • Above-knee amputation

(*continued on next page*)

Table 1
(*continued*)

Nerve	Motor Function	Sensory Function	Clinical Presentation	Potential Injury Causes
Saphenous (*branch of femoral*)	No motor function	Supplies skin of medial leg and foot	Pain and numbness on medial leg and knee	• Total knee arthroplasty • Above-knee amputation
Infra-patellar (*branch of saphenous nerve*)	No motor function	Sensation over anteromedial aspect of knee and anteroinferior knee joint capsule	Anteromedial knee pain commonly associated with lateral knee numbness	• Total knee arthroplasty • Knee arthroscopy
Common peroneal (*also known as common fibular nerve*)	Innervates biceps femoris muscle (knee flexion). Also gives off terminal branches to innervate peroneus longus, peroneus brevis, and tibialis anterior.	Two cutaneous branches: sural communicating nerve (lower posterolateral leg) and lateral sural cutaneous nerve (upper lateral leg). Terminal branches also contribute to sensory function (below).	Pain and numbness. Footdrop (loss of dorsiflexion and eversion) and loss of sensation on dorsum of foot and lateral side of leg	• Varicose vein surgery • Short saphenous vein surgery • Above-knee amputation
Superficial peroneal	Innervates peroneus longus and brevis	Sensation over dorsum of foot (except webspace between hallux and second digit)	Pain and altered sensation	• Tibia/fibula fracture surgery
Deep peroneal	Innervates tibialis anterior	Sensation over webspace between hallux and second digit	Pain and altered sensation	• Tibia/fibula fracture surgery
Sural	No motor function	Sensation over posterolateral aspect of distal leg and lateral aspect of foot, heel, and ankle	Pain and altered sensation and pain over the sensory distribution	• Bunionectomy (lateral sural) • Calcaneus surgery • Knee arthroscopy
Pudendal	Innervates bulbospongiosus, ischiocavernosus, levator ani muscles, external urethra, and anal sphincter (voluntary control of fecal and urinary continence)	Sensation over perineum (perineal nerve), skin around anus (inferior rectal nerve), and external genitalia (dorsal nerve of penis/ clitoris)	Pain and altered sensation in perineum and genital area, with possible fecal/urinary incontinence.	• Hip arthroscopy • Hip arthroplasty

Lateral femoral cutaneous	No motor function	Sensation over anterior and lateral thigh (anterior branch) and lateral aspect of greater trochanter to midthigh region (posterior branch)	Pain and altered sensation and pain over the sensory distribution	• Blind femoral vessels cannulation • Delivery in lithotomy position • Hip arthroplasty and arthroscopy
Posterior femoral cutaneous	No motor function	Sensation over glutes (via gluteal branches), superomedial thigh and part of external genitalia (perineal branch), and posterior thigh (perforating cutaneous branches)	Pain and altered sensation and pain over the sensory distribution	• Above-knee amputation • Tight thigh belt • Hip surgery • Posterior thigh skin graft
Greater trochanteric sensory	No motor function	Sensation over lateral hip	Greater trochanteric pain syndrome: lateral hip pain, localized to greater trochanter	• Hip arthroplasty • Femur neck fracture surgery
Superior gluteal	Innervates gluteus medius, gluteus minimus, tensor fascia latae	No sensory function	Trendelenburg gait (lesion is contralateral to hip that drops)	• Hip arthroplasty
Inferior gluteal	Innervates gluteus maximus	No sensory function	Decreased hip extension, difficulty climbing stairs, and standing from a seated position	• Hip arthroplasty

Abbreviations: IP joint, interphalangeal; MCP, metacarpophalangeal.

DIAGNOSIS

In most of the cases, the diagnosis is clinical and can be confirmed by a diagnostic nerve block. However, in some challenging presentations, nerve conduction studies and magnetic resonance (MR) neurogram may be needed. Four diagnostic modalities can be helpful:[21,22]

- Electrophysiological studies: both electromyography (EMG) and nerve conduction studies can help determine the site, severity, and chronicity of the injury and monitor for nerve recovery. The main disadvantage is its discomfort to the patient.
- Autonomic nerve studies: sweat test, wrinkle test, and thermography.
- Ultrasonography: may show a hypoechoic, swollen nerve or neural interruptions and compressions. A repeatable ultrasonic Tinel sign over swollen nerves can be beneficial diagnostically (ie, the patient feels the pain reproduced as the transducer moves over the nerve). Individual fascicles can be scanned in the larger nerves looking for specific injuries.
- MR neurogram: can indicate the site and severity of the injury. For example, Sunderland grade I appears as hyperintense nerve; grade II and III appears as hyperintense, thickened with prominent fascicles; grade IV appears as heterogeneous nerve; and grade V appears as complete nerve transection.[23] MR neurogram also shows denervated muscles. The main disadvantage of MR neurogram is its lower sensitivity for milder forms of nerve injury (namely neurapraxia).

Pain medicine doctors typically evaluate patients for acute postoperative surgical complications after the surgeon's assessment. If not, a consultation with the surgeon is necessary. If the pain is at the site of surgery and lasts more than 3 months, then the diagnosis of chronic (persistent) postsurgical pain is fulfilled.

MANAGEMENT

Conservative treatment with antineuropathic medications is the first line. Examples of antineuropathic medications include anticonvulsants such as gabapentin and pregabalin; serotonin-norepinephrine reuptake inhibitors such as duloxetine and venlafaxine; and tricyclic antidepressants such as nortriptyline and amitriptyline.[24] Physical therapy and rehabilitation are crucial for nerve injury rehabilitation.[25] Interestingly, a ketogenic diet—very low in carbohydrates, high in healthy fat, and moderate in protein content—and intermittent fasting have been suggested for patients with persistent postsurgical pain for their potential role in reducing nociception and inflammation.[26]

At this point in time, we have various tools to identify injured nerves in the setting of persistent postoperative pain: history and physical examination, ultrasound-guided nerve examination and diagnostic block, electrophysiological studies (eg, EMG/nerve conduction velocity), and MR neurogram. Once identified, treatment depends on the duration and severity of pain combined with the sensory and motor function of the injured nerve. Most importantly, ongoing, actively compressed, or impinged nerves need surgical consultation and release. Once the need for surgical intervention is ruled out, more severe and longer-duration neuropathic pain may require more invasive treatment options. As the damaged peripheral nerve fires ectopic C- and A-delta fibers, the central nervous system is flooded with action potentials releasing glutamate and creating allodynia and hyperalgesia around the injury site. If this pathway is interrupted early with local anesthetic block, then perhaps we can reduce the long-term potentiation that can occur and reduce the chance for development of chronic neuropathic pain. The goal is to identify very early complex regional pain syndrome and prevent it from becoming a central pain syndrome.

In the first few weeks after nerve injury, blocks with or without steroids are the mainstay of treatment of all nerves: mixed, sensory, and motor. It is important to note that all blocks are temporary. The goal of the block is to reduce the glutamate load to the spinal cord for sufficient duration to allow the neuropathic symptoms to abate and ideally not return. The steroids may decrease C-fiber transmission and extend the duration of the local anesthetic block without requiring an indwelling catheter. If a nerve block results in only 6 to 12 hours of analgesia with no residual effect, then neuromodulation (eg, ablation or stimulation) is needed. If the nerve block provides numbness for 6 to 12 hours but analgesia and reduction in allodynia for days to weeks, then repeat block is very reasonable (**Fig. 3**).

If the nerve block is insufficient for relief, then the next step depends on neural target. Small sensory nerves could be targets for ablation. Cryoablation has the capacity to freeze an individual nerve without damaging surrounding tissue. Once frozen, the nerve loses all sensory and motor function, then regenerates down the neural sheath over 3 to 6 months with return of sensation and normal function again. Cryoablation will generally be reversible. Radiofrequency ablation can kill nerves using heat but with the downside of also damaging surrounding tissue and thus being more irreversible with a chance of worsening pain. That stated, ablations are likely best reserved for severe pain of longer duration, as a successful

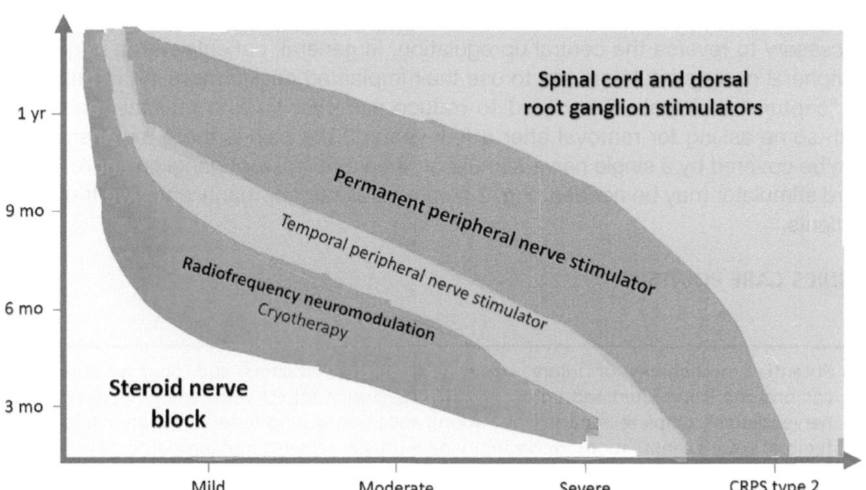

Fig. 3. Interventional "nonsurgical" pain management approach to chronic pain due to perioperative nerve injury. This approach mainly depends on 2 main variables: the severity (x-axis) and the duration of chronic pain (y-axis). We recommend always to start with nerve block that can be repeated based on the patient's response. This is also important as a diagnostic step. The thickness of the color correlate with the potential long-term benefit that patient is expected to have based on our experience. For example, the more severe the pain, and the longer the duration, the less we expect the long-term benefit of a steroid block to be. Another example, if the patient has moderate pain and it has been more than 6 months, we recommend radiofrequency neuromodulation. We typically recommend the implantable stimulator devices for patients with more severe pain with longer duration, typically, more than 1 year. However, we always start from the less invasive to the more invasive options. CRPS, complex regional pain syndrome; mo, months; yr, year.

ablation will have loss of function, and all ablations will have risk of new neuropathic pain.

For most other nerves, including mixed and motor nerves, pulsed radiofrequency neuromodulation can be attempted. Pulsed radiofrequency neuromodulation is nonablative and should be considered a one-time nerve stimulation rather than an ablation-like procedure. Postsurgical electrical stimulation has been shown to improve nerve recovery after surgery.[27,28] Activating the A-beta fibers enhances their transmission at the expense of the damaged C-fibers, and in some ways, this somehow simulates classic complex regional pain syndrome physical therapy desensitization treatment. We intend to activate the normal sensory parts of the nerve, whether we use physical therapy or direct neuromodulation when treating complex regional pain syndrome. Researchers have shown that pulsed radiofrequency neuromodulation seems to work better for younger and less severe neuropathic pain.

Once the injured nerve pain pathway has become more entrenched, nerve blocks and one-time neuromodulation may be insufficient. These injured nerves become candidates for temporary peripheral nerve stimulation using indwelling wires that can stay for 30 to 60 days. These wires replace the incoming pathologic C-fiber nociception with A-beta fiber paresthesia for the duration of treatment, in some ways mimicking an indwelling nerve block. If the spinal cord responds favorably to this new medical grade electricity, then the central phenomena such as allodynia and hyperalgesia continue to abate and reduce, with almost 70% of patients maintaining analgesia 12 months after stimulation has stopped.[29–31]

If the pain returns after temporary stimulation, or if the pain is long-standing and severe, then permanent peripheral nerve stimulation may provide as many weeks as necessary to reverse the central upregulation. In general, patients with a permanent peripheral nerve stimulator tend to use their implanted device more in the beginning to "capture" their pain. They tend to reduce use over time to maintain analgesia, with some asking for removal after a few years. If the pain is more expansive than can be covered by a single nerve stimulator, then a dorsal root ganglion and/or spinal cord stimulator may be needed. **Fig. 3** summarizes our approach when we treat such patients.

CLINICS CARE POINTS

- Potential mechanisms of injury are nerve stretch (retractors and poor positioning), compression (tourniquet and tight belts), hypoperfusion (direct vascular injury), direct nerve trauma (complete or partial laceration), and injury during vessel cannulation (eg, blind femoral vessels cannulation). Nerve injury pain usually presents as neuropathic pain that ranges from mild to severe mononeuropathy and extending to CRPS type 2.
- Common findings include allodynia, primary and secondary hyperalgesia, and hyperpathia, with hypoesthesia to touch and pinprick.
- In most cases, the diagnosis is clinical and can be confirmed by a diagnostic nerve block. However, in some challenging presentations nerve conduction studies and MR neurogram may be needed.
- Neuropathic pain medications and desensitization physical therapy are common first-line treatments.
- Interventional, nonsurgical management range from steroid nerve block to peripheral, dorsal root ganglion, and spinal cord stimulators—based on the severity and duration of the pain.

DISCLOSURE

A.S. Terkawi: None, O.K. Altirkawi: None, V. Salmasi: Consultant for AppliedVR. Funding from NINDS as K23 (1K23NS120039–01A1). E. Ottestad: Consultant for BioVentus, Nalu, SPR Therapeutics, Coloplast, Invicta (equity), Abbott, and Medtronic. Grants and research support from Bioness.

REFERENCES

1. Borsook D, Kussman BD, George E, et al. Surgically Induced Neuropathic Pain. Ann Surg 2013;257(3):403–12. https://doi.org/10.1097/SLA.0b013e3182701a7b.
2. Sonia Menezes RRRTSMKGTM. Injuries resulting from positioning for surgery: incidence and risk factors. Acta Med Port 2013;26:12–6.
3. Lalkhen AG, Bhatia K. Perioperative peripheral nerve injuries. Cont Educ Anaesth Crit Care Pain 2012;12(1):38–42. https://doi.org/10.1093/bjaceaccp/mkr048.
4. Welch MB, Brummett CM, Welch TD, et al. Perioperative peripheral nerve injuries: a retrospective study of 380,680 cases during a 10-year period at a single institution. Anesthesiology 2009;111(3):490–7. https://doi.org/10.1097/ALN.0b013e3181af61cb.
5. Sawyer RJ, Richmond MN, Hickey JD, et al. Peripheral nerve injuries associated with anaesthesia. Anaesthesia 2000;55(10):980–91. https://doi.org/10.1046/j.1365-2044.2000.01614.x.
6. Hewson DW, Bedforth NM, Hardman JG. Peripheral nerve injury arising in anaesthesia practice. Anaesthesia 2018;73(Suppl 1):51–60. https://doi.org/10.1111/anae.14140.
7. Abolkhair AB, El-Kabbani AO, Al-Mulhem A, et al. Psychometric and accuracy comparison of three commonly used questionnaires for the diagnosis of neuropathic pain. Saudi J Anaesth 2021;15(4):409–18. https://doi.org/10.4103/sja.sja_352_21.
8. Harden RN, McCabe CS, Goebel A, et al. Complex Regional Pain Syndrome: Practical Diagnostic and Treatment Guidelines 5th edition. Pain Med. 2022;23(Suppl 1):S1-S53. doi:10.1093/pm/pnac046
9. Castelli G, Desai KM, Cantone RE. Peripheral Neuropathy: Evaluation and Differential Diagnosis. Am Fam Physician 2020;102(12):732–9.
10. Mohammed A, Miniato NN. Anatomy, bony pelvis and lower limb, sural nerve. Bethesda, MD: StatPearls Publishing; 2022.
11. Kevin J, Kinter BWN. Anatomy, abdomen and pelvis, pudendal nerve. Bethesda, MD: StatPearls Publishing; 2022.
12. Matthew Koh B.M., Anatomy, abdomen and pelvis, obturator nerve, 2022, StatPearls Publishing, Bethesda, MD.
13. Marina Basta T.S.M.V., Anatomy, shoulder and upper limb, suprascapular nerve, 2022, StatPearls Publishing, Bethesda, MD.
14. Henry BM, Graves MJ, Pękala JR, et al. Origin, Branching, and Communications of the Intercostobrachial Nerve: a Meta-Analysis with Implications for Mastectomy and Axillary Lymph Node Dissection in Breast Cancer. Cureus 2017. https://doi.org/10.7759/cureus.1101.
15. Kenia A, Maldonado PT. Anatomy, thorax, medial pectoral nerves. Bethesda, MD: StatPearls Publishing; 2022.
16. Manolakos K, Zygogiannis K, Mousa C, et al. Anatomical Variations of the Iliohypogastric Nerve: A Systematic Review of the Literature. Cureus 2022. https://doi.org/10.7759/cureus.24910.

17. Chrona E, Kostopanagiotou G, Damigos D, et al. Anterior cutaneous nerve entrapment syndrome: management challenges. J Pain Res 2017;10:145–56. https://doi.org/10.2147/JPR.S99337.
18. Rachel E, Becker BM. Anatomy, shoulder and upper limb, ulnar nerve. Bethesda, MD: StatPearls Publishing; 2022.
19. Sharp E, Roberts M, Żurada-Zielińska A, et al. The most commonly injured nerves at surgery: A comprehensive review. Clin Anat 2021;34(2):244–62. https://doi.org/10.1002/ca.23696.
20. Terkawi AS, Romdhane K. Ultrasound-guided pulsed radiofrequency ablation of the genital branch of the genitofemoral nerve for treatment of intractable orchalgia. Saudi J Anaesth 2014;8(2):294–8. https://doi.org/10.4103/1658-354X.130755.
21. Yasusuke Hirasawa. Chapter 2: Diagnosis of Peripheral Nerve Injury and Entrapment Neuropathy, Pages 13-20. Treatment of Nerve Injury and Entrapment Neuropathy. (2002).
22. Christian Bischoff JK, WSMattler. State-of-the-Art Diagnosis of Peripheral Nerve Trauma: Clinical Examination, Electrodiagnostic, and Imaging. Modern Concepts of peripheral nerve Repair 2017;11–25.
23. James F. Grifth and Roman Guggenberger. Chapter 18: Peripheral Nerve Imaging, Pages 259-268. Musculoskeletal Diseases 2021-2024 Diagnostic Imaging. (2021).
24. Fradkin M, Batash R, Elmaleh S, et al. Management of Peripheral Neuropathy Induced by Chemotherapy. Curr Med Chem 2019;26(25):4698–708. https://doi.org/10.2174/0929867326666190107163756.
25. Andersen Hammond E, Pitz M, Steinfeld K, et al. An Exploratory Randomized Trial of Physical Therapy for the Treatment of Chemotherapy-Induced Peripheral Neuropathy. Neurorehabil Neural Repair 2020;34(3):235–46. https://doi.org/10.1177/1545968319899918.
26. Susan A. Masino and David N. Ruskin. Chapter 8: Nutritional Recommendations to Address Pain: Focus on Ketogenic/Low-Carbohydrate Diet, Pages 69-71. Minimally Invasive Surgery for Chronic Pain Management. An Evidence-Based Approach. (2020).
27. Power HA, Morhart MJ, Olson JL, et al. Postsurgical Electrical Stimulation Enhances Recovery Following Surgery for Severe Cubital Tunnel Syndrome: A Double-Blind Randomized Controlled Trial. Neurosurgery 2020;86(6):769–77. https://doi.org/10.1093/neuros/nyz322.
28. Chu XL, Song XZ, Li Q, et al. Basic mechanisms of peripheral nerve injury and treatment via electrical stimulation. Neural Regen Res 2022;17(10):2185–93. https://doi.org/10.4103/1673-5374.335823.
29. Deer TR, Gilmore CA, Desai MJ, et al. Percutaneous Peripheral Nerve Stimulation of the Medial Branch Nerves for the Treatment of Chronic Axial Back Pain in Patients After Radiofrequency Ablation. Pain Med 2021;22(3):548–60. https://doi.org/10.1093/pm/pnaa432.
30. Gilmore CA, Kapural L, McGee MJ, et al. Percutaneous Peripheral Nerve Stimulation for Chronic Low Back Pain: Prospective Case Series With 1 Year of Sustained Relief Following Short-Term Implant. Pain Pract 2020;20(3):310–20. https://doi.org/10.1111/papr.12856.
31. Gilmore C, Ilfeld B, Rosenow J, et al. Percutaneous peripheral nerve stimulation for the treatment of chronic neuropathic postamputation pain: a multicenter, randomized, placebo-controlled trial. Reg Anesth Pain Med 2019;44(6):637–45. https://doi.org/10.1136/rapm-2018-100109.

Pragmatic Comparative Effectiveness Trials and Learning Health Systems in Pain Medicine: Opportunities and Challenges

Vafi Salmasi, MD, MS(Epi)*, Abdullah Sulieman Terkawi, MD, MS(Epi), Sean C. Mackey, MD, PhD

KEYWORDS

- Pragmatic effectiveness trials • Pain medicine • Informed consent
- Learning health care system • CHOIR

KEY POINTS

- Large pragmatic effectiveness trials generate evidence for real-world applications of treatment modalities by enrolling a large number of patients at a lower cost; the findings can be generalized to a wider population.
- Alteration or waiver of a traditional informed consent discussion is crucial in successful application of large pragmatic effectiveness trials in pain medicine.
- Learning health care systems can provide a dynamic and adaptable infrastructure that can facilitate data collection for routine clinical care; this is a crucial step for efficiently collecting subjective outcome measures needed for studying chronic pain treatments.

INTRODUCTION TO PRAGMATIC COMPARATIVE EFFECTIVENESS TRIALS

Despite increased available pain therapies, more than 50 to 100 million people in the United States still live with pain and 20 million live with high-impact chronic pain that frequently limits life or work activities.[1–3] We know little about which treatments are best for which patient under their particular circumstances or the efficacy and safety of various treatments over time. There is a lack of empirical evidence regarding the effectiveness of the various approaches to anesthesia, perioperative medicine, and pain management, which are barriers to effective and consistent care. Without this empirical evidence to match the patient's unique characteristics with the relative effectiveness of different treatment options, clinicians are likely to rely on what they

Financial Support: None.
Department of Anesthesiology, Perioperative and Pain Medicine, Stanford University School of Medicine, Palo Alto, USA
* Corresponding author. 1070 Arastradero Road, Suite 200, Palo Alto, CA 94305.
E-mail address: vsalmasi@stanford.edu

Anesthesiology Clin 41 (2023) 503–517
https://doi.org/10.1016/j.anclin.2023.03.010 anesthesiology.theclinics.com

learned in their training from mentors. Consequently, this phenomenon can therefore perpetuate unwarranted variability in their practice. Therefore, we require reliable high-quality clinical evidence to improve patient outcomes continuously and ultimately tailor the most effective therapy for a specific patient and their needs.

Large randomized clinical trials or aggregates of multiple large trials are considered the gold standard of clinical evidence.[4] The results of large randomized clinical trials are more reliable because they minimize different sources of confounding and bias. When well conducted, randomized controlled trials have excellent internal validity. However, these clinical trials are not problem free. They are costly, labor intensive, and time-consuming to conduct such trials. The results of these randomized trials have limited generalizability (ie, limited external validity) unless they enroll participants in diverse clinical settings and include patient-centered outcomes.[5–9] Indeed, generalizability of randomized controlled trial data is problematic, as classic trials exclude up to 90% of patients.[10–12] Our recent literature review on the impact of exclusion criteria on clinical trials revealed frequent use of psychosocial exclusions in clinical trials.[13] The fact that many patients with chronic pain have psychosocial distress implies that the patients most in need of being enrolled in clinical trials are those most likely to be excluded. Furthermore, concerns about growing health care costs further limit the resources necessary to conduct these clinical trials successfully with reasonable generalizability. Therefore, we must focus on more novel and efficient designs—such as large pragmatic randomized trials—to generate clinical evidence of similar quality that can be generalized to a larger portion of our population.[14–24]

Pragmatic randomized clinical trials are a valuable alternative to conventional explanatory clinical trials with inevitable trade-offs. These pragmatic trials better assess the "effectiveness" of a treatment in "real-world" settings, thus offering higher generalizability. Pragmatic effectiveness trials are larger, embedded into routine clinical care, and can investigate simple or complex treatments or treatment paths. Patients are still randomized to receive different treatments but are not necessarily blinded to their allocation. Applying proper randomization, more objective data collection measures, and appropriate statistical methods preserves protection against different confounding and bias sources. The treatment protocols should be more flexible, allowing adjustment when necessary for the clinical care of individual patients. Outcome measures should better reflect what is essential in clinical practice. These trials can enroll large numbers of patients over a shorter period of time and at a fraction of the cost compared with conventional explanatory trials.[14,25–31] The ultimate aim of pragmatic effectiveness trials is to "inform real-world decision-making process."[25,31,32]

Despite numerous advantages, pragmatic effectiveness trials are not the perfect solution for all circumstances. Delivering a treatment and collecting data in a "real-world" setting increases heterogeneity. It is, therefore, difficult to estimate the treatment effect under optimal conditions. The treatment effect is also less uniform in the study population, necessitating more precise clarification about different subgroups and the range of treatment effects.[14]

Considering the pros and cons, large pragmatic effectiveness trials are optimal trial design choices in various clinical settings. At the end of the pragmatism spectrum, pragmatic effectiveness trials use outcome data collected in routine clinical. Clinicians and automatic recording systems gather a wealth of data in perioperative period. Anesthesia and perioperative medicine have the luxury of using these data to conduct large pragmatic effectiveness clinical trials; these trials are well embedded within routine clinical care with minimal to no individual patient contact.[14,33–40] However, embedding large pragmatic effectiveness trials within clinical care is more challenging in pain medicine.

APPLICATION OF PRAGMATIC COMPARATIVE EFFECTIVENESS TRIALS IN PAIN MEDICINE

Application of large pragmatic effectiveness trials provides multiple opportunities in pain medicine: (1) researchers can investigate more complex treatment modalities or treatment paths while giving the clinicians the flexibility to tailor the treatment to the needs of their patients; (2) this trial design also focuses on outcome measures that are more important to clinicians, for example, disability, social function, quality of life, or even cost-effectiveness instead of a simple pain score; and (3) simplicity of these trials and their lower burden allow longer follow-up periods.[25] When studying chronic diseases such as patients with chronic pain, assessing how treatment effect changes over a longer course of therapy is crucial. The results of pragmatic effectiveness trials can guide long-term, real-world application of different treatment modalities for patients with chronic pain.[14,25]

Application of large embedded pragmatic effectiveness trials in pain medicine poses its unique challenges: (1) the outcome measures required for these studies are not routinely collected in all clinical settings, thus limiting the application of this design. Collecting all necessary outcome measures promptly and with an acceptable compliance rate requires a unique clinical infrastructure poised to streamline this process. (2) Even in practices that collect these outcome measures, they record them during clinical visits. These clinical visits are not necessarily synchronous with the time intervals important for studying a specific intervention. More advanced statistical methods can partially overcome the limitations of asynchronous data collection; however, this method cannot perfectly substitute proper data gathering at predefined intervals. (3) Obtaining more objective outcome measures on disability and physical function is very difficult in these pragmatic trials. Use of commercial and research-grade actigraphy devices might overcome this limitation soon. (4) Finally, waiver of informed consent process or simplification of the process is routinely acceptable in pragmatic clinical trials that rely on registries and medical records to collect more objective outcome measures with no participant contact. However, collecting more subjective patient-reported outcomes makes this streamlined research process more challenging.[41] This process is more complicated for pharmacologic therapies considering that most medications used to treat chronic pain are "off-label." Most of the pragmatic clinical trials in pain medicine investigate nonpharmacological therapies, for example, behavioral therapies, physical therapy techniques, treatment pathways, and so forth.[25]

These challenges have significantly limited the application of pragmatic effectiveness trials in pain medicine. A more recent systematic review could only identify 57 clinical trials that met the criteria to be considered as "pragmatic trials." The average PRECIS-2 score for these trials was 3.8 ($\pm$0.6), which is comparable to other fields (eg, 3.83 $\pm$ 0.78 in cardiology).[42] However, domain-specific scores were lower for recruitment and follow-up.[25] The investigators of this systematic review also suggested several areas of improvement for future pragmatic effectiveness trials in pain medicine: (1) better reporting of the nature of the study center; (2) better reporting of qualifications and expertise of providers; (3) indicating the nature of pain condition, for example, duration of pain, pain diagnosis, location of pain, and so forth; (4) providing more detailed information on comparator groups and how "usual clinical care" is defined; (5) better reporting of other pain treatments participants received; and (6) better justifying of the choices made in trial design.[25] It is essential to know if the choice of delivery method of intervention, outcome measures, and follow-up period are made based on clinical reasons, patient preferences, clinician, preferences, or feasibility of the study.[14,25]

These challenges and shortcomings should not discourage pain researchers from application of this novel design to investigate long-term, real-world applications of chronic pain treatments. Conversely, understanding these challenges and areas for improvement can guide pain researchers to design and conduct more robust pragmatic effectiveness trials by improving the infrastructure for recruitment and data collection and being more diligent in explaining their methods and findings.[25]

INFORMED CONSENT

The first step in successfully conducting pragmatic effectiveness trials in pain medicine is improving the ability to systematically recruit more patients while minimizing the research burden for study participants and clinicians. The traditional informed consent process can be burdensome for both participants and researchers and thus hamper the streamlined recruitment process. The traditional informed consent discussion involves explaining at least 3 important factors to the potential participants: (1) the purpose of the study; (2) specifics of the research process including randomization, data collection, additional visits or tests, and so forth; and (3) potential risks and benefits of participating in research, including those of the experimental treatment.[41,43,44] By design, pragmatic, effective trials do not involve "experimental treatment," and additional visits/test while trying to minimize alterations to "usual clinical care" of the participants. Therefore, the waived or streamlined informed consent process may be necessary for the successful conduct of pragmatic effectiveness trials.[41,45]

The traditional informed consent process can cause significant distress and confusion for patients. The decision-making process can cause anxiety for some patients and have adverse emotional consequences. For patients trying to decide about the next steps of a treatment plan, adding a vast amount of information (many informed consent forms are 15 pages or more) and another decision point about participation in a research study leads to information overload and significant anxiety.[41,43]

The ethical principle that advocates the necessity of a traditional informed consent discussion is based on patient autonomy. The common assumption is that we give the patients full autonomy by providing them with as much information as possible at any decision point.[41,43,46–48] However, we challenge this assumption, as it is beloieved that information overload—the state in which increasing the amount of information decreases the ability to make a rational decision—fails to improve autonomy and minimize harm because it poses an unnecessary burden and distress for patients. This process is not only an obstacle to autonomous decision-making but also tends to be more confusing for the participants when used in pragmatic effectiveness trials; the participants of these trials will receive some form of efficacious "usual clinical care" in either arm of the study.[41,43] We argue that the actual research intervention in these pragmatic effectiveness trials is the process of randomization and not the treatment modalities the participants will receive, as no "experimental" treatment option is available in these studies.[41,43]

The controversy about informed consent in pragmatic clinical trials dates to 1980s.[41,49,50] Although Vickers and colleagues argue that traditional research informed consent can be even counterproductive for explanatory clinical trial[43]; when applied for pragmatic clinical trials it can compromise trial integrity or even make it impossible to conduct.[41] At best, experts doubt whether traditional informed consent is ethically necessary when we are studying existing medical practice in large pragmatic effectiveness trials. At worst, others argue that legalistic long informed consent documents for minimal risk trials may result in an "injurious misconception";

potential participants then reject being in a trial because of an exaggerated projection of risk.[41,43,51]

Symons and colleagues summarized 6 models that represent a spectrum of simplified, altered, or waived informed consent.[41] They discussed the acceptability of these models in different research ethics environments of the United States, Australia, and the United Kingdom.[41] They also represented 3 examples showing how large pragmatic trials became feasible using these models.[36,40,41,52] They also emphasized that nearly all research regulatory bodies allow waiver of informed consent if "the research would not be feasible or practicable to carry out without the waiver, the research has important social value, and the research poses no more than minimal risks toward participants." Most large pragmatic effectiveness trials meet the criteria for being impactful and posing no more than minimal risk; the main question is what makes a trial "impracticable."[41,53–55]

The United States Secretary's Advisory Committee on Human Research Protections defines trial impracticability as follows: "Appropriate ethical or scientific rationales might include, for example: (i) scientific validity would be compromised if consent were required because it would introduce bias to the sample selection; or (ii) subjects' behaviors or responses would be altered, such that study conclusions would be biased; or (iii) the consent procedure would itself create additional threats to privacy that would otherwise not exist; or (iv) there is risk of inflicting significant psychological, social or other harm by contacting individuals or families. Once the IRB has determined that the waiver or alteration does not adversely impact the research's ethical nature or scientific rigor, logistical issues (eg, cost, convenience, speed) may be considered."[53] This paragraph provides useful framework about how ethics committees can assess overall balance of risks, burden, and benefit when making decisions about alteration or waiver of informed consent process. Some further argue that consideration of cost is an important factor in determining the impracticability of a pragmatic trial; this consideration is more important for high-impact, publicly funded, investigator-led clinical trials.[41,56,57]

Some opponents to this concept argue that in some cases the risks of the disclosure of data may be more harmful than the minimal risks posed by randomization in large effectiveness trials. Waiving consent for observational and retrospective studies, considering excessive cost but not taking into account the same consideration for clinical trials, would seem a double standard.[41] During times of major economic rationalization and progressively more limited health care system resources, allocating valuable resources to obtaining individual consent could be unethical.[41,58]

This debate has gained momentum after the Institute of Medicine advocated applying a "Learning Healthcare System" for more effective knowledge generation.[59] As we will describe in detail later, a learning health care system embeds clinical research into routine clinical practice to continually improve care and deliver value; altered or waived consent models are essential for this integration.[41,59] Different pioneer groups have proposed different models to adapt informed consent to learning health care systems: integrating research consent with the routine clinical discussion with patients; routine randomization as the default position followed by post-hoc consent or opt-out models; and integrating a rigorous, systematic evaluation into normal practice and waiving individual consent where patients and the public are better informed.[35,36,39–41,43,45,51,52,59–61]

Many large pragmatic effectiveness trials leverage flexible approaches to use altered or waived informed consent. Most experts now agree that these flexible models are essential for successfully implementing "Learning Healthcare Systems"[59] to embed pragmatic trials in routine clinical practice. Most also agree that the application of altered or waived consent is not only ethically defensible but also can promote *beneficence* and *justice* by more effective use of limited resources to maximize knowledge generation.

THE LEARNING HEALTH SYSTEM AND HIGH-QUALITY, REAL-WORLD DATA COLLECTION

Effective systems to help practitioners integrate relevant measures and monitor patient outcomes have not existed until recently. The United States Institute of Medicine (IOM; now the National Academy of Medicine [NAM]) called for developing learning health care systems. As envisioned by the IOM, a Learning Health System (LHS) leverages an integrated digital infrastructure to provide data-based driven and coordinated care that is available just in time to the clinician and that is centered on the patient. LHSs combine science, informatics, data science, incentives, and culture that are then aligned for continuous improvement and innovation. The NAM and National Science Foundation extolled the virtues of LHSs[62] and declared that LHSs can rapidly inform decisions that have transformative effects on improving health.[63] Properly implemented, LHSs can be used to optimize and tailor care as well as their future potential to help achieve the goal of precision medicine.

A defining attribute of an effective LHS is to have a data collection system that is (1) already embedded in routine clinical practice; (2) simple and short enough that minimize time and mental burden for participants and clinicians; and (3) valid for measuring the intended outcomes.[14,64] In perioperative medicine, available objective measures meet all these criteria, and we can easily extract them from medical records without frequent patient contact; this has resulted in the more widespread use of larger-scale pragmatic clinical trials in anesthesiology.[14,33–40] Although an anesthesiologist relies heavily on objective data while delivering care intraoperatively, routine clinical practice of a pain physician involves seeking several patient-reported outcome measures through asking subjective questions.

More pain clinicians and academic centers are using standardized patient intake forms or questionnaires to collect more uniform pieces of information about their patients that can better guide their practice.[25] Streamlined integration of these data collection systems into routine clinical care requires that these instruments are simple enough and provide value for clinicians and patients.[25,64] Vickers and colleagues have been using an embedded system for more than a decade.[64,65] They believe that their success is because of following these 10 golden rules:

1. What seems obvious to an engineer (or informatics manager) may not be obvious to a patient.
2. What seems quick and easy may strike the patient as burdensome.
3. Questionnaires developed for research may not be appropriate for clinical practice.
4. Many words used by doctors and researchers can be replaced by something simpler.
5. Mandatory fields and open text cause problems.
6. Do not ask questions for clinical care unless you are prepared to act.
7. Patients have to see that completing the questionnaire is in their best interests.
8. A subgroup of users can cause a great deal of additional work, but, unlike Amazon and Uber, you cannot ignore those users.
9. Watch patients use your tool and ask about their experiences.
10. Patient trust is hard to gain and easy to lose.[65]

Once we implement such a system and integrate it into routine clinical practice, we can apply it to conduct larger-scale pragmatic effectiveness trials.[64,66,67] A dynamic learning health care system allows the researchers to adapt data collection points to gather outcome measures necessary to test their hypotheses. Reporting findings based on high-quality subjective data is valuable and represents the measures clinicians use to make decisions when delivering care in routine clinical practice.

THE STANFORD LEARNING HEALTH SYSTEM MODEL AND FUTURE DIRECTIONS

In recognizing the societal problem of pain, the IOM *Relieving Pain In America* report called for "greater development and use of patient outcome registries that can support point-of-care treatment decision making, as well as for aggregation of large numbers of patients to enable assessment of the safety and effectiveness of therapies."[1] Similarly, in the Health and Human Services *National Pain Strategy* (Mackey; Co-Chair), the committee stated, "better data are needed to understand the problem and guide action." In response to these calls, Stanford University Division of Pain Medicine developed CHOIR (http://choir.stanford.edu; Principle Investigator: Mackey) as an innovative, open-source, highly flexible, and free learning health care system (LHS).

CHOIR (**Fig. 1**) was developed to provide high-quality, point-of-care data to optimize care and for real-world research discovery. Using a Web-based interface, CHOIR captures patient-reported outcome data at each clinic visit, graphically displays real-time results that inform point-of-care decisions, and tracks patient treatment responses longitudinally. CHOIR emphasizes tracking of patient-generated information as a core component of clinical practice, allowing for individualized improvements in the health care delivery process over time, and guiding precision medicine. As a flexible platform, CHOIR has also been tailored for other medical specialties, including Preoperative Anesthesia Assessment, Pediatric Pain,[68] Orthopedics Hand and Joint Replacement, Interventional Radiology,[69] Chronic Fatigue, Psychiatry, and Primary Care/Family Medicine.[70]

CHOIR integrates NIH Patient-Reported Outcomes Measurement Information System (PROMIS) measures to efficiently and rapidly capture 15 to 20 domains of physical, psychological, and social functioning. The role that psychological and social

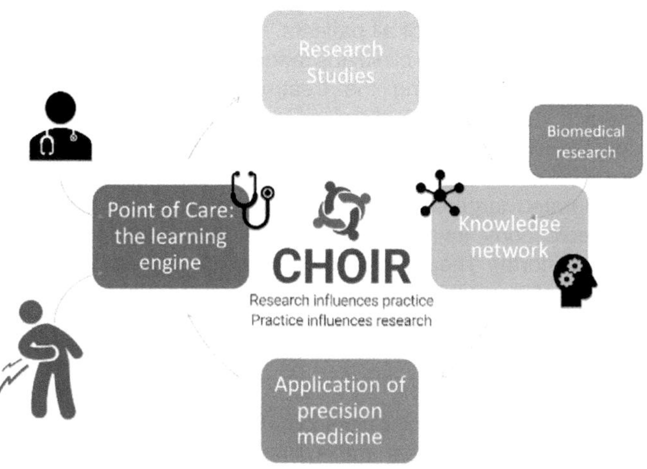

Fig. 1. CHOIR.

factors play in the incidence, magnitude, and persistence of pain, as well as the associated costs of care, have increasingly come to light and, as noted earlier, is frequently a basis for exclusions in clinical trials. Consequently, there has been a demand to measure and monitor psychological and social factors to manage these complex interactions better. Another strength of PROMIS measures is that they allow comparisons of individual patients against national population norms. CHOIR also has a built-in computer adaptive testing engine (CHOIR-CAT) to deliver both legacy and more modern item response theory (IRT) surveys, such as those used by PROMIS. The use of computerized adaptive testing (CAT) reduces participant burden. Overall and after several hundred thousand administrations of PROMIS surveys, CHOIR-CAT reduces subject burden by approximately 75% compared with instruments based on classic testing theory. CHOIR also features an interactive, validated pain body map (CHOIR Body Map) available in CHOIR and separately as a library within Research Electronic Data Capture (REDCap).[71,72]

In addition to its clinical utility, CHOIR has been an invaluable research tool to capture real-world research evidence, which has been a high priority by the Food and Drug Administration, the National Institutes of Health, and NAM.[73,74] Furthermore, CHOIR addresses the need for generation of systematic practice-based evidence by allowing low-cost, large, prospective, observational studies on thousands (or more) of patients in a "real-world" clinic setting. From real-world data collected from patients with chronic pain and using CHOIR, we have gained critical insights about the effects and impacts on chronic pain from tobacco,[75] cannabis,[76] social functioning and social isolation,[77–80] fatigue,[81] perceived injustice,[82,83] pain catastrophizing,[84–86] opioid misuse,[87–91] multiple overlapping pain conditions,[92,93] cancer,[94,95] and symptom severity.[96] More than 30 manuscripts (full list at https://choir.stanford.edu/publications/) have been published using CHOIR data across multiple sites, providing unique insights into the characteristics and treatment responses of "real-world" patients with pain and other conditions.

We have successfully adapted CHOIR to conduct large-scale pragmatic effectiveness trials more effectively and at a lower cost by applying these modifications.

1. We have successfully worked with our institutional board review to implement a 2-step informed consent process. Before a clinical encounter, the patients read a one-page simplified informational sheet about pragmatic effectiveness trials and randomization. We follow with a more formal informed consent for patients who are randomized later instead of all patients.
2. If there is a true equipoise, the clinicians randomize the patients to a treatment arm instead of randomly choosing the treatment themselves. This point-of-care randomization[97] step allows the clinicians to initiate treatment immediately without waiting for the process of randomization to be completed by a research coordinator.
3. We have integrated targeted questionnaires in CHOIR for each general type of treatment (medications, invasive interventions, behavioral interventions, physical therapy, and so forth). The patients receive and complete these questionnaires as a component of their clinical care at time intervals relevant to each specific treatment modality.[97]
4. A research coordinator contacts the patients to obtain formal research informed consent to use the patient information in our clinical trials.

We believe that successful implementation of this model will allow academic centers to maximize the process of generating knowledge by transforming each clinical encounter into a research opportunity.

This model has limitations including the following: (1) successful research recruitment requires the constant engagement of the clinicians in our research process. It is essential to constantly remind clinicians during their busy and stressful clinical days until this process becomes a habitual step of their routine clinical practice; (2) we still lack objective data to characterize and improve the participants' physical and social functioning. More widespread application of wearable devices might be an opportunity to overcome this limitation in the future and is a future goal for integration within CHOIR[98–101]; and (3) ethics committees might still be hesitant to accept this altered method of consenting participants, especially when investigating more invasive interventions. An ongoing dialogue and collaboration between investigators and ethics committees is necessary to better educate members of ethics committees about these advances in clinical trials and benefits of applying them; this is only feasible if we demonstrate that our research teams are fully committed to always protecting rights of all patients and research participants and advocating for them.

SUMMARY

Application of large pragmatic effectiveness clinical trials in pain medicine poses certain unique challenges, considering the lack of more uniform, objective outcome measures. These challenges have limited the number of these trials in our literature. Pain researchers are thinking more creatively to build a better infrastructure of learning health care systems to streamline the informed consent process and embed data collection into routine clinical care. We can then successfully leverage these systems' benefits to design and conduct larger scale pragmatic effectiveness trials. These trials are essential for understanding our treatments' effectiveness in real-world application.

CLINICS CARE POINTS

- When reading research papers, we should consider eligibility criteria more carefully to assess if the results can be applied to our patient population.
- When reading research papers, we should pay attention to outcome measures and decide if they represent what is important for our clinical practice.

CONFLICT OF INTEREST STATEMENT

The authors do not have any conflict of interest about the material discussed in the article.

REFERENCES

1. IOM. Relieving Pain in America: A Blueprint for Transforming Prevention, Care, Education, and Research. In: Relieving Pain in America: A Blueprint for Transforming Prevention, Care, Education, and Research. Washington (DC)2011.
2. Dahlhamer J, Lucas J, Zelaya C, et al. Prevalence of Chronic Pain and High-Impact Chronic Pain Among Adults - United States, 2016. MMWR Morb Mortal Wkly Rep 2018;67(36):1001–6.
3. Von Korff M, Scher AI, Helmick C, et al. United States National Pain Strategy for Population Research: Concepts, Definitions, and Pilot Data. J Pain 2016;17(10): 1068–80.

4. Devereaux PJ, Yusuf S. The evolution of the randomized controlled trial and its role in evidence-based decision making. J Intern Med 2003;254(2):105–13.
5. Collins R, MacMahon S. Reliable assessment of the effects of treatment on mortality and major morbidity, I: clinical trials. Lancet 2001;357(9253):373–80.
6. Hennekens CH, Demets D. The need for large-scale randomized evidence without undue emphasis on small trials, meta-analyses, or subgroup analyses. JAMA 2009;302(21):2361–2.
7. Myles PS. Why we need large randomized studies in anaesthesia. Br J Anaesth 1999;83(6):833–4.
8. Tunis SR, Stryer DB, Clancy CM. Practical clinical trials: increasing the value of clinical research for decision making in clinical and health policy. JAMA 2003; 290(12):1624–32.
9. Feldman AM. Bench-to-Bedside; Clinical and Translational Research; Personalized Medicine; Precision Medicine-What's in a Name? Clin Transl Sci 2015;8(3): 171–3.
10. C. G, J. S, R. E.. Large simple trials and knowledge generation in a learning health system. Washington DC: Institute of Medicine; 2013.
11. Fiore LD, Lavori PW. Integrating Randomized Comparative Effectiveness Research with Patient Care. N Engl J Med 2016;374(22):2152–8.
12. Fortin M, Dionne J, Pinho G, et al. Randomized Controlled Trials: Do They Have External Validity for Patients With Multiple Comorbidities? Ann Fam Med 2006; 4(2):104–8.
13. Salmasi V, Lii TR, Humphreys K, et al. A literature review of the impact of exclusion criteria on generalizability of clinical trial findings to patients with chronic pain. Pain Rep 2022;7(6):e1050.
14. Sessler DI, Myles PS. Novel Clinical Trial Designs to Improve the Efficiency of Research. Anesthesiology 2020;132(1):69–81.
15. Reith C, Landray M, Devereaux PJ, et al. Randomized clinical trials–removing unnecessary obstacles. N Engl J Med 2013;369(11):1061–5.
16. Jackson N, Atar D, Borentain M, et al. Improving clinical trials for cardiovascular diseases: a position paper from the Cardiovascular Round Table of the European Society of Cardiology. Eur Heart J 2016;37(9):747–54.
17. Macleod MR, Michie S, Roberts I, et al. Biomedical research: increasing value, reducing waste. Lancet 2014;383(9912):101–4.
18. Hadorn D, Wilson N, Edwards R, et al. How to substantially increase recruitment in cancer trials in New Zealand. N Z Med J 2013;126(1381):57–68.
19. Berry DA. Adaptive clinical trials in oncology. Nat Rev Clin Oncol 2011;9(4): 199–207.
20. Ford I, Norrie J. Pragmatic Trials. N Engl J Med 2016;375(5):454–63.
21. Calvo G, McMurray JJ, Granger CB, et al. Large streamlined trials in cardiovascular disease. Eur Heart J 2014;35(9):544–8.
22. Concato J. Is it time for medicine-based evidence? JAMA 2012;307(15):1641–3.
23. Concato J. When to randomize, or 'Evidence-based medicine needs medicine-based evidence. Pharmacoepidemiol Drug Saf 2012;21(Suppl 2):6–12.
24. Vollert J, Kleykamp BA, Farrar JT, et al. Real-world data and evidence in pain research: a qualitative systematic review of methods in current practice. Pain Rep 2023;8(2):e1057.
25. Hohenschurz-Schmidt D, Kleykamp BA, Draper-Rodi J, et al. Pragmatic trials of pain therapies: a systematic review of methods. Pain 2021;5(2):e878.

26. Chalkidou K, Tunis S, Whicher D, et al. The role for pragmatic randomized controlled trials (pRCTs) in comparative effectiveness research. Clin Trials 2012;9(4):436–46.
27. Moore RA, Derry S, McQuay HJ, et al. Clinical effectiveness: an approach to clinical trial design more relevant to clinical practice, acknowledging the importance of individual differences. Pain 2010;149(2):173–6.
28. Roland M, Torgerson DJ. What are pragmatic trials? Bmj 1998;316(7127):285.
29. Williams HC, Burden-Teh E, Nunn AJ. What is a pragmatic clinical trial? J Invest Dermatol 2015;135(6):1–3.
30. Loudon K, Treweek S, Sullivan F, et al. The PRECIS-2 tool: designing trials that are fit for purpose. Bmj 2015;350:h2147.
31. Treweek S, Zwarenstein M. Making trials matter: pragmatic and explanatory trials and the problem of applicability. Trials 2009;10:37.
32. Zwarenstein M, Thorpe K, Treweek S, et al. PRECIS-2 for retrospective assessment of RCTs in systematic reviews. J Clin Epidemiol 2020;126:202–6.
33. Guidet B, Leblanc G, Simon T, et al. Effect of Systematic Intensive Care Unit Triage on Long-term Mortality Among Critically Ill Elderly Patients in France: A Randomized Clinical Trial. JAMA 2017;318(15):1450–9.
34. Smit-Fun VM, de Korte-de Boer D, Posthuma LM, et al. TRACE (Routine posTsuRgical Anesthesia visit to improve patient outComE): a prospective, multicenter, stepped-wedge, cluster-randomized interventional study. Trials 2018; 19(1):586.
35. Kopyeva T, Sessler DI, Weiss S, et al. Effects of volatile anesthetic choice on hospital length-of-stay: a retrospective study and a prospective trial. Anesthesiology 2013;119(1):61–70.
36. Kurz A, Kopyeva T, Suliman I, et al. Supplemental oxygen and surgical-site infections: an alternating intervention controlled trial. Br J Anaesth 2018;120(1): 117–26.
37. Semler MW, Self WH, Wanderer JP, et al. Balanced Crystalloids versus Saline in Critically Ill Adults. N Engl J Med 2018;378(9):829–39.
38. Panjasawatwong K, Sessler DI, Stapelfeldt WH, et al. A Randomized Trial of a Supplemental Alarm for Critically Low Systolic Blood Pressure. Anesth Analg 2015;121(6):1500–7.
39. Sessler DI, Turan A, Stapelfeldt WH, et al. Triple-low Alerts Do Not Reduce Mortality: A Real-time Randomized Trial. Anesthesiology 2019;130(1):72–82.
40. Myles PS, Dieleman JM, Forbes A, et al. Dexamethasone for Cardiac Surgery trial (DECS-II): Rationale and a novel, practice preference-randomized consent design. Am Heart J 2018;204:52–7.
41. Symons TJ, Zeps N, Myles PS, et al. International Policy Frameworks for Consent in Minimal-risk Pragmatic Trials. Anesthesiology 2020;132(1):44–54.
42. Sepehrvand N, Alemayehu W, Das D, et al. Trends in the Explanatory or Pragmatic Nature of Cardiovascular Clinical Trials Over 2 Decades. JAMA Cardiol 2019;4(11):1122–8.
43. Vickers AJ, Young-Afat DA, Ehdaie B, et al. Just-in-time consent: The ethical case for an alternative to traditional informed consent in randomized trials comparing an experimental intervention with usual care. Clin Trials 2018; 15(1):3–8.
44. Simes RJ, Tattersall MH, Coates AS, et al. Randomised comparison of procedures for obtaining informed consent in clinical trials of treatment for cancer. Br Med J 1986;293(6554):1065–8.

45. Aaronson NK, Visser-Pol E, Leenhouts GH, et al. Telephone-based nursing intervention improves the effectiveness of the informed consent process in cancer clinical trials. J Clin Oncol 1996;14(3):984–96.
46. Jones DS, Grady C, Lederer SE. Ethics and Clinical Research"–The 50th Anniversary of Beecher's Bombshell. N Engl J Med 2016;374(24):2393–8.
47. The Belmont Report. Ethical principles and guidelines for the protection of human subjects of research. J Am Coll Dent 2014;81(3):4–13.
48. World Medical Association Declaration of Helsinki ethical principles for medical research involving human subjects. 2013.
49. Chalmers I, Silverman WA. Professional and public double standards on clinical experimentation. Control Clin Trials 1987;8(4):388–91.
50. Chalmers I. Double standards on informed consent to treatment, Informed Consent in Medical Research. In: Doyal T, editor. *Informed consent in medical research.* London, UK: BMJ Books; 2000. p. 266–75.
51. Goldstein CE, Weijer C, Brehaut JC, et al. Ethical issues in pragmatic randomized controlled trials: a review of the recent literature identifies gaps in ethical argumentation. BMC Med Ethics 2018;19(1):14.
52. Huang SS, Septimus E, Kleinman K, et al. Chlorhexidine versus routine bathing to prevent multidrug-resistant organisms and all-cause bloodstream infections in general medical and surgical units (ABATE Infection trial): a cluster-randomised trial. Lancet 2019;393(10177):1205–15.
53. U.S. Department of Health and Human Services website: Office for Human Research Protections, Attachment D: Informed Consent and Waiver of Consent. In: Protections USDoHaHSwOfHR, ed2013.
54. U.S. Department of Health and Human Services website: Office for Human Research Protections, Attachment B: Recommendations on Regulatory Issues in Cluster Randomized Studies. SACHRP recommendations on regulatory issues in cluster randomized studies. In: U.S. Department of Health and Human Services website: Office for Human Research Protections AB, ed2016.
55. National Health, Medical Research Council (NHMRC). The National Statement on Ethical Conduct in Human Research. Council AGNHaMR; 2018.
56. Kalkman S, Kim SYH, van Thiel G, et al. Ethics of Informed Consent for Pragmatic Trials with New Interventions. Value Health 2017;20(7):902–8.
57. Kalkman S, van Thiel G, van der Graaf R, et al. The Social Value of Pragmatic Trials. Bioethics 2017;31(2):136–43.
58. Zeps N, Iacopetta BJ, Schofield L, et al. Waiver of individual patient consent in research: when do potential benefits to the community outweigh private rights? Med J Aust 2007;186(2):88–90.
59. Institute of Medicine Roundtable on Evidence-Based M. In: Olsen L, Aisner D, McGinnis JM, editors. The learning healthcare system: Workshop summary. Washington (DC): National Academies Press (US) Copyright © 2007, National Academy of Sciences.; 2007.
60. Coyne CA, Xu R, Raich P, et al. Randomized, controlled trial of an easy-to-read informed consent statement for clinical trial participation: a study of the Eastern Cooperative Oncology Group. J Clin Oncol 2003;21(5):836–42.
61. Modi N. Ethical pitfalls in neonatal comparative effectiveness trials. Neonatology 2014;105(4):350–1.
62. (IOM) IoM. Characteristics of a Continuously Learning Health Care System Available at: http://www.iom.edu/Reports/2012/Best-Care-at-Lower-Cost-The-Path-to-Continuously-Learning-Health-Care-in-America/Table.aspx. Published 2012. Updated 9/12. Accessed2014.

63. Friedman C, Rubin J, Brown J, et al. Toward a science of learning systems: a research agenda for the high-functioning Learning Health System. J Am Med Inf Assoc 2014;22(1):43–50.
64. Vickers AJ, Scardino PT. The clinically-integrated randomized trial: proposed novel method for conducting large trials at low cost. Trials 2009;10:14.
65. Vickers AJ, Chen LY, Stetson PD. Interfaces for collecting data from patients: 10 golden rules. J Am Med Inform Assoc 2020;27(3):498–500.
66. Lin J, Bunn V. Comparison of multi-arm multi-stage design and adaptive randomization in platform clinical trials. Contemp Clin Trials 2017;54:48–59.
67. Parmar MK, Sydes MR, Cafferty FH, et al. Testing many treatments within a single protocol over 10 years at MRC Clinical Trials Unit at UCL: Multi-arm, multi-stage platform, umbrella and basket protocols. Clin Trials 2017;14(5):451–61.
68. Bhandari RP, Feinstein AB, Huestis SE, et al. Pediatric-Collaborative Health Outcomes Information Registry (Peds-CHOIR): a learning health system to guide pediatric pain research and treatment. Pain 2016;157(9):2033–44.
69. Hoang NS, Hwang W, Katz DA, et al. Electronic Patient-Reported Outcomes: Semi-Automated Data Collection in the Interventional Radiology Clinic. J Am Coll Radiol 16(4 Pt 1), 2018. 472-277.
70. Harle CA, Listhaus A, Covarrubias CM, et al. Overcoming barriers to implementing patient-reported outcomes in an electronic health record: a case report. J Am Med Inform Assoc 2016;23(1):74–9.
71. Harris PA, Taylor R, Thielke R, et al. Research electronic data capture (REDCap)–a metadata-driven methodology and workflow process for providing translational research informatics support. J Biomed Inform 2009;42(2):377–81.
72. Cramer E, Ziadni M, Scherrer KH, et al. CHOIRBM: An R package for exploratory data analysis and interactive visualization of pain patient body map data. PLoS Comput Biol 2022;18(10):e1010496.
73. Sherman RE, Anderson SA, Dal Pan GJ, et al. Real-World Evidence - What Is It and What Can It Tell Us? N Engl J Med 2016;375(23):2293–7.
74. ElZarrad MK, Corrigan-Curay J. The US Food and Drug Administration's Real-World Evidence Framework: A Commitment for Engagement and Transparency on Real-World Evidence. Clin Pharmacol Ther 2019;106(1):33–5.
75. Khan JS, Hah JM, Mackey SC. Effects of smoking on patients with chronic pain: a propensity-weighted analysis on the Collaborative Health Outcomes Information Registry. Pain 2019;160(10):2374–9.
76. Sturgeon JA, Khan J, Hah JM, et al. Clinical Profiles of Concurrent Cannabis Use in Chronic Pain: A CHOIR Study. Pain Med 2020;21(11):3172–9.
77. Ross AC, Simons LE, Feinstein AB, et al. Social Risk and Resilience Factors in Adolescent Chronic Pain: Examining the Role of Parents and Peers. J Pediatr Psychol 2018;43(3):303–13.
78. Karayannis NV, Baumann I, Sturgeon JA, et al. The Impact of Social Isolation on Pain Interference: A Longitudinal Study. Ann Behav Med 2018;53(1):65–74.
79. Sturgeon JA, Carriere JS, Kao MJ, et al. Social Disruption Mediates the Relationship Between Perceived Injustice and Anger in Chronic Pain: a Collaborative Health Outcomes Information Registry Study. Ann Behav Med 2016;50(6): 802–12.
80. Sturgeon JA, Dixon EA, Darnall BD, et al. Contributions of physical function and satisfaction with social roles to emotional distress in chronic pain: a Collaborative Health Outcomes Information Registry (CHOIR) study. Pain 2015;156(12): 2627–33.

81. Sturgeon JA, Darnall BD, Kao MC, et al. Physical and psychological correlates of fatigue and physical function: a Collaborative Health Outcomes Information Registry (CHOIR) study. J Pain 2015;16(3):291–8.e291.
82. Ziadni MS, You DS, Sturgeon JA, et al. Perceived Injustice Mediates the Relationship Between Perceived Childhood Neglect and Current Function in Patients with Chronic Pain: A Preliminary Pilot Study. J Clin Psychol Med Settings 2020; 28(2):349–60.
83. Sturgeon JA, Ziadni MS, Trost Z, et al. Pain catastrophizing, perceived injustice, and pain intensity impair life satisfaction through differential patterns of physical and psychological disruption. Scand J Pain 2017;17:390–6.
84. Ziadni MS, Sturgeon JA, Darnall BD. The relationship between negative metacognitive thoughts, pain catastrophizing and adjustment to chronic pain. Eur J Pain 2018;22(4):756–62.
85. Feinstein AB, Sturgeon JA, Darnall BD, et al. The Effect of Pain Catastrophizing on Outcomes: A Developmental Perspective Across Children, Adolescents, and Young Adults With Chronic Pain. J Pain 2017;18(2):144–54.
86. Sharifzadeh Y, Kao MC, Sturgeon JA, et al. Pain Catastrophizing Moderates Relationships between Pain Intensity and Opioid Prescription: Nonlinear Sex Differences Revealed Using a Learning Health System. Anesthesiology 2017;127(1): 136–46.
87. You DS, Cook KF, Domingue BW, et al. Customizing CAT administration of the PROMIS Misuse of Prescription Pain Medication Item Bank for patients with chronic pain. Pain Med 2021;22(7):1669–75.
88. Hettie G, Nwaneshiudu C, Ziadni MS, et al. Lack of Premeditation Predicts Aberrant Behaviors Related to Prescription Opioids in Patients with Chronic Pain: A Cross-Sectional Study. Subst Use Misuse 2021;1–6.
89. You DS, Hah JM, Collins S, et al. Evaluation of the Preliminary Validity of Misuse of Prescription Pain Medication Items from the Patient-Reported Outcomes Measurement Information System (PROMIS)(R). Pain Med 2019;20(10): 1925–33.
90. Gilam G, Sturgeon JA, You DS, et al. Negative Affect-Related Factors Have the Strongest Association with Prescription Opioid Misuse in a Cross-Sectional Cohort of Patients with Chronic Pain. Pain Med 2019;21(2):e127–38.
91. Hah JM, Sturgeon JA, Zocca J, et al. Factors associated with prescription opioid misuse in a cross-sectional cohort of patients with chronic non-cancer pain. J Pain Res 2017;10:979–87.
92. Hah JM, Aivaliotis VI, Hettie G, et al. Whole Body Pain Distribution and Risk Factors for Widespread Pain Among Patients Presenting with Abdominal Pain: A Retrospective Cohort Study. Pain Ther 2022;11(2):683–99.
93. Barad MJ, Sturgeon JA, Hong J, et al. Characterization of chronic overlapping pain conditions in patients with chronic migraine: A CHOIR study. Headache J Head Face Pain 2021;61(6):872–81.
94. Wilson JM, Schreiber KL, Mackey S, et al. Increased pain catastrophizing longitudinally predicts worsened pain severity and interference in patients with chronic pain and cancer: A collaborative health outcomes information registry study (CHOIR). Psycho Oncol 2022;31(10):1753–61.
95. Azizoddin DR, Schreiber K, Beck MR, et al. Chronic pain severity, impact, and opioid use among patients with cancer: An analysis of biopsychosocial factors using the CHOIR learning health care system. Cancer 2021;127(17):3254–63.

96. Gilam G, Cramer EM, Webber KA 2nd, et al. Classifying chronic pain using multidimensional pain-agnostic symptom assessments and clustering analysis. Sci Adv 2021;7(37):eabj0320.
97. Petrou PA, Leong MS, Mackey SC, et al. Stanford Pragmatiec Effectiveness Comparison (SPEC) protocol: Comparing long-term effectiveness of high-frequency and burst spinal cord stimulation in real-world application. Contemp Clin Trials 2021;103:106324.
98. Anchouche K, Elharram M, Oulousian E, et al. Use of Actigraphy (Wearable Digital Sensors to Monitor Activity) in Heart Failure Randomized Clinical Trials: A Scoping Review. Can J Cardiol 2021;37(9):1438–49.
99. Moore SA, Da Silva R, Balaam M, et al. Wristband Accelerometers to motiVate arm Exercise after Stroke (WAVES): study protocol for a pilot randomized controlled trial. Trials 2016;17(1):508.
100. Furness C, Howard E, Limb E, et al. Relating process evaluation measures to complex intervention outcomes: findings from the PACE-UP primary care pedometer-based walking trial. Trials 2018;19(1):58.
101. Kyle SD, Madigan C, Begum N, et al. Primary care treatment of insomnia: study protocol for a pragmatic, multicentre, randomised controlled trial comparing nurse-delivered sleep restriction therapy to sleep hygiene (the HABIT trial). BMJ Open 2020;10(3):e036248.

Chronic, Noncancer Pain Care in the Veterans Administration

Current Trends and Future Directions

Rena Elizabeth Courtney, PhD[a,*], Mary Josephine Schadegg, MA[b]

KEYWORDS

- Interdisciplinary • Whole health • Veteran • Chronic pain • Stepped care model
- Pain education • Implementation • Complementary and integrative health

KEY POINTS

- The Veterans Health Administration (VHA) uses the evidence-based stepped care model of pain management (SCM-PM) to provide cost-effective, population-based care, and there have been several innovations and strong practices at each level of care in the last several years.
- Step one trends: consultation for primary care providers, use of electronic dashboards to identify and intervene for high-risk patients, use of peer support specialists and technology to assist with patient education, infusion of complementary and integrative health (CIH) modalities to support wellness, and primary care provider education.
- Step 2 trends: establishment of pain management teams and evidence-based behavioral health interventions that are being disseminated through nationwide provider rollout trainings.
- Step 3 trends: increasing the number of intensive pain rehabilitative programs available nationwide.
- Whole Health includes 3 components (Pathway, Well-Being and CIH, and Clinical Care), which have the potential to significantly affect chronic pain care within the VHA, with exciting opportunities for further research.

INTRODUCTION/HISTORY/DEFINITIONS/BACKGROUND

Chronic pain is a debilitating condition that is more prevalent in veterans than in the general population.[1] The Veterans Health Administration (VHA) has implemented programs and policies to ensure veterans are offered evidence-based care at the highest standard. VHA Directive 2009-053[2] provided policy and a foundation for the stepped care

[a] Salem VA Medical Center, Virginia Tech Carilion School of Medicine, 1970 Roanoke Boulevard (Building 143, 3H), Salem, VA 24153, USA; [b] University of Mississippi, 207 Peabody Hall University, MS 38677, USA
* Corresponding author.
E-mail address: rena.courtney2@va.gov

Anesthesiology Clin 41 (2023) 519–529
https://doi.org/10.1016/j.anclin.2023.02.004
1932-2275/23/Published by Elsevier Inc.

model for pain management (SCM-PM) are to be implemented across the VHA. This model established a population-based method for ensuring that veterans are connected with the appropriate level of pain care in a timely and cost-effective manner, with cases that are lower risk and with fewer comorbidities being managed in primary care, and those with more complex needs referred to specialty services. The SCM-PM ensures patient-centered care and is based on the evidence-based biopsychosocial model.[3–5] The SCM-PM suggests that there are 3 levels of intervention: level 1 primary care, level 2 specialty care, and level 3 interdisciplinary pain rehabilitation program (IPRP) and advanced pain medicine diagnostics. Building on the foundation set by VHA Directive 2009-053[2] and in the spirit of the SCM-PM,[3] several innovative approaches have been created although implementation of this method varies widely from facility to facility. This article provides a narrative review of recent trends and describes strong practices in Veterans Administration (VA) pain care for each of these levels of treatment as well as a discussion of future directions for research.

DISCUSSION

Trends in Veterans Administration Stepped Model of Pain Care

Level 1 trends

This foundational level of care, which is most suited for low-complexity cases involving less comorbidity, tends to involve patients' active self-management of their chronic pain (eg, diet, exercise, sleep) with interventions provided by primary care, or patient aligned care teams (PACT) in the VA.

Support for primary care providers. Primary care providers are often tasked with managing several complex chronic health conditions within a short patient visit, including chronic pain, despite some providers feeling they have not been adequately trained in pain care.[6,7] To equip PACT providers with more information about chronic pain, the Minneapolis VA Medical Center (VAMC) implemented a course of Pain Neuroscience Education to the PACT teams.[8] Investigators found that the completion of these courses was associated with an increase in pain knowledge and had an overall positive impact on clinical practice even 1 year following the classes.[8] The VA has also invested in the development of technology-based programs that provide education and specialist support for primary care providers. For example, the Extension for Community Healthcare program uses telementoring to provide clinical education and support for primary care providers related to chronic pain.[9] The use of this program is associated with an increased utilization of pain services and provider initiation of non-opioid medications.[9] Nationally, VA also implemented the Opioid Safety Initiative.[10,11] Among several other programmatic components, the Opioid Safety Initiative includes the use of an electronic dashboard that utilizes the information from the electronic medical record (EMR) to identify patients who have been prescribed a high morphine equivalent daily dose (MEDD), and/or concurrent prescriptions for opioids and benzodiazepines. Academic detailers, tasked with facilitating provider education within VA, use these dashboards in collaboration with administration to discuss these trends with frontline providers and discuss alternative methods for addressing the patient's needs. Finally, the VA also supported the creation of Stratification Tool for Opioid Risk Mitigation, which uses EMR information to identify patients with chronic pain at risk for overdose and/or suicide-related adverse events.[11,12] Interdisciplinary teams (IDTs) then review the veteran's EMR and provide individualized treatment recommendations in the chart to alert the veteran's providers about methods for reducing risk, leading to a reduction in all-cause mortality.[13] This interdisciplinary case review intervention is now required of all VAMCs per VHA Directive 2021-21.[14]

Patient interventions. Although pain care typically involves provider-led services, the VA has begun to pilot peer support interventions to encourage veterans to self-manage their pain. Matthias and colleagues[15] utilized a biweekly intervention involving pairs of peer-support specialists and veterans interacting during 4 months. The results suggested an increase in veterans' self-efficacy and the degree to which veterans viewed pain as a dominant feature in their life and/or identity (ie, pain centrality). Technology has also increased access to level 1 pain care services, which might have been previously inaccessible to veterans experiencing barriers to care (eg, full-time work schedules, living in remote locations, childcare responsibilities). For example, the Puget Sound VAMC utilized telehealth to educate veterans at community-based outpatient clinics in rural locations.[16] This intervention included education in pain, acupuncture, and opioid safety, as well as components of cognitive-behavioral therapy (CBT). The team found that treatment delivery in this format was feasible and acceptable for their rural veterans. Further, a team at the Palo Alto VAMC has been utilizing telehealth to provide yoga to veterans in their homes to increase access to Complementary and Integrative Health (CIH) modalities and decrease clinical barriers.[17] Veterans participating in these services reported high satisfaction and improvements in their chronic pain and mental health symptoms.

Level 2 trends

Level 2 of the stepped care model in the VA focuses on interventions for higher levels of patient distress, risk, comorbidity, and complexity that requires more specialized care than is possible through primary care.[3] In order to address each component of the established biopsychosocial model, treatment by several providers is often necessary.[18] Within the VHA, this may include referrals to specialty providers working independently in separate departments within that VAMC, or referrals to a pain management team (PMT). For those referring to specialty services, the VA has supported research into evidence-based practices in behavioral medicine for chronic pain (eg, Cognitive Behavioral Therapy for Chronic Pain [CBT-CP]; Acceptance and Commitment Therapy [ACT]). This research has demonstrated that CBT-CP with veterans effectively decreases pain intensity and interference and improves functioning across domains.[19,20] VA-driven research also demonstrated that the inclusion of acceptance and valued living into psychotherapy with veterans decreases pain interference and decreases time to pain cessation and time to opioid cessation.[21–23] Through rollout trainings, the VA has effectively increased access to evidence-based psychotherapy for veterans through educating, mentoring, and certifying psychotherapists in CBT-CP.[24] Additionally, the VA has launched research programs focusing on varying treatment lengths to decrease the time burden on patients, providers, and the health-care system.[21]

Some VAs have found it more efficient to have specialty providers serving together using the PMT model. These teams may use an interdisciplinary or a multidisciplinary approach[27] because the implementation of PMTs has varied widely across the VHA. For example, the San Francisco VA Healthcare System established an integrated pain team model, which involves an interdisciplinary team (psychology, pharmacy, and primary care provider) meeting with a veteran simultaneously and the team providing recommendations on how to optimize the patient's pain treatment plan.[28] These teams also offer follow-up appointments because they take over opioid prescribing from the veterans' primary care providers and provide education on nonpharmacological treatment options. In order to support further innovation, the VA supported a Rapid Process Improvement Workshop in Connecticut.[29] The workshop resulted in the development of another integrated pain clinic and an opioid reassessment clinic that centered on assessing and monitoring patients prescribed opioids with the intention of increasing safety and efficacy of treatment and decreasing opioid misuse.[29] The integrated pain clinic was housed in PACT and consisted of providers from health psychology, pain medicine, physiatry, and physical therapy meeting with veterans 1:1 sequentially during the course of a 3.5-hour appointment and did not include a follow-up appointment with the team. Outcomes from the workshop indicated higher patient engagement in specialty and multimodal pain care while also increasing the satisfaction in services for both patients and providers. Finally, some VAs have also included pharmacists on PMTs to increase patient safety by having pharmacists address the overprescribing of opioids in chronic pain patients through monitoring, and controlled dosing.[30]

Level 3 trends

Level 3 of the SCM-PM pertains to advanced care for individuals suffering from chronic pain that have high levels of comorbidity and complexity, as well as symptom resistance to lower levels of care. IPRPs are one example of how the VHA provides this level of care. The IPRP model typically involves intensive, multimodal, interdisciplinary treatment during the course of several weeks and typically 60 to 100+ hours of provider-led services.[25] Murphy and colleagues[26] found that there has been significant growth in the number of IPRPs between 2009 and 2019 within the VHA. Veterans without access to a regional IPRP can be referred to some programs, such as the Tampa VAMC, which accept referrals from VAs all over the country. The Tampa VAMC offers both an inpatient IPRP and a fully virtual outpatient IPRP, which provides rehabilitative services using telehealth.[31] IPRPs, such as PMTs, have a significant variability among the programs in several factors, including number of providers, disciplines involved, service line offering the service, length of the program, and inclusion of and format for a shared medical appointment.[26] Despite these differences, Murphy and colleagues[26] found that these higher level of care programs resulted in increased functioning and decreased pain catastrophizing and sleep difficulties.

Trends in Whole Health

The VA Whole Health model encourages approaching health care through empowerment of the patient and equips the veteran with the skills needed to take control of their health and well-being while living a value-based life.[32] This approach works to shift the culture of the VHA to focus less on "what is the matter with you?" to "what matters to you?".[33] Consequently, in 2011, the VA created the Office of Patient Centered Care and Cultural Transformation and charged this office with facilitating and sustaining a cultural change.[34] The premise of the Whole Heath model is to use individualized, proactive, and patient-driven methods in health care that emphasize and orbit around the veterans' values and provider collaboration to facilitate healthy living and well-being.[34] Hence, the VA has focused on implementing practices that fulfill the 3 interconnected arms of the Whole Health approach that include: (1) Pathway, (2) Well-Being and CIH, and (3) Clinical Care.[32–35] The potential benefits of this Whole Health approach include not only provide the veteran with the skills and support to make sustainable life changes but also increase health outcomes, improve quality of care, provide more cost-effective options, and increase satisfaction for the patient and provider.[34] Specifically for chronic pain, the Whole Health approach has the potential for decreasing opioid use[29] and increasing implementation of best pain practices.[28]

The Pathway portion of the WH model focuses on the exploration of veterans' values and goals associated with their health and well-being.[32] Exploration of values is promoted through peer-led programs to increase proactive health and well-being and to motivate veterans to be engaged in their own health.[33,35] One such VA-initiated peer-led group program is the Taking Charge of My Life and Health (TCMHLH) group, which aims to guide patients in the exploration of their values and goals. The TCMHLH group has been shown to increase patient engagement in treatment and identification with reasons for living, improve mental health and quality of life, and decrease perceived stress.[36] The foundational focus on connection to peers and overall well-being in the TCMHLH group is then used as a bridge to the network of practitioners provided by the VA through the second arm of the Whole Health model (Well-Being). This arm of Whole Health focuses on the development and promotion of skills associated with self-care, well-being, and engagement in evidence-based CIH,[32] such as acupuncture, chiropractic, meditation, massage therapy, biofeedback, clinical hypnosis, guided imagery, yoga, and tai chi.[33] Research supported these CIH programs across various domains of health, including chronic pain.[37] For example, research on veteran has shown decreases in pain for acupuncture,[30,38] yoga,[17] massage,[39] and biofeedback.[40] The VA has funded and published several evidence maps that guide the reader through the support for many of these CIH modalities.[39,41]

The final arm of the Whole Health model, Clinical Care, focuses on the provision of conventional treatment and CIH. Aiming to foster independence and efficacy in the management of their health and well-being, these treatments should be informed by the veterans' personal values and goals.[32,35] This arm of Whole Health intends to integrate services and to promote imperative access to interdisciplinary teams.[42] VA has supported the development of integrated teams to increase access to pain-focused interdisciplinary care.[42] Similarly, another VA-initiated program is the Whole Health Primary Care Pain Education and Opioid Monitoring Program (PC-POP). The PC-POP uses an interdisciplinary team that facilitates a shared medical appointment with providers (nurse practitioners, psychologists, registered nurses) and patients (maximum of 40 patients) focusing on education and implementation of nonpsychopharmaceutical interventions for chronic pain.[43] This program is intended to run concurrently with treatment as usual.[43] Implementation of the PC-POP has demonstrated positive outcomes including increased engagement, documentation of substance-related provider queries, and decreased MEDD among patients.[43]

The VA established several flagship sites that were tasked with implementing WH.[33] These flagship sites have shown positive preliminary results.[33] The Well-Being and CIH arm of the Whole Health model was furthest along in terms of implementation across the flagship sites, whereas the Clinical and Pathway arms were slower to develop.[33] The Whole Health model lowered rates of burnout and turnover and increased motivation and job enjoyment for VA employees who had engaged in Whole Health services.[33] Increased engagement in Whole Health services by veterans with chronic pain decreased opioid use and improved life engagement, well-being, and perceptions of care. Further, results of VA flagship evaluations indicated that the early implementation of Whole Health resulted in higher utilization of services for veterans with comorbid Posttraumatic Stress Disorder (PTSD) and chronic pain, as compared with those with chronic pain alone.[44] Hence, in these preliminary findings Whole Health seems to present as an efficient method to reach complex patients with chronic pain who are in need of integrated care.

Model pain programs that have adopted Whole Health

The following programs, although varying widely in their structure and approach, were launched within VHA with the goals of integrating Whole Health into VAMCs that were already utilizing SCM-PM (**Fig. 1**).

WH PC-POP at Salt Lake VA Healthcare System: One of the goals of the previously discussed PC-POP was to increase consults to their Whole Health Program.[43] While providing patient education, the team also includes information on the WH approach, and referrals to the Whole Health Program may also be included in the treatment plans. Of note, veterans participating in this program are called once every 3 months by a nurse.

Integrative Health Clinic in Salt Lake City VA Healthcare System: Veterans referred to the Integrative Health Clinic complete an intake, which includes psychoeducation on the biopsychosocial model of chronic pain.[45] Veterans then select at least one treatment offered by the clinic (see **Fig. 1**) although the number of classes and the duration of program participation are based on the patient.[45] Typically, veterans are seen for follow-up after 6 months and then annually from that point on if the veteran chooses to continue to participate.[45]

Empower Veterans Program (EVP) at Atlanta VA Healthcare System: EVP consists of veterans participating in Whole Health and self-management groups for 3 hours per week for 10 weeks, although veterans are eligible to repeat the program as many times as requested.[46] Veterans also engage individually with an interdisciplinary team of chaplains, social workers, clinical psychologists, clerks, physical therapy, and a medical doctor. EVP focuses on the integration of Whole Health, mindful movement, and ACT. The program requires approximately 30 hours of engagement for completion and utilizes health coaches for follow-up in both phone and face-to-face formats.

PREVAIL Center for Chronic Pain at Salem VAMC: PREVAIL uses a simultaneous meeting with the veteran, the veteran's support person, and 5 disciplines (interventional pain, psychology, pharmacy, nutrition, and physical therapy). This meeting results in patient-centered treatment plans that focus on increasing active self-management of pain and allows the veteran to choose 3 of the 8 Whole Health self-care areas (ie, Moving the Body; Food and Drink; Recharge; Power of the Mind; Spirit and Soul; Surroundings; Personal Development; and Family, Friends, and Co-Workers) to work on during a 6-month outpatient program.[47] Veterans complete 6 1-hour weekly pain education classes before their IDT meeting. The program utilizes monthly phone coaching to discuss progress toward goals as well as a 6-month follow-up appointment with the 5-discipline team.

FUTURE RESEARCH

There have been several advancements for pain care within the VHA, and there remains a plethora of opportunities for future study. For example, implementation of PMTs has varied widely across the VHA. This variation may result in an increased burden on the patient,[29] confusion about the responsibilities of referring providers,[28] and disruptions to effective research.[42,48] Overall, there is a paucity of research that describes the structure of PMTs across the VHA (eg, disciplines on the team, frequency or presence of follow-up appointments, content of discussions during appointments, presence of a shared meeting with all providers). More information is needed regarding what types of programs exist and which elements maximize patient benefit. Further, replication of similar program models and measurements across VAMCs is essential to facilitate pooling data. This pooled data would assist with analyses on larger sample sizes for larger clinical studies to determine best practices and essential elements of programs that can be put forth as best practices. These opportunities for model and measurement replication also exist for IPRPs in the VHA with the overarching goal of determining the most effective methods of higher level care of chronic pain. Finally, effective methods for implementing and disseminating model programs into VAMCs are needed. Future

Name of Program	PC-POP[43]	Integrative Health Clinic[45]	EVP[46]	PREVAIL[47]
Location	Salt Lake City VAMC	Salt Lake City VAMC	Atlanta VAMC	Salem VAMC
Program Duration (Weeks)	24	Depends on Veterans' preference	10	24
Total Program Duration (Hours)	1	Depends on Veterans' preference	30	10
Inclusion of Follow-up	Yes- phone call every 3 months	Yes- seen once every 6 months	No- May repeat the program as often as desired	Yes
Types of Providers	2 Nurse Practitioners, 1 Psychologist, 2 Registered Nurses	Nurse Practitioner, Medical Doctor (for intake)	Chaplains, Social Workers, Clinical Psychologists, Clerks, Physical Therapy, and a Medical Doctor	Interventional Pain, Psychology, Physical Therapy, Pharmacy, and Nutrition
CIH Modalities	Referrals to nonpharmacological treatments	acupuncture, aquatic bodywork, Choose to Heal Stress management, herbal/nutritional supplement/drug interaction education and counseling, medical hypnosis, meditation, qigong, tobacco cessation, weight management, and yoga	Mindfulness, Mindful Movement	Mindfulness, referral to yoga and acupuncture
Simultaneous Meeting with Providers and Patient	No- shared medical appointment model	No	Yes	Yes
WH Integration	Education on whole health approach and referral to WH Pathway as indicated	Provides referrals to CIH	Whole Health group education	Referral to WH Pathway and educate on WH model, Veterans choose from 8 WH self-care areas to develop treatment plans
Setting	Outpatient	Outpatient	Outpatient	Outpatient

Fig. 1. Overview of components within model pain programs adopting WH.

research to determine the efficacy of such models in civilian populations and effective dissemination and maintenance strategies in nonmilitary health-care systems is imperative. The established RE-AIM (reach, efficacy, adoption, implementation, and maintenance) framework[49,50] may offer a useful model for planning and evaluating such dissemination research because it is designed to address the implementation of interventions in real-world, complex settings (eg, VAMCs).

In addition to more extensive research on the programs and interventions mentioned for each level of the SCM-PM, there is also a critical need to understand how the WH Clinical Care framework can be most effectively translated into interventions that are disseminated across the VHA. There is also an urgent need to understand how each arm of the Whole Health model may be used in isolation, sequentially, or simultaneously to provide the maximum benefit to veterans suffering with chronic pain. Similar to PMTs and IPRPs in VHA, VA programs integrating the Whole Health vary and it is crucial to understand and replicate model programs. Thankfully, there are some partnerships (eg, NIH-DoD-VA Pain Management Collaboratory) and several funding mechanisms (eg, DoD Congress Directed Medical Research Program; NIH HEAL Initiative; VA HSR&D) that may contribute to these research endeavors.

SUMMARY

The VHA has been a leader in pain care and continues to support innovation to provide excellent care for veterans suffering from chronic pain. Overarching trends in recent years have been the use of technology to decrease barriers to care for veterans, as well as the increase and expansion in the use of interdisciplinary, stepped care, and Whole Health models. Exciting opportunities exist for researchers to deepen our understanding of implementing and disseminating these models across the VHA, with the potential for eventual application in civilian and active-duty health-care systems.

CLINICS CARE POINTS

- The VHA offers evidence-based approaches that address each critical component of the established biopsychosocial model for chronic pain across each level of the SCM-PM.
- The Whole Health model in VHA is effective in the treatment of chronic pain and may provide a framework for organizing elements of the biopsychosocial model with proven active self-management strategies.
- PMTs and IPRPs vary widely across the VHA and may benefit from replicating model programs to assist with research efforts.
- Simultaneous meeting with veterans and providers from several disciplines may offer a more efficient way for patients to interact with their health-care team.

DECLARATION OF INTERESTS

None of the authors has any commercial or financial conflicts of interest nor funding sources for this article.

REFERENCES

1. Van Den Kerkhof EG, Carley ME, Hopman WM, et al. Prevalence of chronic pain and related risk factors in military veterans: A systematic review. JBI Evidence Synthesis 2014;12(10):152–86.

2. Veterans Health Administration. Pain management. VHA directive 2009-053. Washington, DC: Department of Veterans Affairs; 2009. Available at: http://www.va.gov/PAINMANAGEMENT/docs/VHA09PainDirective.pdf. Accessed October, 16, 2022.
3. Rosenberger PH, Philip EJ, Lee A, et al. The VHA's national pain management strategy: implementing the stepped care model. Fed Pract 2011 Aug;28(8):39–42.
4. Gallagher RM. Advancing the pain agenda in the veteran population. Anesthesiol Clin 2016;34(2):357–78.
5. Bruggink L, Hayes C, Lawrence G, et al. Chronic pain: overlap and specificity in multimorbidity management. Aust J Gen Pract 2019;48(10):689–92.
6. Seal K, Becker W, Tighe J, et al. Managing chronic pain in primary care: it really does take a village. J Gen Intern Med 2017;32(8):931–4.
7. Spitz A, Moore AA, Papaleontiou M, et al. Primary care providers' perspective on prescribing opioids to older adults with chronic non-cancer pain: a qualitative study. BMC Geriatr 2011;11:35.
8. Louw A, Vogsland R, Marth L, et al. Interdisciplinary pain neuroscience continuing education in the veterans affairs: live training and live-stream with 1-year follow-up. Clin J Pain 2019;35(11):901–7.
9. Frank JW, Carey EP, Fagan KM, et al. Evaluation of a telementoring intervention for pain management in the Veterans Health Administration. Pain Med 2015;16(6):1090–100.
10. Lin LA, Bohnert ASB, Kerns RD, et al. Impact of the Opioid Safety Initiative on opioid-related prescribing in veterans. Pain 2017;158(5):833–9.
11. Oliva EM, Bowe T, Tavakoli S, et al. Development and applications of the Veterans Health Administration's Stratification Tool for Opioid Risk Mitigation (STORM) to improve opioid safety and prevent overdose and suicide. Psychol Serv 2017;14(1):34–49.
12. Sandbrink F, Oliva EM, McMullen TL, et al. Opioid prescribing and opioid risk mitigation strategies in the veterans health administration. J Gen Intern Med 2020;35(Suppl 3):927–34.
13. Strombotne KL, Legler A, Minegishi T, et al. Effect of a Predictive Analytics-Targeted Program in Patients on Opioids: a Stepped-Wedge Cluster Randomized Controlled Trial [published online ahead of print, 2022 May 2]. J Gen Intern Med 2022;1–7. https://doi.org/10.1007/s11606-022-07617-y.
14. Veterans Health Administration. Conduct of data-based reviews of opioid-exposed or overdose patients with risk factors. VHA Directive 2021-21 Available at: https://www.va.gov/vhapublications/ViewPublication.asp?pub_ID=9554. Accessed October 16, 2022.
15. Matthias MS, McGuire AB, Kukla M, et al. A brief peer support intervention for veterans with chronic musculoskeletal pain: a pilot study of feasibility and effectiveness. Pain Med 2015;16(1):81–7.
16. Glynn LH, Chen JA, Dawson TC, et al. Bringing chronic-pain care to rural veterans: A telehealth pilot program description. Psychol Serv 2021;18(3):310–8.
17. Schulz-Heik RJ, Meyer H, Mahoney L, et al. Results from a clinical yoga program for veterans: yoga via telehealth provides comparable satisfaction and health improvements to in-person yoga. BMC Complement Altern Med 2017;17(1):198.
18. Bevers K, Watts L, Kishino ND, et al. The biopsychosocial model of the assessment, prevention, and treatment of chronic pain. US Neurol 2016;12(2):98–104.

19. Murphy JL, Cordova MJ, Dedert EA. Cognitive behavioral therapy for chronic pain in veterans: Evidence for clinical effectiveness in a model program. Psychol Serv 2022;19(1):95–102.
20. Stewart MO, Karlin BE, Murphy JL, et al. National dissemination of cognitive-behavioral therapy for chronic pain in veterans: therapist and patient-level outcomes. Clin J Pain 2015;31(8):722–9.
21. Cosio D, Schafer T. Implementing an acceptance and commitment therapy group protocol with veterans using VA's stepped care model of pain management. J Behav Med 2015;38(6):984–97.
22. Dindo L, Zimmerman MB, Hadlandsmyth K, et al. Acceptance and commitment therapy for prevention of chronic postsurgical pain and opioid use in at-risk veterans: a pilot randomized controlled study. J Pain 2018;19(10):1211–21.
23. Herbert MS, Malaktaris AL, Dochat C, et al. Acceptance and commitment therapy for chronic pain: does post-traumatic stress disorder influence treatment outcomes? Pain Med 2019;20(9):1728–36.
24. Stewart MO, Karlin BE, Murphy JL, et al. National dissemination of cognitive-behavioral therapy for chronic pain in veterans. Clin J Pain 2015;31(8):722–9.
25. Elbers S, Wittink H, Konings S, et al. Longitudinal outcome evaluations of Interdisciplinary Multimodal Pain Treatment programmes for patients with chronic primary musculoskeletal pain: a systematic review and meta-analysis. Eur J Pain 2022;26(2):310–35.
26. Murphy JL, Palyo SA, Schmidt ZS, et al. The resurrection of interdisciplinary pain rehabilitation: outcomes across a veterans affairs collaborative. Pain Med 2021; 22(2):430–43.
27. Gatchel RJ, McGeary DD, McGeary CA, et al. Interdisciplinary chronic pain management: past, present, and future. Am Psychol 2014;69(2):119–30.
28. Purcell N, Zamora K, Tighe J, et al. The Integrated Pain Team: A Mixed-Methods Evaluation of the Impact of an Embedded Interdisciplinary Pain Care Intervention on Primary Care Team Satisfaction, Confidence, and Perceptions of Care Effectiveness. Pain Med 2018;19(9):1748–63.
29. Dorflinger LM, Ruser C, Sellinger J, et al. Integrating interdisciplinary pain management into primary care: development and implementation of a novel clinical program. Pain Med 2014;15(12):2046–54.
30. Giannitrapani KF, Glassman PA, Vang D, et al. Expanding the role of clinical pharmacists on interdisciplinary primary care teams for chronic pain and opioid management. BMC Fam Pract 2018;19(1):107.
31. Veterans Health Administration. Chronic pain rehabilitation program. Available at: https://www.va.gov/tampa-health-care/programs/chronic-pain-rehabilitation-program/. Accessed November 3, 2022.
32. Kligler B, Hyde J, Gantt C, et al. The whole health transformation at the veterans health administration: moving from "what's the matter with you?" to "what matters to you?". Med Care 2022;60(5):387–91.
33. Bokhour BG, Haun JN, Hyde J, et al. Transforming the veterans affairs to a whole health system of care: time for action and research. Med Care 2020;58(4): 295–300.
34. Krejci LP, Carter K, Gaudet T. Whole health: the vision and implementation of personalized, proactive, patient-driven health care for veterans. Med Care 2014;52(12 Suppl 5):S5–8.
35. Gaudet T, Kligler B. Whole health in the whole system of the veterans administration: how will we know we have reached this future state? J Altern Complement Med 2019;25(S1):S7–11.

36. Abadi MH, Barker AM, Rao SR, et al. Examining the Impact of a Peer-Led Group Program for Veteran Engagement and Well-Being. J Altern Complement Med 2021;27(S1):S37–44.
37. Elwy AR, Johnston JM, Bormann JE, et al. A systematic scoping review of complementary and alternative medicine mind and body practices to improve the health of veterans and military personnel. Med Care 2014;52(12):S70–82.
38. Federman DG, Zeliadt SB, Thomas ER, et al. Battlefield Acupuncture in the Veterans Health Administration: Effectiveness in Individual and Group Settings for Pain and Pain Comorbidities. Med Acupunct 2018;30(5):273–8.
39. Miake-Lye IM, Mak S, Lee J, et al. Massage for Pain: An Evidence Map. J Altern Complement Med 2019;25(5):475–502.
40. Berry ME, Chapple IT, Ginsberg JP, et al. Non-pharmacological intervention for chronic pain in veterans: a pilot study of heart rate variability biofeedback. Glob Adv Health Med 2014;3(2):28–33.
41. Coeytaux RR, McDuffie J, Goode A, et al. Evidence map of yoga for high-impact conditions affecting veterans. Washington (DC): Department of Veterans Affairs (US); 2014.
42. Debar LL, Kindler L, Keefe FJ, et al. A primary care-based interdisciplinary team approach to the treatment of chronic pain utilizing a pragmatic clinical trials framework. Transl Behav Med 2012;2(4):523–30.
43. Marszalek D, Martinson A, Smith A, et al. Examining the effect of a whole health primary care pain education and opioid monitoring program on implementation of VA/DoD-recommended guidelines for long-term opioid therapy in a primary care chronic pain population. Pain Med 2020;21(10):2146–53.
44. Reed DE 2nd, Bokhour BG, Gaj L, et al. Whole health use and interest across veterans with co-occurring chronic pain and PTSD: an examination of the 18 VA medical center flagship sites. Glob Adv Health Med 2022;11. https://doi.org/10.1177/21649561211065374. 21649561211065374.
45. Smeeding SJ, Bradshaw DH, Kumpfer KL, et al. Outcome evaluation of the veterans affairs salt lake city integrative health clinic for chronic nonmalignant pain. Clin J Pain 2011;27(2):146–55.
46. Penney LS, Haro E. Qualitative evaluation of an interdisciplinary chronic pain intervention: outcomes and barriers and facilitators to ongoing pain management. J Pain Res 2019;12:865–78.
47. Courtney RE, Cannizzo F, Dezzutti BP, et al. PREVAIL: development of a whole health interdisciplinary evaluation of chronic pain in a rural VA medical center. oral presentation at pain week 2022. NV: Las Vegas; 2022.
48. Knoerl R, Lavoie Smith EM, Weisberg J. Chronic pain and cognitive behavioral therapy: an integrative review. West J Nurs Res 2016;38(5):596–628.
49. Glasgow RE, Vogt TM, Boles SM. Evaluating the public health impact of health promotion interventions: the RE-AIM framework. Am J Public Health 1999;89(9):1322–7.
50. Kwan BM, McGinnes HL, Ory MG, et al. RE-AIM in the real world: use of the RE-AIM framework for program planning and evaluation in clinical and community settings. Front Public Health 2019;7:345.

9780443183386